PREVENTIVE CARE FOR ELDERLY PEOPLE

PREVENTIVE CARE FOR ELDERLY PEOPLE

DAVID C. KENNIE

Consultant Physician in Geriatric Medicine
Stirling Royal Infirmary

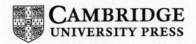

CAMBRIDGE
UNIVERSITY PRESS

Published by the Press Syndicate of the University of Cambridge
The Pitt Building, Trumpington Street, Cambridge CB2 1RP
40 West 20th Street, New York, NY 10011–4211, USA
10 Stamford Road, Oakleigh, Melbourne 3166, Australia

First published 1993

Printed in Great Britain at the University Press, Cambridge

A catalogue record for this book is available from the British Library

Library of Congress cataloguing in publication data
Kennie, David C.
Preventive care for elderly people / David C. Kennie.
p.   cm.
Includes index.
ISBN 0-521-43044-5 (hardback). – ISBN 0-521-43629-X (pbk.)
1. Preventive health services for the aged. 2. Health promotion.
3. Preventive health services for the aged – Cost effectiveness.
I. Title.
[DNLM: 1. Health Services for the Aged. 2. Primary Prevention – in
old age. 3. Preventive Health Services. 4. Health Promotion.
WT 30 K36p 1993]
RA564.8.K45   1993
362.1'9897–dc20
DNLM/DLC 93–3403

ISBN 0 521 43044 5 hardback
ISBN 0 521 43629 X paperback

WD

To the women in my life
Patricia, Fiona, Aileen and Kirsty, for their love, support and
forebearance during this venture
and
Irene Anderson, my secretary, friend and right arm.

Contents

Acknowledgements

I should like to thank the former staff and residents of the Duke–Watts Family Medicine Program, Duke University, North Carolina for their critical approach to medicine and for first raising my interest in the field of preventive care.

I should also like to express my thanks to the members of the health promotion subgroup of the Forth Valley Health Board Joint Development Planning Team for Elderly People. The stimulating discussion engendered in the months that we worked together did much to assist me with this book.

My thanks also go to Mr R. B. Stewart of the audiovisual department of Stirling University for his time and invaluable help with the illustrations.

1

An overall perspective

This book is concerned with promoting the good health of individuals who have already reached old age. This may be achieved by a number of strategies that have been variously described as preventive health care, health promotion or health maintenance. Unlike the situation for younger people, however, interest and knowledge about the preventable problems of old age and strategies to combat these problems are still in their infancy. Irrespective of the age group under consideration, there is also a good deal of emotional controversy surrounding many preventive care strategies. Several of these issues are discussed in detail in later sections of this book. This chapter broadly sets the scene for health promotion and preventive care and begins by defining what is meant by the terms elderly people and old age.

What is meant by old age?

This book concentrates on people who have already reached old age or who are elderly persons. The concept of what is meant by these terms has changed gradually throughout human history and has altered markedly in the last hundred years. In previous centuries, because of the considerably shorter life expectancy, older members of society would be those who, in present day terms, might not yet have reached middle age. However, from the early part of the twentieth century, the age when someone becomes 'elderly' has, for largely political and economic reasons, been considered to start around the age of retiral at 60 to 65 years. Most of this population are, however, relatively fit and vigorous. From a health perspective therefore, a more realistic definition of old age begins around 75 years and upwards. It is this sector of the population that has increasing concomitant medical disorders [1] and resultant physical and mental disability. Even if free from disease, homeostatic reserve in the various

1

organ systems is sufficiently impaired in the majority of this age group [2] to require particular care with their medical intervention and particular effort in the restoration of physical function after illness. A large section of those over 75 years of age have also lost much of their prior system of social support and are at increased risk of institutionalisation [3].

Ideally, old age might best be applied not to the chronological age of an individual but to the extent to which they have aged biologically. The difficulty is in establishing markers that will identify this 'functional age'. For example, Costa and McCrae [4] reviewed data that attempted to use single or multiple criteria for this purpose. This included an analysis of over 600 normal persons in the Boston Normative Study followed over a ten-year period. They concluded that neither anthropometric nor psychosocial variables nor even medical parameters predict ageing changes or death better than does simple chronological age.

In the absence of a precise means of defining 'functional age', this book will allude to elderly people or old age as referring to 'chronological age' from the mid-sixties onwards. It is appreciated, however, that this also is an imperfect definition that results in two broad categories of older person: the relatively fit 'young old'; and an often less fit 'old old' occurring from the mid-seventies onwards.

The potential benefits of health promotion and preventive strategies

A considerable number of benefits have been suggested for preventive care and health promotional strategies in an elderly population. These are now considered separately.

Mortality

An ethical debate could be mounted over the value of prolonging life in old age and certainly few would maintain that prolonging life per se was the primary focus of preventive care and health promotional programmes for this age group. Nevertheless, for many of the fitter members of the elderly population a decrease in mortality and an increase in life expectancy seem reasonable expectations.

The average life expectancy for people entering old age at 65 years has undoubtedly increased, from 11.9 additional years at the turn of this century to 14.3 additional years by 1960 and 16.1 years by 1976 [5]. However, it is difficult to ascribe these changes to preventive care or health promotional measures as these methods were in their infancy prior to the early 1970s. Most of the benefit, therefore, seems attributable to better medical treatment and care. There has also been little further improvement since 1976, suggesting a boundary to upper life expectancy. It is quite likely therefore that, irrespective of the extent to which it is considered desirable, mortality rates for this age group may prove stubbornly resistant to preventive care and health promotional strategies.

Morbidity

Society has long used the adage that health care should be about adding 'life to years' rather than 'years to life'. It is therefore encouraging that there appears to be significant potential to delay the morbidity and disability associated with disease. Fries [5] points out that, when considering the prevention of cardiovascular disease 'in every randomised trial of primary prevention, effects on morbidity have far exceeded effects on mortality'.

Notwithstanding the definite lessening of morbidity that can result from preventive care strategies, there is still no unanimity of opinion about the overall future health of the elderly population. This depends on the *relative* rates of movement between the average age of onset of disease (or disability) and the average age of death (see Fig. 1.1). On the one hand, Fries [5] believes that mortality rates for elderly people in Western societies are now becoming resistant to preventive interventions whilst, as described above, significant potential still exists to delay the onset of disability. A 'compression of morbidity' therefore results in an overall more healthy older population. Alternatively, Kramer [6] and Gruenberg [7] point to the significant fall in mortality in old age that occurred in the 1970s and suggest that this has not been accompanied by much decrease in morbidity but rather is a result of the increase in life expectancy of people with poor health. Kramer [6] therefore predicts increasingly poor health in the elderly population with a subsequent 'pandemic of mental disorders and associated chronic diseases'.

An accurate prediction about the overall health of an elderly population is obviously of importance for the formulation of government policies directed at the provision of services. A resolution to the above debate is therefore currently being attempted using the notion of disability-free [8] or active life expectancy [9]. Review of the current evidence suggests that at the age of 65, men can expect 8 years of disability-free life and women 10, with the life expectancy being respectively 14 and 19 years. There are also significant disparities in these figures between various socioeconomic groups (see p. 231).

Wellbeing

The above benefits of preventive care are largely 'medically' orientated and carry with them an implicit message that old age is about illness and disability. This is, however, a false stereotype. Illness and disability usually do not occur until old age is well advanced and even then affect only a minority. Hence, in the above discussion about old age, the importance of the distinction between the 'young old' and the 'old old' was emphasised. Furthermore, Laslett [10], in considering the traditional 'ages of man', suggests that the 'young old' are in a *third age*, which should be one of positive development, of personal

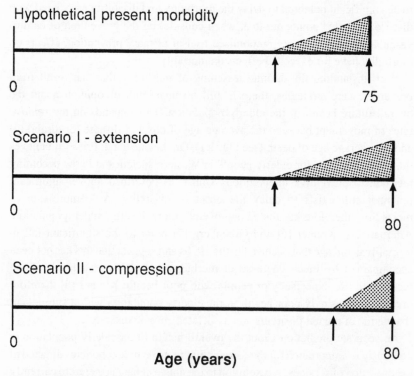

Fig. 1.1. The association between average age of death and average age of onset of morbidity. In the hypothetical present model, average age of onset of morbidity occurs at age 60, increasing in frequency to a maximum (indicated by the shaded area) at average age of death at 75. Extension of lifespan, without change in the average age of onset of morbidity (scenario II), results in a larger population in poor health. If there is still the potential to delay the onset of morbidity [5], without changing average age of death, then a smaller proportion of elderly people are in poor health (scenario II). Adapted from ref. [5]

achievement and fulfilment. This is then followed by a *fourth age* of 'dependence, decrepitude and death'.

Health promotion (as distinct from preventive care practice) has been seen as a major vehicle in helping the elderly population to realise and achieve the more positive aspects of health in old age. On the one hand, health promotion places considerable personal responsibility on elderly individuals through advice and exhortation that they adopt healthy lifestyles and practice regular 'body maintenance'. Some of these self-care programmes have been evaluated in randomised controlled trials and have resulted in improved psychological wellbeing, confidence and some coping skills [10a, 11]. On the other hand, health promotion should be concerned about activities that enable and empower older people to achieve their full potential. Minkler and Pasick [12] rightly express concern that in the USA, health promotion has previously been unduly focussed on individual *responsibility* for health at the expense of ignoring the individual's *response-ability*, that is their capacity for responding effectively to the challenges posed by the environment. *Response-ability* requires consideration of the elderly person's housing and transportation needs, level of income, access to services and many other social issues. Real success therefore requires mechanisms that enable society to focus on individual behaviours and enable it to supply social choices. If Filner and Williams' [13] definition of health as 'the ability to live and function effectively in society and to exercise self reliance and autonomy to the maximum extent feasible' is accepted, then the remit of health promotion must encompass 'any combination of health education and related organizational, political and economic interventions designed to facilitate behavioural and environmental changes conducive to health'.

Carer burden and stress

Until recently, the role of preventive care and health promotion in minimising caregiver stress has been neglected. Research and service programmes have had delayed institutionalisation and financial savings as their primary focus, rather than the wellbeing of carers. However, the continued ageing of society, an improved knowledge of the problems experienced by family carers and the heightened awareness of these problems amongst service providers as they have been brought to their attention through various advocacy groups, is changing the situation. Now, the emphasis has shifted towards accepting that family carers have rights of their own to a certain quality of life and to the limit of stress to which they may be subjected. The preventive care and health promotional strategies outlined later in this book are therefore based on these latter assumptions (see also p. 26).

Societal burden

A healthier elderly population might benefit society in a number of ways: for example, society might use its more active sapiental authority, or its workforce may have a lengthened potential activity. Overwhelmingly, however, the societal benefits of preventive care and health promotion have been seen in the context of a reduced need for resources and accompanying cost savings. This issue has had such political backing that it is discussed separately in the following section.

Health promotion and cost savings

There have been many notable advocates of using health promotion and preventive care as ways of reducing health care costs. Indeed the logic of the allegory of health promotion refocussing upstream, to where people are being thrown into a river, rather than conventional health care, which merely tries to pull them out downstream, is superficially attractive. However, the situation is far more complex than is immediately apparent. Refocussing upstream is efficient only when the point at which people are entering the water is within reachable distance. They must also be entering the water at an identifiable and limited number of sites and something must be able to be done to stop them taking the plunge. Whilst redirecting resources to refocus upstream, it must also be accepted that a number of people will drown as they are allowed to float past farther downstream.

The idea that preventive strategies will save costs is, therefore, far too simplistic. Several economists have reviewed the evidence [14, 15] and are mostly in agreement. Russell [14] summarises this by saying 'even when the financial cost of the preventive measure looks small, careful evaluation often shows that the full costs are rather large, larger than any savings'. In fact, prevention usually adds to medical expenditure. A detailed discussion on the costs of health promotion and preventive strategies is provided in Chapter 14.

Risks and disadvantages

Despite the many advantages of health promotion and preventive care for elderly people, there are also several potential risks and disadvantages.

1. One of the commonest preventive measures is screening for early un-detected disease. However, the screening process identifies a number of entirely healthy individuals who, because of the inadequacies of the screening test, are wrongly identified as having a problem or risk factor. These individuals who show 'false positive' must then be subjected to further (and usually more complex) investigation before being proven to be well. Inherent in any screening programme, then, is the need to incon-venience a few to benefit the majority. No matter how much this problem is minimised, some continue to feel that screening can be achieved only by coercion and deception and that this is invariably an infringement of an individual's personal liberty. Practically, screening programmes for elderly people must ensure that any benefit outweighs any harm and that, ethically, each elderly person must be accurately informed of the balance between risks and benefits.

2. A related and particularly important issue is that with age there is a decline in physiological functioning in almost every organ system, particularly after the eighth decade of life. Consequently, the elderly person has a signifi-cantly decreased homeostatic reserve to deal with the stress and challenges imposed by the detection and treatment of early disease and is particularly vulnerable to iatrogenic insult arising from preventive care measures.

3. There is well-documented evidence that certain preventive care strategies such as screening may also do psychological harm by arousing anxiety where none existed before. For example, fear and anxiety in women screened for cervical and breast cancers is well recognised and the same has been found in screening programmes for male hypertensives [16]. Stoate [17] has also shown that general practice patients screened for coronary heart disease scored more highly three months later on a psychological distress scale, as measured by a general health questionnaire, than an age-matched control group.

4. Identifying and highlighting health problems, for example by case finding, in elderly people who are already suffering from chronic incurable illness may be excessively stressful, if not to the older people themselves, then to loving family carers who may already be worrying excessively. This may lead to the loss of the older person's autonomy (for example by being persuaded to go into a nursing home), or worse (if the additional problem identified has no known cure), to the elderly person being taken from doctor to doctor in the hope of some research treatment being available.

5. Health promotional programmes have tended to focus on elderly individuals by placing upon them a responsibility to minimise the risks to their health through their adopting a healthy lifestyle. However, many elderly people do

not wish to change the habits of a lifetime. Consequently, they may be victimised, or blamed as 'deserving' the various ailments from which they suffer, simply because of their obdurate approach.

6. Preventing the health problems that occur in old age can, in extreme cases, be a sign of maladjustment to the ageing process. For example, avoiding grey hair and wrinkles, or baldness may for many be an expression of choice, yet for a few it can also be a sign of concern or even denial of the ageing process. Rather than preventive measures, some form of psychological counselling may be more appropriate.

7. It is possible that an emphasis on health promotion or preventive care becomes merely a highly publicised, token gesture of interest in the health problems of old age while the real problems of neglect and inequity of resource distribution are left unaddressed. This fear mirrors some of the previous concern in the USA about screening black races for sickle cell anaemia [18].

8. Health maintenance of elderly people is a relatively attractive concept for clinicians. However, it allows them to concentrate on the relatively more attractive 'young old' and salves their conscience about their relative neglect of a wide range of more pressing health problems in those who are more frail [19].

9. The increased awareness of health issues (brought about in part by health promotion programmes) has been suggested as a reason for a decline in people's subjective sense of healthiness in the USA. Health is becoming so industrialised and commercialised that it may enhance many people's dissatisfaction with their health.

Variance

There is considerable variation around the world in the degree to which countries have adopted health promotion and preventive strategies. In some it may be a matter of timescale, in that the country is still struggling to generate wealth or to introduce political stability, public health measures or an adequate health care system and does not yet consider preventive strategies as a priority. In more affluent societies, the variation may be partly cultural depending on the extent to which its individuals believe in scrutiny by other individuals or believe in taking responsibility for their own destiny. Variation will also depend on the stoicism that individuals have developed from their life's experiences. This latter aspect is particularly important for an elderly population that has experienced the hardship and traumas of war. As younger generations age, their expectations will no doubt increase, yet their acceptance of the tribulations of old age may at the same time be less well tolerated. The affluence of society itself further explains variation in interest in preventive care, and there becomes a thin dividing line between the adoption of appropriate health promotional strategies and a society's narcissistic pursuit of hedonism.

Politics is a further reason why the adoption of health promotion varies from country to country. For example, its comprehensive adoption in the USA may in part have been due to the Carter Administration (1976–80) which was retreating from introducing a national health insurance policy because it was considered too expensive. 'Raising the banner of prevention therefore, coincided very nicely with the retreat from national health insurance; presumably, it was both cheaper and better.' [20] However, politics also operate within the health care arena and health promotion is still used vociferously as a way of leading health services away from its intensely biotechnological stance towards a more holistic approach. It is also used as a means of promoting community versus institutional or hospital care. Interestingly, the strength of these political reactions seem in direct proportion to the perceived imbalance of the existing health care system, which again may explain the influence of the preventive care movement in the USA.

Lastly, variation in the extent of preventive care in a country depends on the nature of its existing health care system and how it is funded. Perhaps the biggest incentive to implement preventive care measures is the sort of fee-for-service system previously seen operating in the USA. Regrettably, this leads to unacceptably high levels of intervention and iatrogenic insult, particularly in elderly individuals. Conversely, in a relatively underfunded 'blanket' national health service, such as that in the UK, health promotional measures are viewed far more sceptically; the existing distribution of scarce resources within health care are often maintained at the expense of introducing useful preventive strategies.

Primary, secondary and tertiary prevention

Traditionally, preventive strategies have been considered in three categories. *Primary* prevention consists of those measures designed to reduce the incidence of disease in a population by delaying the age of onset. *Secondary* prevention consists of those measures designed to reduce the prevalence of a disease in a population by shortening its course and duration. *Tertiary* prevention consists of interventions to minimise the resultant distress, disability or handicap.

Over the years this categorisation has served well in clarifying thinking and serving as an operational basis for preventive strategies with younger populations. Regrettably, however, the distinctions between primary, secondary and tertiary prevention fit poorly into the language of chronic disease because there is so much overlap and duplication. For example, a risk factor for hip fracture, such as falls, is also a symptomatic health problem in its own right that requires preventive measures. Also, because hypertension is a risk factor for cerebrovascular disease, a tertiary preventive strategy, such as a reduction of high blood pressure, becomes at the same time a primary preventive strategy for stroke.

Kane [21] has also tried classifying traditional preventive activity according to the World Health Organization's classification for chronic disease [22]. This defines three points in a continuum: *impairment* of an organ system created by disease; *disability* that results in dysfunction; and social *handicap* that results despite compensatory efforts. Nevertheless, significant difficulties were encountered in using even this system because of 'blur and overlap' that required somewhat arbitrary decisions to be made in categorisation.

In view of these problems, little attempt is made throughout the remainder of this book to consider separately strategies concerned with primary, secondary or tertiary prevention. Instead, as actually happens in caring for elderly people, a mix of these strategies is considered together.

Separation versus integration

'Preventive care' and 'health promotion' are not synonymous terms nor necessarily similar activities. Each has a different focus in relation to the types of strategy employed and the evolutionary stage of the health problem at which they are targeted. Regrettably, an uneasy tension is often seen between those who espouse preventive health care and those who propound the benefits of health promotion.

Some of the reasons for this are immediately apparent. Health promotion tends to be conducted outwith the health care arena. However, preventive health care is an integral part of the training and daily practice of health care professionals. Health promotion finds lay personnel, government departments and public health professionals in its ranks of advocates, whereas preventive health care traditionally includes doctors and nurses among its supporters. Health promotion espouses a more social model of care, preventive health care a more disease orientated one.

Some of the reasons for the tensions between health promotion and preventive care are less obvious but more distressing. Essentially it comes down to the proponents of one philosophy trying to gain control over the proponents of the other. Health promotion is frequently advocated as a means of preventing more and more funds being thrown into the apparently bottomless pit of health service delivery. Often health promotion is perceived as promoting a more community oriented, less institutionalised, type of care. Health promotion, by enabling and empowering elderly people, may be considered more desirable than having them succumb to a health care delivery system that often robs them of their autonomy.

Yet, this schism is artificial and it is unfortunate that health promotion and preventive health care are sometimes viewed as competitive. They are manifestly complementary. Therefore, whilst accepting that many important and effective strategies to promote the health and wellbeing of an elderly population are best funded and conducted outwith health service delivery, I have tried, in this book, to minimise the differences in approach by discussing preventive care strategies and health promotion together. Roemer [20] summarises the situation well by stating 'The demonstrable achievements of prevention, combined with the continued escalation of the costs of therapy, led naturally to political and social pressures for containment of the rising costs of medical care, creating an artificial dichotomy between prevention (with high value and low cost) and treatment (with low value and high cost). Unfortunately, such a dichotomy not only overlooks the many benefits derived from medical care, but also ignores the great value of the medical care process as a major channel for the delivery of preventive health service.'

In some health care systems, however, and particularly in the USA, it is difficult to endorse such a statement entirely, for preventive medicine is often a mere marketing front designed to draw the elderly person into complex biotechnological investigation and research. Also, the medical care process can only be a 'major channel for the delivery of preventive health service' to elderly people if it is holistic in nature emphasising functional restoration and the maintenance of social support as well as offering treatment and cure. With these caveats, however, 'a health care system that makes integrated preventive/ therapeutic services accessible . . . (to the elderly population) . . . would have the greatest human and economic value' [20].

Starting early versus starting late

The optimum time for applying strategies to affect the health of elderly people is largely unknown. Conventionally, and currently, the view tends to be held that this is best started early in the life-cycle. It is logically comforting to believe in intervention before troubles arise and much emphasis has been placed on early and mid-life programmes for cardiovascular fitness, hypertension screening and efforts to combat postmenopausal osteoporosis. A further reason for starting early is that certain risk factors (such as the effects of obesity on the risk of disease) may become immutable after some duration of time [21]. A further boost to early intervention has come from the report of Tatara et al. [23] showing an inverse relationship between the uptake of health check ups in middle aged adults and hospital use by those 70 years and over. However, the authors themselves caution against assuming this relationship to be causal.

Alternatively, Fries [5] points out that it may be in early and later old age that the greatest impact from health promotional practices may be obtained. If they are begun earlier than this, the health problem to be countered is still a long time in coming and the health promotional gains may have evaporated by the time in life when the elderly person is significantly at risk. If, as the evidence seems to indicate, it takes only a few years to build stronger bones or achieve cleaner arteries or reduce the risks from smoking, health promotional practices to achieve these aims could still be very effective even if begun in later life when the events to be prevented are only a few years away. Even small changes in the older population might yield big and rapid differences in health and economic endpoints. From this perspective, programmes for cardio-vascular fitness or cancer prevention might be switched from the young to the old.

It is likely that during life there will be 'windows of opportunity' for applying preventive strategies that will have maximal effect on an older population. It is clear, however, that before any intergenerational transfer of resources is undertaken, more research needs to be carried out on the relative impact of preventive strategies at various phases of the life-cycle.

References

1. Akhtar AJ, Broe GA, Crombie A et al. Disability and dependence in the elderly at home. Age Ageing 1973; **2**: 102.
2. Shock NW. Systems integration. In: Finch CE, Hayflick L (eds) Handbook of Biology of Aging, pp. 639–61. New York: Van Nostrand Reinhold, 1977.
3. Sinclair I. Residential Care: The Research Reviewed, National Institute of Social Work. London HMSO, 1988; p. 246.
4. Costa PT, McCrae RR. Functional age: conceptual and empirical critique. In: Haynes SJ, Feinleib M (eds) Second Conference on the Epidemiology of Aging, US Department of Health and Human Services. Washington, DC: National Institutes of Health, 1977.
5. Fries, JF, Green LW, Levine S. Health promotion and the compression of morbidity. Lancet 1989; **1**: 481–3.
6. Kramer M. Rising pandemic of mental disorders and associated chronic diseases and disabilities. Acta Psychiatr Scand 1980; **62**: 282–97.

7. Gruenberg EM. The failures of success. Millbank Mem Fund Quart 1977; **55**: 3–24.
8. Robine JM, Ritchie K. Healthy life expectancy: evaluation of global indicator of change in population health. Brit Med J 1991; **302**: 457–60.
9. Katz S, Branch L, Branson MH et al. Active life expectancy. N Engl J Med 1983; **309**: 1218–24.
10. Laslett P. A Fresh Map of Life: The Emergency of the Third Age, London: Weidenfeld and Nicolson, 1989.
10a. Dean K, Holstein BE. Health promotion among the elderly. In: Badura B, Kickbusch I (eds) Health Promotion Research. Geneva: WHO Regional Publications European Series No. 37, 1989.
11. Nelson EC. Medical self-care education for elders: a controlled trial to evaluate impact. Amer J Pub Health 1984; **74**: 1357–62.
12. Minkler M, Pasick RJ. Health promotion in the elderly: a critical perspective on the past and future. In: Dychtwald K (ed) Wellness and Health Promotion for the Elderly, pp. 39–51. Rockville, MD: Aspen Publications, 1986.
13. Filner B, Williams TF. Health promotion for the elderly: reducing functional dependency. In: Healthy People. Washington, DC: US Government Printing Office, 1979.
14. Russell LB. Is Prevention Better Than Cure? Washington DC: The Brookings Institution, 1986.
15. Cohen DR, Henderson JB. Health Prevention and Economics. Oxford: University Press, 1988.
16. Haynes RB, Sackett DL, Taylor DW et al. Increased absenteeism after detection of labelling of hypertensive patients. N Engl J Med 1978; **299**: 741–4.
17. Stoate HG. Can health screening damage your health? J Roy Coll Gen Pract 1989; **39**: 193–5.
18. Bergman AB. The menace of mass screening. Amer J Pub Health 1977; **67**: 601–2.
19. Kennie DC. Health maintenance of the elderly. J Amer Geriatr Soc 1984; **32**: 316–23.
20. Roemer MI. The value of medical care for health promotion. Amer J Pub Health 1984; **74**; 243–8.
21. Kane RL, Kane RA, Arnold SB. Prevention in the elderly: risk factors. Health Services Research 1985; **19**: 945–1005.
22. World Health Organisation. International Classification of Impairments, Disabilities and Handicaps. Geneva: WHO, 1980.
23. Tatara K, Shinso F, Suzuki M et al. Relation between the use of health check ups starting in middle age and demand for inpatient care by elderly people in Japan. Brit Med J 1991; **302**: 615–18.

2

What is health in old age?

The health of a nation is one of its most valuable resources, and is one foundation for the generation of economic wealth. This idea begs the questions: what exactly is health, and in particular, what does it mean to elderly people? Several concepts have been propounded. One of the most commonly quoted is that of the World Health Organization (WHO) who took a broad perspective and defined health as 'a state of complete physical, mental and social wellbeing' [1]. There are, however, several problems with this type of definition. Firstly, it is too perfect and may create an inappropriate escalation of demand. Complete physical, mental and social wellbeing means the avoidance of influenza or better access to public facilities for the disabled. It may also mean an increasingly higher pension and better housing or any rights or civil liberties that make the elderly person more content. Taken to its extreme, it can mean virtually any physical goods to keep that person satisfied. Using WHO's definition of perfect health begins to blur the margins between the search for legitimate and feasible health promotional strategies within a society and its narcissistic pursuit of hedonism. Secondly, WHO defines a perfect health that, as we see in Chapter 14, few people even wish to try to attain. The achievement of perfect health is not without a variety of unacceptable costs to many of the individuals concerned. Thirdly, WHO defines health in broad terms that lack the operational precision upon which specific preventive and health promotional strategies for elderly people can be based.

Perhaps a more helpful definition of health in old age around which to base preventive strategies is to describe health as:

a multidimensional matrix of three interwoven components: the absence of disease (including disease symptomatology and iatrogenic disease); an optimal functional status; and an adequate system of social support [2].

The subcomponents of health within this model are now outlined.

14

The absence of disease

Physical health

This consists of freedom from traditional organ-specific disease and the symptoms associated with such disease. In elderly people there is a greater chance of physical disease affecting a greater range of organ systems than in a younger population and of more than one organ system being afflicted simultaneously.

Mental health

The frequency of mental health disorders increases dramatically in later life: the absence of such disorders contributes greatly to the elderly person's health. Mental health consists not only in an absence of psychiatric disease, but also in an absence of psychological morbidity and in a personality that is well adjusted to the vagaries of the ageing process.

An absence of iatrogenic insult

Health in old age also depends on an absence of 'insult' from the interventions of various health care professionals. Traditionally this has focussed on avoiding problems with drugs and minimising morbidity from medical investigation and treatment. However, other types of iatrogenic insult are common, such as the loss of autonomy of an older person if they are inappropriately admitted to institutional care.

An optimal functional status

Many types of bodily function make up the operational components of health in elderly people. These range from the immediate concerns of the rehabilitation process of importance to hospital staff to a broader range of functions required for independent living in the community, and then to a much wider concept of social functioning essential for their psychological wellbeing and quality of life. Functional status therefore consists of the following components.

Mental status

Mental status is probably the most important of all functions for the elderly person to retain in old age, a poor mental status leading in turn to numerous other functional problems. Mental status consists essentially of memory/ cognition and behaviour.

Mobility

Mobility is the key physical function in elderly people. It comprises rising and transferring (i.e. the acts of getting on and off chairs and beds etc.), the ability to maintain balance and an upright posture and the ability to walk and to climb stairs.

Continence and excretion

Continence should be considered as the deposition of urine and/or faeces in appropriate places. Retention of this function is of physical and psychological importance to the elderly person. Other functions within this category include micturition and bowel excretion, both of which often cause problems in old age.

The activities of daily living (ADL)

Traditionally, in the gerontological literature, these wide-ranging activities have been subdivided into ADL and Instrumental Activities of Daily Living (IADL). However, it may be of more practical value to consider these functions in the following three categories.

1. *Personal activities of daily living (PADL)*, such as feeding, toileting, dressing and attending to personal hygiene.
2. *Domestic activities of daily living (DADL)*, for example, cooking and making meals, shopping, cleaning and laundering.
3. *Social activities of daily living (SADL)*, such as interpersonal relationships, work, recreation and the very large diffuse range of human activities that lead to self fulfilment and good psychological health.

Special senses

Included in this category are vision and hearing and, to a lesser extent, taste.

Language and communication

The ability to produce, articulate, phonate and modulate speech are important functions for elderly people in maintaining their independence, social inter-action and morale.

Other functions

Other miscellaneous functions such as sleep and swallowing may be considered here.

An adequate system of social support

A 'support system' for elderly people may be considered as any factor that promotes their independence, dictates a lesser level of care within the living environment and/or improves their quality of life. Four types of support can be identified.

The extent and quality of care provided by others

This consists primarily of the *informal* support system; that is, the range of assistance provided by the nuclear and extended family and by friends. It may also consist of advice, enablement or support from a wide variety of paid *formal* caregivers both in the community and in institutional care. Nurses, bath attendants, home helps, social workers and doctors are common examples.

The nature of the living environment

This includes a consideration of the risk factors within the elderly person's living environment and a consideration of the level of care required to maximise quality of life.

The adequacy of the provisions of care

The provision of personal and domestic aids, home adaptations and the adequacy of financial resources are important considerations for the elderly person's independence and wellbeing.

The operational policies of care

An important but often neglected aspect of an elderly person's health depends on the approach or policy of the main caregiver. Various types of abuse have received publicity, but a more common problem is that of overprotection of elderly persons by their carers.

The main sections of this book now adopt this three-dimensional model of health for health promotion and describe strategies to:

1. Prevent disease and illness;
2. Promote functional independence;
3. Maintain an adequate system of social support.

These preventive strategies must be designed not only to promote health within each component of the health care model but also to avoid adverse effects on the other components of health. For example, gains in health from disease prevention must not be offset by losses in functional status from the iatrogenic insults of the procedures used.

References

1. World Health Organization. Constitution of the World Health Organization: Annexe 1. The First Ten Years of the World Health Organization. Geneva: WHO, 1958.
2. Kennie DC. Health Maintenance of the Elderly. J Amer Geriatr Soc 1984; **32**: 316–23.

3

The goals of health promotion for elderly people

It is important to have explicit, clear goals for health promotion and preventive care that encompass the broad view of health as described in Chapter 2. The needs of carers, and to an extent the needs of society (as a 'corporate carer' for this population), must also be considered. Once these goals are identified, specific measurable and realistic targets can then be formulated for each. The following goals are offered as a starting point in this process.

Health promotion and preventive care for elderly people should:

- catalyse, enable and empower elderly people to continue their self development as individuals and as important members of society
- prevent or palliate physical, psychiatric and psychological disorders and the symptomatic consequences thereof
- prevent iatrogenic insult to health, to functional status and to the social support system
- prolong life where this is desired by the elderly person and is compatible with ethical principles of care
- prolong the period of effective activity and independent living in old age
- ensure a support system adequate to preserve people's autonomy, independence, dignity and quality of life at all levels of care
- avoid institutionalisation as far as is practicable in both humanitarian and economic terms
- support and assist elderly people to adapt to loss when this is inevitable
- ensure that when illness is terminal there is as little distress as possible to patient and caregivers
- minimise the burden on family and other caregivers to improve their quality of life and prolong the period of time they are willing to undertake the caring role

- avoid overprotection, the fostering of dependency and iatrogenic insult in the application of health promotional measures
- achieve the above goals in the most cost effective manner in order that opportunities can exist for funding other services for elderly people.

4

A task for everyone

If preventive strategies and health promotion are to be effective in an elderly population a large number of tasks need to be performed by many sectors of society, both individually and collectively (see Table 4.1). This chapter outlines a number of these tasks. Some are dealt with in more detail in Chapters 12 and 13.

Tasks for elderly people

Health promotion and preventive strategies in old age cannot be fully successful without the willing and active participation of elderly people themselves. They have a number of tasks to fulfil.

Continue self development

Because an older person reaches retirement or some other landmark, chronological age is no reason to lose the drive towards self fulfilment and enjoyment. The nature of activities may change, for this is a time for re-evaluating and re-establishing relationships, but there is considerable opportunity and challenge to utilise the increased amounts of available spare time in a productive, meaningful and satisfying manner.

If older people succumb to the ageist stereotypes prevalent in a community and restrict their activity accordingly it is unlikely they will achieve their optimal psychological and functional health. However, the full realisation of individual self development cannot occur without complementary enabling and empowering activities by other sectors of society.

21

Table 4.1. *The tasks of health promotion*

Tasks for elderly people
Continue self development
Adopt a healthy lifestyle (where appropriate)
Adapt to loss

Tasks for families and carers
Provide informal support
Respect the elderly person's autonomy
Avoid over-protection

Tasks for health care providers
Validate the preventive strategies scientifically
Re-evaluate traditional strategies
Personalise preventive strategies
Reduce iatrogenic insult
Recognise the needs of family carers
Adopt a wider focus

Tasks for public health
Guide organisations that purchase health services in buying appropriate preventive
    strategies
Assist in the appropriate reorientation of funding between traditional health service
    and non-health service organisations
Assess and catalyse the development of local community health strategies
Promote health education for the elderly population

Tasks for government
Provide a nurturing environment for the generation of wealth
Ensure financial manipulation of 'risk goods' to modify health behaviour
Provide legislation to modify health behaviour

Collective tasks
Educate to dispel ageism
Minimise costs

Adopt a healthy lifestyle

A second task for elderly individuals is to adopt a healthy lifestyle. This can involve giving up smoking, taking more exercise, eating a more nutritious and balanced diet or ensuring that the home environment is safer to live in. Many health promotional programmes in the Americas have placed considerable emphasis on these aspects of preventive care [1, 2]. Nevertheless, not all elderly individuals wish to adopt these measures. In Chapter 14 it may be seen that this is because the move towards perfect health is not without some form of cost to the individual concerned.

It is, therefore, appropriate that elderly people should be educated about the advantages of a healthy lifestyle and, as with other sections of society, be persuaded to adopt such a lifestyle. Indeed, it would be ageist to do otherwise. However, information on the advantages should be balanced with information on any costs, the persuasion exerted should not be undue and the elderly individual's autonomy should be respected so that the final decision about adopting a healthy lifestyle rests in their hands.

Adapt to loss

Ultimately, however, it is the elderly individual's ability to adapt to loss that dictates whether or not they will make a success of extreme old age [3]. Almost inevitably, as a people age they experience a variety of losses: initially loss of employment, then possibly loss of health or of a social liberty such as driving; there will be accompanying loss of friends or loved ones; and finally the loss of their own lives, for which everyone must prepare. The coping skills of elderly individuals that are intrinsic to their personality and psychological makeup will in large part dictate the quality of their lives, though as is described in various sections of this book, these skills may be enhanced by training and education.

Tasks for families and carers

Families and other caregivers are inextricably linked with the elderly people whom they support and must also accomplish certain tasks if preventive strategies are to be fully realised.

Provide informal support

An important task that society requires of its families is that they provide support for their elderly relatives. This fortunately seems an inherent social value and in most Western societies the vast majority of all home health care is provided, often very willingly, by family carers [4, 5]. That modern families provide less support for their elderly relatives than did previous generations is now recognised as myth [6].

Respect the older person's autonomy

A second task for families is to respect older people's autonomy. Families must accept that at times the older person may wish to maintain a particular lifestyle or living environment or take a decision about their treatment and care that is not in accordance with the family's views about 'what is best'. In these circumstances, a degree of persuasion is appropriate but, if this fails, the older person's values and wishes must be respected and adhered to. This can often create considerable anxiety in a family and make the job of keeping 'hands off' a painful option for them. In these circumstances it is often the family, rather than the older person, that requires counselling and support.

Avoid overprotection

Another temptation for a family, as they see someone they care for deteriorate and become more frail, is to overprotect that person. Overprotection can take many forms: excessive visiting; opting to carry out chores that could otherwise be done by the older person; keeping the elderly person in bed for an unnecessarily long period after an illness; or requesting an excessive input from community services. If overprotection persists for long, the health of elderly people suffers. They learn a dependent, submissive role and end up being functionally less able to look after themselves than if they had been left more alone. The final task for carers, then, is to avoid the trap of overprotection.

Tasks for health care providers

To progress towards a rational and effective preventive approach for elderly people, health professionals must fulfil a number of tasks. The priority given to these tasks depends on the nature of the traditional health care delivery system within which the professionals operate. Because of long standing differences in health care systems, the UK and the USA are often used for comparative purposes.

Validate the strategies scientifically

The first task of health professionals must be to validate their preventive and health promotional strategies scientifically. This is in order to protect an essentially healthy population from iatrogenic insult (see below), to prevent unnecessary costs both to individuals and society, and to maintain the scientific integrity of the individuals concerned. It is particularly important to prove the value of strategies in aged populations and not to rely on results from younger age groups.

Re-evaluate traditional strategies

A further task for health professionals must be their willingness to re-appraise traditional strategies. In the USA and Canada this has taken the form of a re-evaluation of the annual physical examination. Over the last ten years, the Canadian Task Force on the Periodic Health Examination and latterly the United States Preventive Services Task Force have reviewed the available scientific evidence and recommended instead replacement of the annual examination by more restrictive, targeted strategies, implemented at selected times throughout an individual's lifespan. In the UK, the reappraisal task has been different, being one of evaluating the numerous screening and case finding programmes for the elderly population. This is still in progress and is discussed in Chapter 12.

Maintain a balanced approach to preventive activity

I have already pointed out in Chapter 1 that the extent of preventive and health promotional activity for all age groups, but particularly for the elderly population, varies considerably from one country to another. In the USA, health professionals must guard against an uncritical, overzealous invasive approach to prevention. In the UK, they must guard against ignorance, apathy and inactivity. Ideally then, a balanced approach should be adopted between the Scylla of overzealous activity and the Charybdis of nihilistic inertia.

Personalise preventive strategies

The elderly population is not homogeneous; they have widely varying levels of illness and disability. Elderly people themselves vary considerably in their health care values and their wishes about future care. Whilst it is important to define various preventive strategies precisely, it is important to personalise each measure to suit the individual concerned. This topic is discussed in Chapter 11.

Reduce iatrogenic insult

The elderly population is one in which there is a decline in functioning in almost every organ system, resulting in impaired homeostasis and a vulnerability to iatrogenic insult. A major goal of health promotion in elderly people must therefore be a reduction in the various types of iatrogenic insult. As some of the detection manoeuvres employed in preventive care carry with them an inherent risk, reduction of iatrogenic insult should not only be a goal of health promotion, but should also be a principle in the application of preventive care. The risk of iatrogenic insult is, unfortunately, greatest in the most interventionist and biotechnologically orientated health care systems such as that of the USA.

Recognise the needs of family carers

An important task of health promotion in the elderly population is to address the needs of family carers. Traditionally, the emphasis on supporting them has been to encourage them to continue with their caring role for as long as possible, either because there were inadequate institutional places into which to admit the older person or because of perceived financial savings by keeping that person in the community longer. Nowadays, meeting the needs of carers also means promoting *their* health, giving them a choice about the extent of their caring role and trying to relieve their burden so that they no longer fall foul of the various physical and psychological disorders associated with the caring role.

Adopt a wider focus

Health in old age is a matrix of three interwoven components; freedom from disease and disease symptoms, an optimal functional status, and an adequate system of social support [7]. Optimal health for elderly people therefore requires a broad, balanced approach with emphasis on each of these three sectors. Successful health promotion for elderly people must use a wider focus than in other age groups, with equal emphasis on preventing disease, implementing strategies that enhance functional status and implementing strategies that strengthen systems of social support.

Tasks for Public Health

The role of Public Health in preventive and health promotional programmes for elderly people include: guidance to organisations that purchase health services in buying appropriate preventive strategies that will have maximum impact on the health of an older population; assisting in the appropriate reorientation of funding between traditional health service and non-health service organisations; assisting and catalysing the development of local community health strategies; and promoting health education for the elderly population.

Tasks for government

It should be appreciated that when attempting to plan and implement health promotional policies, one sector of government not only may be vying for funds with another, but also may be in direct conflict with another sector's policies. For a government to implement health promotion successfully, it must therefore ensure an authoritative overview on policy and activity in all relevant departments and give responsibility to someone of sufficient standing that the policy can be effected in spite of internal conflicts.

The government has three roles in health promotion. Firstly, it must create a nurturing environment for public and private firms to generate the income that is necessary if health promotional measures are to be funded, in part, out of the public purse. Secondly, it has the power to modify healthy behaviour and the purchase of 'risk goods' by financial incentives and disincentives (such as favourable pricing of lead-free petrol and taxing of cigarettes). Thirdly, government can provide legislation that either restricts unhealthy behaviour (for example, strict drink–driving laws) or enables and empowers elderly people to lead a full and healthy life in society. This last role is important because central and local government must provide a framework within which public and private organisations are forced to take responsibility for planning and funding changes in the social institutions (employment, housing, education, leisure and recreation etc.) necessary to meet the health needs of an ageing population.

Collective tasks

The various sectors of society must also work *together* to complete the two following major tasks without which health promotional strategies would be singularly unsuccessful.

Set an appropriate allocation for funding

Society in general acts to support its elderly population by contributing a high proportion of its Gross National Product to the public funding of care of elderly people. The extent of the resources placed at the disposal of elderly people for promoting their health may be perceived by many as a governmental decision and, in the final analysis, this may be so. However, in most countries it is merely a response by government to implicit or explicit messages given to it by various sectors of society. It is often the minimal response that a government considers society will allow it to take without jeopardising its position.

Deciding on an appropriate allocation of funding for health promotional measures in old people is, therefore, a task incumbent on all of us and one that stretches the limits of society's altruism. Within this framework, it is nevertheless quite appropriate for society to ensure it gets the best value for any *additional* money it is intending to spend and to seek more effective ways of spending *existing* health care funds so that it better promotes the overall health of the elderly population.

Educate to dispel ageism

Perhaps the most important collective task is for society to educate itself to remove its ageist views about health in old age. Often elderly people are under-referred or referred late for health care, with the result that potentially remediable problems have become too far advanced by the time anything is done about them. There are many reasons for these nihilistic views: treatable health problems may be considered an irremediable part of the normal ageing process; elderly people are relatively stoic and put up with many problems, not wishing to bother others; all health care and preventive strategies in old age may wrongly be considered to be of no value; and there may be problems of geographical and financial access to health services. Elderly people themselves are often ageist and under-report illness for precisely the above reasons. They should therefore be targeted about the potential of preventive strategies and early treatment. For the frail elderly it is often family carers that are the main procurers of services. They too may have negative views about what can be achieved and may require education. Sadly, many health and social service professionals also require to be educated, a task that the remainder of this book sets out to accomplish.

References

1. Minkler M, Pasick RJ. Health promotion and the elderly: a critical perspective on the past and future. In: Dychtwald K (ed) Wellness and Health Promotion for the Elderly, pp. 39–51. Rockville, MD: Aspen Publications, 1986.
2. Estes CL, Fox S, Mahoney CW. Health care and social policy. In: Dychtwald K (ed) Wellness and Health Promotion for the Elderly, pp. 55–65. Rockville, MD: Aspen Publications, 1986.
3. Christiansen D. Dignity in aging: notes on geriatric ethics. J Humanistic Psychol 1978; **18**: 41–54.
4. Home care for persons 55 and over, US July 1966–June 1968. Vital and Health Statistics Series 10 No. 73 Department of Health Education and Welfare. PBN HSM 72–1–620. National Center for Health Statistics, 1972.

5. Kane RL, Kane RA. Care of the aged: old problems in need of new solutions. Science 1978; **200**: 913–19.
6. Muir Gray JA. The prevention of family breakdown. In: Muir Gray JA (ed) Prevention of Disease in the Elderly, pp. 38–50. Edinburgh: Churchill Livingstone, 1985.
7. Kennie DC. Health maintenance of the elderly. J Amer Geriatr Soc 1984; **32**: 316–23.

5

Critique of strategies

In order to safeguard an essentially healthy population from iatrogenic insult, to prevent unnecessary costs both to individuals and to society, and to maintain the scientific integrity of the health professionals concerned, a number of rules or principles have been evolved over the years to define acceptable strategies for the screening of 'normal' populations [1–3]. Rogers et al. [4] have further refined these criteria so they become relevant to the elderly population with chronic illness. Despite this emphasis on screening criteria, the relevant principles are also pertinent to a wide range of other preventive care and health promotional strategies. In those countries where preventive care programmes have been widely practised, national 'task forces' have been set up to critique the various strategies and to make reliable recommendations on good practice. Most noticeable of these was firstly the Canadian Task Force on the Periodic Health Examination [5] and subsequently the United States Preventive Services Task Force [6]. These working parties have further developed the above principles to establish new international standards.

The preventive care and health promotional strategies outlined in this book are therefore discussed in the context of these accepted principles. For ease of presentation, each health problem is therefore considered under the following headings.

- Importance
- Feasibility of detection
- Effectiveness of preventive strategies
- Cost of applying detection and prevention strategies

These aspects are now considered in more detail.

The importance of the health problem

The importance of a health problem will be considered in a number of ways. The first is its impact on the individual elderly person so afflicted. The parameters used here should include not just its effect on mortality but also the associated morbidity it incurs in terms of suffering from symptom complexes (such as pain) and functional disability.

Other important outcomes are also considered. The various types and degrees of burden imposed on those families and other persons caring for elderly people with the problem influence the importance of the problem. In a wider sense, the impact of the problem on society, as assessed by the community and institutional resources (and the associated costs) required to provide care to those afflicted is also a factor.

The feasibility of detection

Wherever feasible, primary, secondary and tertiary preventive strategies should be considered for each health problem. For primary prevention, the issue under consideration in this section will be the feasibility of *targeting* those elderly people who have, or exhibit, the appropriate risk factors. For tertiary prevention, the issue under consideration will be the feasibility of *increasing the awareness* of health care professionals so that they take greater cognisance of the problem that requires amelioration.

Secondary prevention usually revolves around the issue of screening, and here the issue under consideration will be to assess how feasible it is to detect the problem in its early stages. It is in this area of screening detection manoeuvres (usually for disease states) that the most stringent criteria need to be applied.

The suitability of a screening test depends in part on its *reliability*; that is, its ability to be accurately reproduced between different laboratories or observers, or by the same observer or laboratory at different times. The suitability of a screening test also depends on its *accuracy*, which is measured in terms of four indices: sensitivity, which refers to the proportion of persons with the problem who test positive; specificity, which refers to the proportion of persons without the problem who test negative; the positive predictive value, which refers to the proportion of persons with a positive test who have the problem; and the negative predictive value, which refers to the proportion of persons with a negative test who do not have the problem. The mathematical relationship between these indices is shown in Table 5.1.

When evaluating any benefit that may accrue from screening populations of

Table 5.1. *Relationship between indices that measure the accuracy of screening tests*

		Health problems	
		Present	Absent
Test	Positive	*A* (True positive)	*B* (False positive)
	Negative	*C* (False negative)	*D* (True negative)
Sensitivity	=	Proportion of persons with problem who test positive	$\dfrac{A}{A+C}$
Specificity	=	Proportion of persons without problem who test negative	$\dfrac{D}{B+D}$
Positive predictive value	=	Proportion of persons with positive test who have problem	$\dfrac{A}{A+B}$
Negative predictive value	=	Proportion of persons with negative test who do not have problem	$\dfrac{D}{C+D}$

frail elderly who are vulnerable to iatrogenic insult, it is important to realise that the benefits of early detection to those afflicted are often counterbalanced by the suffering imposed on a far greater number of relatively healthy individuals who do not have the disorder. This suffering includes the inconvenience of screening, the iatrogenic insult of any further tests required to make a confirmatory diagnosis and, sometimes, further iatrogenic insult from unnecessary surgery.

Some estimate of this adverse impact of screening can be obtained by considering the specificity of the screening test. A test with poor specificity will result in healthy persons being told that they have the condition. These persons are known as false positives and it is they who will require further diagnostic assessment to exclude the condition. The likely rate of achieving false positives with a test will also vary, depending on the prevalence of the condition in the elderly population being screened: the indicator that best reflects this problem being the positive predictive value of the test.

The effectiveness of preventive strategies

The effectiveness of any preventive care or health promotional strategy is vitally important and therefore, for each health problem, a comprehensive

Table 5.2. *Effectiveness of intervention*

Grade	Criteria
I	Evidence obtained from at least one properly randomised controlled trial
II-1	Evidence obtained from well designed cohort of case-control analytic studies, preferably from more than one centre or research group
II-2	Evidence obtained from comparisons between times or places with or without the intervention. Dramatic results in uncontrolled experiments (such as the results of the introduction of penicillin in the 1940s) could also be regarded as this type of evidence
III	Opinions of respected authorities, based on clinical experience, descriptive studies or reports of expert committees

The effectiveness of intervention can be graded into one of four categories according to the quality of the evidence obtained. Adapted from ref. [5].

review of the available scientific evidence is provided wherever possible. Particular attention is given to data obtained from studies on aged populations, rather than relying on extrapolation of results from younger age groups.

Both the Canadian Task Force on the Periodic Health Examination and the United States Preventive Services Task Force developed strict grading criteria according to the quality of the scientific evidence available (see Table 5.2). Although such a formal grading of the evidence is not provided in this book, the interested reader may wish to interpret the research in the light of the particular weighting suggested by these august bodies.

Unfortunately, it will be seen that, for many health problems afflicting elderly people, and particularly for those relating to functional difficulties and the social support system, relatively little scientific evidence is offered for scrutiny. These measures should therefore not be adopted wholeheartedly without further evaluation, particularly if they are costly or incur iatrogenic insult. Nevertheless, it is important to realise that lack of *evidence* for a strategy does not necessarily imply lack of *efficacy*. Research evidence may be lacking because the ageist bias of the scientific community has excluded elderly people from scientific trials for no particularly good reason. Additionally, the practicalities and variables involved in mounting research, particularly psychosocial research, in an older population can be extremely difficult to manage. These problems are set against a background where there is little incentive to carry out evaluative studies, the research funds for study of ageing usually being only a small fraction of the national budget. Simply because a strategy lacks a foundation in scientific information, it should not necessarily be excluded from a recommended health maintenance protocol.

Lastly, the words efficacy and effectiveness are used frequently in the text and should be noted to have rather different meanings. Efficacy implies the usefulness of a particular strategy when tested in the rather artificial situation of a research trial. Effectiveness tends to be used when extrapolating this potential usefulness to the population as a whole. Sometimes, strategies of considerable apparent value fail to bring about benefit in a wider population because of the practicalities involved. Conversely, a preventive strategy that has only a minor impact on reducing relative risk in a research study may nevertheless have significant impact on a population, in terms of absolute risk, if the target condition is common and associated with a significant morbidity and mortality.

The cost of applying detection and prevention strategies

The cost of targeting health promotional strategies or of detecting a disorder and applying preventive care is an important consideration that receives detailed consideration in Chapter 14. The evidence suggests that the majority of preventive strategies add to costs rather than create savings [7] and therefore the choice between such strategies as well as the choice between health promotion and traditional health care delivery is partly economic. The ultimate decision on any allocation of funds should only be made once health professionals and the general public have been fully informed on these issues.

Discussion about the costs of various strategies will, wherever possible, be based on cost effectiveness or cost–benefit analyses. These economic yard-sticks (as well as the inherent ageist bias that they contain) are also discussed in Chapter 14.

References

1. Cuckle HS, Wald NJ. Principles of Screening in Ante-natal and Neo-natal Screening. Oxford: University Press, 1984.
2. Cochrane AT, Holland WW. Validation of screening procedures. Br Med Bull 1971; **27**: 3–8.
3. Wilson JMG, Jungner G. Principles and Practice of Screening for Disease. Geneva: World Health Organisation, 1968.
4. Rogers, J, Supino P, Grower R. Proposed evaluation for screening programmes for the elderly. Gerontologist 1986; **26**: 564–70.
5. Canadian Task Force on the Periodic Health Examination. Can Med Assoc J 1979; **121**: 1193–1254.

6. Report of the US Preventive Services Task Force. Guide to Clinical Preventive Services. Baltimore, MD: Williams and Wilkins, 1989.
7. Russell LB. Is Prevention Better Than Cure? Washington, DC: The Brookings Institution, 1986.

6

Cancer prevention

Cancer is the second most common cause of death in the elderly population [1]. Table 6.1 shows the annual incidence of the ten most common cancers in England and Wales and the proportions of these cases that occur in men and women aged over 70 and over 80 years [2]. The reasons for the increased rate of cancer in old age is unknown, though it may be due to a decrease in immune surveillance or to an increasing frequency of DNA damage resulting in more frequent malignant transformation of normal cells.

Despite cancer being so common, surprisingly little is known about its behaviour in older patients. Previously, older patients have tended to be excluded from clinical trials because of negative ageist bias, misperceptions about the ageing process or, on occasions, the sheer impracticality of including very frail elderly individuals in such research. Despite this, cancer has been closely scrutinised by the biomedical industry for many years and more is probably known about the prevention of cancer than the prevention of many other health problems in old age.

This chapter therefore reviews the importance of each of the major cancers afflicting the elderly population, evaluates the worth of screening programmes, and makes recommendations for practising clinicians based on current evidence. Where appropriate, comment is also made about primary preventive strategies.

Breast cancer

Importance

Breast cancer is the commonest cancer in women (except skin cancer) and has only just been ousted by lung cancer as the commonest cause of cancer *deaths* in women. Of all breast cancers, 50 per cent occur in women over 65 years of age [3]. The age-specific incidence (number of cases per year per hundred

36

Table 6.1. *Annual incidence of the ten most common malignancies in England and Wales by age*

	Women				Men		
Type	n	>70 yr (%)	>80 yr (%)	Type	n	>70 yr (%)	> 80 yr (%)
Breast	21363	36	14	Lung	26203	50	12
Skin	10576	58	25	Skin	11678	49	15
Lung	9840	48	14	Prostate	9524	72	25
Colon	8192	64	29	Bladder	6886	54	15
Ovary	4539	35	12	Stomach	6788	56	16
Stomach	4465	71	34	Colon	6648	54	17
Rectum	4308	62	27	Rectum	5269	50	15
Cervix	4043	20	6	Pancreas	2926	51	15
Uterus	3329	37	12	Oesophagus	2436	47	14
Pancreas	2772	66	28	Leukaemia	2319	46	15
Total		48	19	Total		53	16

n is the number of new cases for each type of cancer per annum in England and Wales.
Source: Fentimen et al. Lancet 1990; 335: 1020–2.

thousand females for each age group) of breast cancer rises progressively (see Fig. 6.1) [4]. In the US, by 75 years the cumulative prevalence reaches between 6 and 10 per cent.

Research from Sweden has shown that survival rates are lower with increasing age. Adami [5], using data relating to age at diagnosis and the relative survival from a computerised registry of 50068 women, showed that women aged 40 to 49 years of age had the best prognosis. The difference in relative survival between those older than 75 and those 45 to 49 increased from 8.6 per cent at two years, to 12.2, 20.3 and 27.5 per cent after five, ten and fifteen years of follow up, respectively.

There are several risk factors for breast cancer. Perhaps the most important of these is a family history of the disease in the elderly person's mother or sister which increases the chance two- to threefold [6].

Detection

Three types of detection manoeuvre are available.

Breast self examination (BSE)

In Britain, breast self examination is carried out by only 24 per cent of those over 75 years of age, compared with 55 per cent of those younger than 65 years

[7]. The technique may be a worthwhile precaution that will increase the probability of detecting breast cancer at an early age, but its estimated sensitivity is low (20 to 30 per cent), and is lower in older women. So far the technique has not been shown to reduce mortality rates [8]. Its future role awaits the outcome of several trials [9, 10].

Clinical breast examination (CBE)

This is an effective method of detection, though it now identifies fewer carcinomas than the technique of mammography [11]. However, without mammography the majority of tumours could still be detected clinically. The precise role of CBE alone as a screening tool has recently been reported in women aged 50 to 59 years [12] and is discussed below. Evidence from the USA again suggests a decline in the use of CBE with increasing age. Forty per cent of women aged 75 years and older were receiving annual CBE from their physicians, compared with 75 per cent in those younger than 65 years [13].

Mammography

This now seems the most effective form of screening. Originally there was some concern over the potential carcinogenic effect of the radiation dose from this procedure, but the dose currently used for plain film mammography is low and the carcinogenic effect is estimated to be lower for older women [14]. The probability that ten mammogram examinations will cause breast cancer in the remaining years of an elderly woman's life is probably less than 1 in 50 000. However, a major concern about mammography is the number of women without cancer who present with falsely positive results at each examination and then require surgical consultation to exclude the lesion. In one trial this occurred in 2 per cent of women 50 to 65 years of age [15]. The chance of needing such an additional workup rises to 20 to 30 per cent after ten mammograms.

A serious concern with all current screening techniques is the potential lack of lead time. Based on cell doubling times, up to 90 per cent of tumours can metastasise by the time they are 6 mm in diameter and many will have disseminated by the time they are clinically apparent. Nevertheless, the interval between the first development of malignant cells and onset of symptoms is long, perhaps as many as ten years. Although the percentage of elderly patients presenting with only local disease may be similar to those for younger age groups [16], there are conflicting reports on whether the overall extent of tumour mass is greater in older age groups [16].

Acceptance of invitation for screening declines with age; for example, in one study 60 per cent accepted in their fifties but only 22 per cent accepted in their eighties [17]. In the UK, older women are excluded from routine call and recall mainly because it was thought that their response to invitation would be so low that the expected benefit would not justify the effort. However, Hobbs et al. [18] have recently shown that there is a potential for high attendance at routine screening by older women if they are invited in the same way as younger women. Response rates for invitation to screening for women 65 to 79 years were 54.5 per cent, 58.4 per cent and 60.7 per cent for the indices of crude population coverage ratio, crude invitation population coverage ratio, and

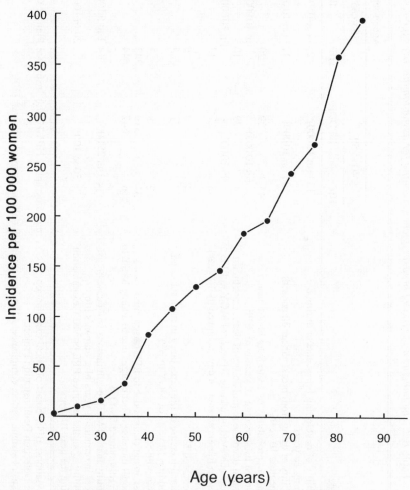

Fig. 6.1. Age-specific incidence of breast cancer in Sweden in 1970. Adapted from ref. [5].

Table 6.2. *The benefits and risks of breast cancer screening for asymptomatic average-risk women of various ages*

	Age group					
	40 to 50		55 to 65		65 to 75	
Variable	HIP	BCDDP	HIP	BCDDP	HIP	BCDDP
Probability of developing breast cancer during the coming 10 years	133 (in 10000)		233 (in 10000)		279 (in 10000)	
Probability of dying from breast cancer diagnosed in the next 10 years	86 (in 10000)		123 (in 10000)		120 (in 10000)	
Decrease in probability of death from breast cancer achieved by screening 10 years with BPE	15	29 (in 10000)	20	41 (in 10000)	21	42 (in 10000)
Additional decrease in probability of death from breast cancer achieved by adding 10 years of MGY to BPE	8	29 (in 10000)	10	41 (in 10000)	10	42 (in 10000)
Increase in life expectancy in days achieved by 10 years of BPE	13	27	13	26	10	18
Discounted 5%	4	8	6	10	5	9
Additional increase in life expectancy in days achieved by adding 10 years of MGY to BPE	7	27	7	26	5	18
Discounted 5%	2	8	3	10	2	9
Increase in net charges due to BPE (discounted 5%), $	331	319	243	232	233	226
Additional increase in net charges due to adding MGY to BPE (discounted 5%$), $	666	647	644	621	616	598
Probability that 10 MGY examinations will cause breast cancer in remaining years of a woman's life	< 1 in 25 000		< 1 in 50 000		< 1 in 50 000	
Probability of a false positive BPE or MGY examination during the next 10 years	30 in 100		20 in 100		20 in 100	

Abbreviations: BPE, breast physical examination; MGY, mammography; HIP, Health Insurance Plan of Greater New York; BCDDP, Breast Cancer Detection Demonstration Project.
All answers assume perfect compliance. All prices are in US dollars. Adapted from ref. [30].

corrected invited population coverage ratio, respectively. The acceptability of this screening service to elderly women has also been reported in detail [19].

Compliance with screening can be improved by including a definite appointment time in the letter of invitation to screen [20]. There is some suggestion that screening studies may self select those with a higher incidence of breast problems and symptoms.

Effectiveness

Theoretically, the early detection of breast cancer in elderly individuals should bring about significant benefits. Five and ten-year absolute postoperative survival rates following mastectomy are as good in patients older than 70 years as in younger patients [21]. The frequency of oestrogen-receptor-positive breast cancers increases with age [22] and, in most studies, adjuvant systemic therapy with hormonal agents has proven significantly more efficacious in older than in younger patients [23]. Elderly women may be rather less responsive to chemotherapy, but they do tolerate it well provided appropriate dosage adjustments are made.

The above theoretical benefits for elderly women have now been realised in seven carefully controlled studies [8, 24–29] and one uncontrolled study [15], which have shown a reduction in mortality achieved by breast cancer screening with CBE, mammography or both. Whether these benefits will be sustained if extrapolated to routine service screening on a country-wide basis remains to be seen.

Eddy [30] has made detailed calculations of the benefits, risks and costs of breast cancer screening for asymptomatic average-risk women of various ages. To do this, a computerised model was applied to the results of two screening programmes from the USA, the Health Insurance Plan Study (HIP) and the Breast Cancer Detection Demonstration Project (BCDDP). These studies were chosen as representing an underestimate of the effectiveness of screening (HIP) and an overestimate of the effectiveness of screening (BCDDP). Based on this lower and upper limit, Eddy [30] calculated the data shown in Table 6.2. The data in this table can be used to estimate answers to questions that apply to average-risk, asymptomatic women of different ages who are contemplating annual breast cancer screening with CBE or mammography or both for the coming ten years. The projections in the table assume a full ten years of screening, full compliance and lifetime follow up. The reductions in mortality are therefore higher than may be achieved in practice.

Further work by Mandelblatt et al. [30a], using a decision analysis model, suggested that screening had the potential to save lives even in the very old, that

Table 6.3. *Marginal cost of adding a year of life calculated for various strategies used in screening for breast cancer*

Age group and strategy	Cost ($)	
	BCDDP	HIP
40 to 50 years		
Annual BPE[a]	14 509	33 000
Annual BPE and MGY[b]	29 427	134 081
55 to 65 years		
Annual BPE[a]	8113	15 536
Annual BPE and MGY[b]	21 717	83 830
65 to 75 years		
Annual BPE[a]	9597	17 173
Annual BPE and MGY[b]	25 395	92 412

BPE, breast physical examination; MGY, mammography; BCDDP, Breast Cancer Detection Demonstration Project; HIP, Health Insurance Plan of Greater New York. All prices are in US dollars.
Health effects and costs discounted 5%. All estimates are approximate; significant digits are retained to avoid roundoff error, not to imply precision.
[a] Compared with no screening.
[b] Compared with annual breast physical examination.
Adapted from ref. [30].

savings were highest for black women and that these savings decreased with increasing age and comorbidity. For women aged 85 years and older (with or without comorbidities), the short term morbidity of anxiety or discomfort associated with screening may have outweighed the benefits.

The optimal frequency of screening examinations for the elderly population is still to be identified but depends on the interval between a cancer's initial detectability and the development of obvious signs of the disease. In younger women the preclinical interval appears to be less than two years and therefore more frequent screening is advocated. However, in elderly people the preclinical interval appears longer and screening every two years may be adequate.

Primary prevention

In view of the success of tamoxifen in reducing the incidence of contralateral tumours among women with breast cancer, a number of large trials are currently being mounted in healthy women 'at risk' of the disease using this drug as a means of chemoprevention. At least one of these trials has expanded its high risk category to include all women over 60 years old. However, there has been criticism of the rationale of the strategy and of the potential toxicity of the drug as a primary prevention measure [30b].

Cost

The cost of preventing one cancer by mammographic screening has been estimated as varying between £2750 and £80 000 [31, 32]. The variability in estimation depends on whether only the screening procedure is taken into account or whether the screening procedure plus additional investigational and surgical outlay is estimated. For example, Holnberg [33] has estimated a 150 per cent increase in operations and inpatient days during the initial screening round. Holnberg believed this increased workload would be temporary, but others [34] have put forward cogent reasons why it is more likely to be ongoing.

The detailed calculations on screening elderly women for breast cancer performed by Eddy [30] both in terms of the marginal cost of adding a year of life to an individual and the financial impact of population screening are shown in Table 6.3. It is obvious that screening requires considerable resources and finance. The costs of screening and workups outweigh, by a factor of about 100, any savings achievable through reduced treatment costs.

Cervical cancer

Importance

Cancers of the female reproductive tract are the fourth most common cause of cancer deaths among women. Although morbidity and mortality from this disease are declining, this is not the case in older women, where 25 per cent of the cervical cancer incidence and 41 per cent of all cervical cancer deaths occur [35]. For white women the age-specific rates for invasive carcinoma of the cervix remain constant after age 45, while for black women the age-specific rates for invasive carcinoma continue to increase after age 45 and may well do so into the 80s [36]. Conversely, the incidence of carcinoma in situ of the uterine cervix is very low after age 65 years (see Fig. 6.2). It is also recognised that urban black and hispanic populations have a high incidence of carcinoma as do those with multiple sexual partners, those with prior venereal disease and those in lower income groups [36]. Smokers have also been found to have a 50 per cent higher risk than non-smokers [37].

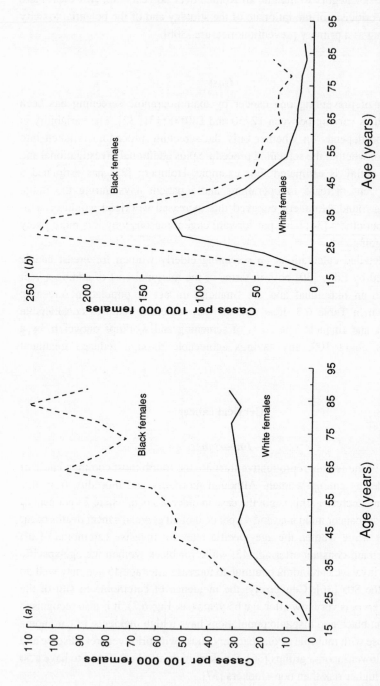

Fig. 6.2. (a) Incidence of invasive carcinoma of the cervix in white and black populations. Note the contrasting rates after age 45. (b) Incidence rates of carcinoma of the cervix in situ for the same populations, showing the sharp decline after age 35. Adapted from ref. [36].

Detection

The commonest manoeuvre is the Papanicolaou (Pap) smear. The yield from this test varies depending on the nature of target population and on its previous screening history. Siegler [38] reported only 33 invasive carcinomas in 30 000 women over 65 years, an incidence of 0.001 per cent. However, Mandelblatt [39], screening an outpatient population 65 years and over in New York, found an overall prevalence rate of 13.5 per thousand abnormal Pap smears in this age group. These figures suggest a need for screening in urban ethnically diverse populations. Conversely, it is important to remember that, in an aged population, women who have never been sexually active are not at risk for the development of cervical cancer. The policy for cervical screening in very frail elderly people also needs careful consideration. For example, in a US nursing home population 1130 smears were performed on 420 asymptomatic elderly women over a three-year period. This screening programme revealed only two women with smears positive for invasive carcinoma. One of these refused any further diagnostic workup [40]. Elderly women who have had hysterectomies cannot automatically be excluded from screening, since many of them had their surgery at a time when partial hysterectomies, which left the cervix in place, were still popular. In a recent study, one-third of all elderly women who had had hysterectomies in the past were found to have cervixes [41]. Also, between 4 and 8 per cent of cervical cancers arise in the cervical stump [42] and women who have had hysterectomies for malignant disease are at higher risk for the development of vaginal cancer, which can be detected by vaginal smear [43].

By itself, the Pap smear carries virtually no risk (though often some inconvenience and embarrassment). The main risks are those of a false negative result, creating a false sense of security and of a false positive result necessitating further workup and treatment. False negative rates for women of all age groups have been estimated as varying between 7 and 60 per cent [44]. Similarly, relative false positive rates for carcinoma in situ or invasive cancer have been estimated as 0.24 per cent to 0.6 per cent [45]. The sensitivity of the test in elderly women is not known in detail, but there is potential for both greater false negative and false positive rates. Roberts [46] has suggested that reduced exfoliation of cells from the cervix of postmenopausal women may result in false negative results. However, false positive results are also a concern in this population. Reduced levels of oestrogen can cause mild inflammation that can mimic all degrees of dysplasia and malignancy [47].

There are also major problems with both the performance and the interpretation of the test in older women. Poor accessibility, due to atrophy of supporting structures, makes sampling in this population difficult. After the menopause, the squamocolumnar junction (where cervical cancer arises) moves back into the endocervical canal [48] and is frequently not visible. Consequently, when a smear is taken it is difficult to know if the area at risk has been adequately sampled or not. In addition to scraping with an Ayre's spatula, the examination may be better performed by inserting into the cervical canal a sterile cotton swab or 'cyto' brush moistened with saline [49].

All reports that have investigated screening histories have shown that increasing age correlates with decreased likelihood to have been screened recently or to have ever been screened at all. For example, compared with 66 per cent in younger age groups only 7 per cent of those over 75 years in the UK have had a Pap smear in the last five years and most of these have been taken in gynaecological wards or at out-patient clinics because of specific gynaecological problems [7]. In the USA 15 per cent of women aged 65 to 74 years and 38 per cent of women 75 years and older report never having had a Pap smear. However, Mandelblatt et al. [49a] have reported that a major reason for non-use of the screening test in elderly black women in the USA is that a physician hasn't recommended it and that levels of knowledge about cervical cancer are low suggesting that patient education might enhance the use of early cancer detection.

Nevertheless, the Pap smear is clearly perceived as an unacceptable or irrelevant procedure to many of the very old. Several studies have estimated the non-participation rate in screening to vary between 50 and 85 per cent. In one study [39], 47 per cent of potential participants either refused to have a Pap smear or did not keep their follow up appointment.

Effectiveness

No randomised controlled trial of the effects of the Pap smear has ever been conducted. Nevertheless, there is strong indirect evidence from various parts of the world that cervical cancer screening reduces the mortality from this disease. This evidence comes from a number of historical studies [50–55], from case-control studies [56–62] and from analysis of data from large screening programmes [63].

In many of these studies, elderly women have been excluded from these screening programmes. Fletcher [64] has discussed in detail many of the reasons for this and argues that this policy is not consistent with the evidence. In regions in which elderly women have also been aggressively screened, their rates of death have declined as well [59]. In Iceland, the decline for women over the age of 75 years was actually greater than that for any other age group [50], mortality falling by 60 per cent in those over 60 years of age. Fletcher [64]

Table 6.4. *Cervical smear conversion rates*

Age group (years)	Age-specific incidence conversion rate (per 1000 women)
50–59	0.39
60–64	0.21
65–69	0.11
70–79	0.08
> 79	0.0

Source: ref. [38].

argues that women over 65 might in fact benefit most from screening, with a 63 per cent improvement in five-year mortality.

The extent of any screening programme for elderly women depends on their previous screening history, their relative risk of developing cervical cancer and the resources available. It has been suggested that one negative smear (or ideally two negative smears) for a woman of average risk at 65 years of age would obviate the need for further screening because the age-specific incidence of conversion of negative to positive smears becomes much less with increasing age [65] (see Table 6.4).

Recently, some concern has been expressed that the population from which these conversion rates have been taken may have been at relatively low risk of cervical cancer, but further evidence for a more conservative policy in the elderly population comes from a recent prospective study in Sweden of a large unselected female population [66]. It found that the incidence of cervical cancer among women over 70 years of age who had at least one normal Pap smear in the previous ten years was only 3 cases per 100 000 [66].

Eddy [67] has recently provided more detailed estimates of continuing with a further four triennial examinations after age 65 years and after age 74 years. The results are shown in Table 6.5. Continuing screening in a (previously screened) 65 year old will increase life expectancy by about three days and decrease the chance of death from cervical cancer by about 18 in 10 000. If a woman has never been screened previously the effect is roughly twice as great.

As Eddy [67] also points out, there is a good deal of leeway in advising a frequency for screening: the effectiveness of screening is not very sensitive to this variable. Any interval from one to four years will deliver virtually the same benefits. The fear that there is a group of women who progress rapidly from dysplasia to carcinoma in situ to invasive carcinoma (and who therefore require more frequent screening) may be no less a consideration for older than for younger women [63] but is, so far, not substantiated by existing evidence.

Cost

Table 6.5 also shows the marginal discounted net cost per year of life expectancy compared with no further screening as calculated by Eddy [67] for an older population. These calculations assumed a cost of $75 for the Pap smear (unless otherwise noted, dollar prices are in US dollars). Any proportional change in this would result in a proportional change in the marginal cost.

When screening an elderly population of mixed ethnicity it has been estimated that early detection of cervical neoplasia saved $5907 and 3.7 years of life per 100 Pap tests. When average medical costs per year of life extended by screening were included, the programme cost $2874 per year of life saved [68].

Colorectal cancer

Importance

Cancer of the colon and rectum are the second most frequently occurring cancers and the second most common cause of cancer deaths. Sixty per cent of colorectal cancers occur in persons 65 years or older [69] and the peak of incidence is in those over 80 years old [70]. A 65-year-old man without previously diagnosed colorectal carcinoma has about a 6 per cent chance of ultimately developing the disease and about a 3 per cent chance of eventually dying from it [71].

There are several groups known to be at particular risk of developing colon cancer [72]. A particularly important risk factor for colon cancer is a family history of the disease. The risk may be two- to threefold higher if a first degree relative has colorectal cancer [73]. Although patients with pernicious anaemia have been suspected of having an increased risk of colorectal cancer, one study showed that this did not reach statistical significance in the five years after diagnosis [74]. A particularly controversial category of elderly people at risk of colonic cancer are those with colonic polyps. Although it is known that 5 to 10 per cent of such polyps become malignant [75], that the greater the number of polyps the greater the risk of cancer [76], that larger polyps are associated with a higher incidence of malignant change [77] and that even if removed, the afflicted person remains at increased risk for cancer in other areas of the bowel [76], nevertheless other considerations make the general application of screening measures debatable. Firstly, necropsy studies of asymptomatic patients show prevalence rates of adenomas of 40 to 60 per cent in those over

Table 6.5. *Estimated outcomes of cervical cancer screening for a previously screened average-risk asymptomatic woman screened every three years for four additional examinations*

	Starting at	
Estimated outcome	age 65	age 74
Decrease in probability of developing invasive cervical cancer[a] per 10000	45.7	17.7
Decrease in probability of dying from invasive cervical cancer[b] per 10000	17.9	6.2
Increase in life expectancy (days)	3.1	1.1
Increase in life expectancy, discounted 5% (days)	1.6	0.5
Net costs, discounted 5%, $	229	220
Marginal cost per year of life expectancy (compared with no further screening)[c] $	52241	160000

All estimates are approximate. Decimal points are retained to avoid roundoff errors. It is assumed that the woman was screened previously every three years for at least 12 years (at least five previous examinations). All prices are in US dollars.

[a]Reference probability without screening: 94.5 in 10000 for women age 65; 61.2 in 10000 for women age 74.

[b]Reference probability without screening 39.8 in 10000 for women age 65; 24 in 10000 for women age 74.

[c]Health effects and costs are discounted 5%.

Adapted from ref. [67].

75 years [78]. This compares with incidence and prevalence rates of colorectal cancer in this age group of 3 and < 7 per 10000 respectively. Thus most polyps cannot give rise to cancers. Furthermore, Stryker [79] estimates the cumulative risks of a diagnosis of cancer at the site of the index polyp at 5 years, 10 years and 20 years as 2.5 per cent, 8 per cent and 24 per cent respectively. More recently, Atkin et al. [80] assessed the long term risk of colorectal cancer after polypectomy for rectosigmoid adenomas and found the incidence of rectal cancer in these patients to be the same as in the general population. Moreover, in patients with only a single small tubular adenoma that is only mildly or moderately dysplastic, future screening surveillance was probably of little value because the risk of colon cancer was so low. Koretz [80a] has also recently provided evidence that polyps that are already cancerous can behave in a benign biological fashion and remain clinically silent for several years. In addition to this evidence it has to be remembered that polypectomy has not yet been evaluated in a controlled clinical trial, that colonoscopy and polypectomy carry small but significant risks of haemorrhage and perforation, and that the procedure is inconvenient and costly.

Detection

The commonest detection manoeuvre used in screening has been the faecal occult blood test (FOBT) performed using a proprietary kit such as Haemoccult ii. There are problems with the specificity of such a method, since Haemoccult testing has been shown positive to some non-blood compounds in the bowel. A new immunological technique for detecting faecal haemoglobin has been reported as more specific and sensitive, identifying more adenomas and carcinomas than the Haemoccult kit [81]. However, its utility in large screening programmes has not yet been shown.

There are many other problems with FOBT as a screening procedure. It fails to detect 20 to 40 per cent of 'curable' cancers and 75 per cent of adenomas [82]. Although the positive predictive value of FOBT increases with age [83], it still has a low predictive accuracy for cancer. Numerous false positives may arise due to asymptomatic diverticular disease, peptic ulcer disease or haemorrhoids (however, Pye et al. [84] have recently shown that bleeding from the use of non-steroidal anti-inflammatory drugs should not be implicated). In two controlled studies evaluating FOBT, cancer was found in only 9 to 12 per cent of positive cases [85, 86]. In a further population referred to a tertiary cancer care centre, analysis of positive tests in people over 70 years of age showed that 23 per cent were due to colorectal cancer and 37 per cent to adenomas. A further complication in the evaluation of FOBT results from screening programmes is that many of the individuals may not be asymptomatic but may already have complaints relating to potential cancer pathology. This certainly was the case in one study described by Kurnick et al. [87]. They found that of 5595 patients screened, only two additional cases of colorectal cancer were identified by FOBT that could not have been detected by history alone.

A wide range of acceptance rates of FOBT has been reported in the literature, reflecting differences in both the population studied and the method of approach. Generally, compliance with FOBT tends to drop off significantly with increasing age [88]. For example, in one study the compliance rate for those 45 to 60 years of age was 65 per cent, whilst it was 25 per cent for those over 75 years. In another study, where invitation to screen came by letter from the primary care physician and was predated by a home visit, the rate for those aged 45 to 64 years was 50 to 55 per cent whilst for those over 70 it was 43 per cent [89]. When the FOBT screen has been offered opportunistically during routine consultation with the family practitioner, 54.3 per cent of patients 70 years or over have complied [90]. There is some evidence, however, that if elderly people are willing to be tested with FOBT then only about a fifth will be non-compliant with further diagnostic work to evaluation of a positive FOBT [91].

A further sign of poor acceptance of this test by elderly patients and possibly by physicians is shown in the study by Klos et al. [92]. They examined the utility of FOBT in nursing home patients in the USA. They found that the use of FOBT in this population increased with age, but that this was secondary to increased use of the test as a diagnostic tool. There was little change with age in use of FOBT for screening. Irrespective of the reason for use, 14 per cent of those tested had at least one positive test, yet 58 per cent of the patients with positive tests underwent no additional diagnostic testing. No cause for the positive FOBT was found in 68 per cent of patients receiving the test for routine screening. They concluded that many patients either refused diagnostic workup or were deemed inappropriate candidates for further workup.

The problem is that FOBT is *not* an innocuous test. A positive result mandates an extensive workup, from sigmoidoscopy to double contrast enema and colonoscopy, which the physician feels morally bound to perform. The morbidity in elderly people from these procedures, from the required bowel preparation, and from any accompanying hospitalisation, is significant. After one of the most extensive reviews of this screening procedure Frank [93] concludes 'its routine application to asymptomatic patients represents premature enthusiasm rather than thoughtful medical practice' and 'the risks of occult blood screening could outweigh the benefits at any age-group'.

Other screening tests for colorectal cancer are sigmoidoscopy and colonoscopy. These methods have improved detection rates of cancer and adenomas over the FOBT but they are obviously more invasive and expensive to use and must have limited acceptability as first line screening methods in general population screening. A comprehensive review of the role of these procedures has recently been provided by the US Preventive Services Task Force [94].

Of the more invasive tests, flexible sigmoidoscopy is increasingly considered the screening method of choice, being more sensitive in picking up lesions than is the rigid sigmoidoscope, being more rapid to perform, and being more acceptable to elderly individuals. It is also a reasonably safe procedure provided it is done by an experienced operator.

Effectiveness

No randomised trial of sigmoidoscopic screening has as yet shown a reduced mortality from colorectal cancer. However, studies have shown an improved stage distribution for tumours detected by screening sigmoidoscopy compared with that of tumours diagnosed after onset of symptoms and recently, a case control study of screening by rigid sigmoidoscopy showed that participants (mean age at diagnosis of 66 years) who had undergone one or more screening examinations in the preceding ten years had a 60 to 70 per cent reduction in the risk of death [95]. In another controlled trial of sigmoidoscopy in younger patients in which 20 cm of the colon was examined, a reduction in colorectal cancer mortality was suggested [96]. However, the investigators concluded that the reduction in mortality could not be attributed to sigmoidoscopic screening.

There is little evidence on the efficacy or lack of efficacy on screening with FOBT, although cancers detected by screening are found to be at a less advanced pathological stage [97]. Five controlled trials of FOBT are under-way; two of these are in the USA [86, 98], one in England [99], one in Denmark [100] and one in Sweden [101]. Preliminary mortality data from two of these show a handful of fewer deaths from colorectal cancer in the screened groups, but the numbers were very small in relation to the large number of persons studied; it seems unlikely, therefore, that untargeted FOBTs will prove a highly effective or efficient strategy for decreasing mortality from colorectal cancer [101a].

There is some evidence, however, that in people of high risk some benefit may accrue from sigmoidoscopic screening. Studies indicate that removal of a polyp using rectosigmoidoscopy decreases the expected incidence of sub-sequent carcinoma of rectum and sigmoid. A family history of colonic cancer can be used to identify those at risk and target appropriate screening. Colonoscopy can detect a higher number of premalignant colonic polyps in this high risk group but a modelling approach suggests that barium enema is the most cost effective screening approach in this situation [102].

Primary prevention

Although there is fairly strong epidemiological evidence linking diet with colonic cancer, the exact constituents responsible are still under debate [103, 104]. However, for some time there has been a belief that high fat diets (because of their increased effect on bowel microflora, bile acids and carcinogen production) and low fibre content in the diet (which slows transit time, thus increasing exposure to potential carcinogens) may predispose to colonic cancer. Recent interest in this hypothesis has been fuelled by a study in which younger nurses who consumed more animal fat and less crude fibre (and a greater proportion of red to white meat) were at increased risk of developing colon cancer during a six-year follow up period [105]. The American Cancer Society recommends a diet to minimise the risk of colonic cancer, though a randomised prospective study of the benefit of this diet has not yet been completed. It is also suggested that calcium supplementation in subjects at high risk of familial colonic cancer reduces epithelial cell proliferation to levels seen in subjects at low risk [106].

Recently, some hope has arisen that primary prevention may be achieved through the use of low-dose aspirin. Three out of four recent trials [107–109] have shown decreased death rates from colon cancer associated with more frequent aspirin and/or other non-steroidal anti-inflammatory drug use. In one of the studies the relative risk of those using aspirin 16 or more times per month was 0.60 in men and 0.58 in women.

Cost

Despite the absence of hard data on the benefits of screening, a more detailed assessment of the cost effectiveness of a periodic screening programme for colorectal carcinoma in elderly people has recently been attempted by Wagner et al. [110]. They concluded that a programme of annual FOBT in an elderly population would detect at least 17 per cent of expected cases of cancer and could cost $35 000 per year of life saved (1991 prices). Screening schedules that include period sigmoidoscopy would prevent more cases of cancer but could cost between $43 000 and $47 000 per year of life saved.

Other estimations for screening the population in the USA have suggested considerable resource utilisation for this preventive strategy. For example, screening the population over 50 years with annual FOBT and flexible sigmoidoscopy every 3 to 5 years would amount to over $1.1 billion [111]. It has further been estimated that for every 1 per cent increase in false positives there would be an increase to the financial cost of that nation of $2 million annually.

Prostatic cancer

Importance

The average annual age-adjusted incidence rate of prostatic carcinoma per 100 000 men over 65 years is 635.2 [112]. Prostatic cancer is the second most common cause of cancer mortality in men 75 years and older [113]. It is also responsible for considerable, but less quantified morbidity.

Detection

There is no satisfactory detection manoeuvre for screening for prostatic cancer [114]. The most widely used strategies of prostate specific antigen (PSA) estimation and digital rectal examination (DRE) were reviewed recently by Oesterling [114a]. Although digital rectal examination lacks specificity, with only 30 per cent of men with suspicious findings having histological evidence of prostate cancer on needle biopsy [115, 116], it can nevertheless detect some lesions that would be missed if reliance were only placed on PSA estimation. The PSA test itself is capable of identifying approximately twice as many prostate cancers as DRE is. However, the PSA test is not specific to prostatic cancer but is produced by all types of prostatic tissue. 'There is a tremendous overlap in the serum PSA values for men with benign prostatic hypertrophy only and patients with early, curable prostate cancer' [114a]. However, unlike the previously used serum marker prostatic acid phosphatase, PSA is not elevated after digital rectal examination [114b] and new techniques such as the rate of change of serum levels of PSA and the relationship of the PSA level to the prostatic volume (the PSA density) are being introduced to improve the specificity of the test.

Effectiveness

Considerable doubt surrounds the effectiveness of early screening and treatment for prostatic cancer. Firstly, the majority of persons suffering from prostatic cancer go to their graves without its being implicated or even being a significant clinical problem [115]. Secondly, the benefit of early intervention is questioned by the apparently favourable outcome shown in some studies in patients with localised cancer who were managed expectantly [116a, 116b]. Thirdly, surgical treatment (particularly radical prostatectomy) carries with it considerable morbidity and its efficacy is in some doubt, the only randomised controlled trial comparing radical prostatectomy with no treatment found it no better than placebo in altering five-year survival [117]. Lastly, published evidence on the benefits of screening are largely descriptive uncontrolled studies that lack conclusive evidence of clinical benefit [114].

Cost

No specific details are available relating to an elderly population.

Lung cancer

Importance

Lung cancer is the leading cause of death in the USA for both men and women [118] and age-adjusted lung cancer mortality rates have increased considerably in recent years [119]. Half of all lung cancers occur in persons 65 years and older [70], the age-specific incidence rates rising with age to 500 per year per 100 000 in men aged 70 years. Beyond 80 years for men and 75 years for women these rates decline somewhat, probably because of a lower smoking prevalence in the oldest age groups.

Detection

The manoeuvres used to detect lung cancer in secondary screening programmes have been radiography and sputum cytology. In general, X-rays and sputum cytology have been considered poorly sensitive or specific on their own but when used in combination and repeated at four-monthly intervals have been shown to pick up nearly 90 per cent of cases.

There is, however, a significant risk of false positive results from such tests. Grzybowski and Coy [120] found that 5.5 per cent of screened men had a suspicious chest X-ray requiring a diagnostic workup before being found to be free of cancer. Higher rates of between 10 and 18 per cent have been reported from the participating centres of the National Cancer Institute (NCI) Program [121] (see below). Likewise, the false positive rate for sputum cytology has been reported around 0.14 per cent [122]. These screening participants may have to be subjected to a fairly extensive battery of investigations including bronchoscopy, bronchial washings and lung biopsy.

A further risk comes from the cumulative dose of irradiation from repeated X-rays, though this is less likely to be significant in the elderly population.

Effectiveness

No data are available relating specifically to screening the elderly for lung cancer, but several screening programmes for a younger population have shown no benefit in overall mortality rates. This may be explained by the 'early' tumours being in reality quite advanced with current treatment not being particularly effective. At least three early non-randomised uncontrolled trials were found to be valueless [123–125]. More recently, the National

Cancer Institute (NCI) in the USA has mounted three fairly intensive and carefully scrutinised randomised controlled trials whose results have become available [126]. A further recent Czechoslovakian study has reached the same general conclusion as the American research [127].

The NCI Early Lung Cancer Detection Program aimed at screening male smokers aged 45 years and older, but 90 per cent were under 65 years [126]. The Program was conducted in three different settings, at Memorial Sloan-Kettering [128], Johns Hopkins University Hospital [129] and the Mayo Clinic [130]. The Mayo Clinic is the longest running and offered the most intensive screening, requiring chest X-rays and sputum cytology from participants on a four-monthly basis over a six-year period. In this arm of the trial, as expected, 46 per cent of cancers detected were resectable in the screened group versus 32 per cent in the control group. However, the lung cancer death rates were virtually similar, 3.2 deaths per 1000 men per year in the screened group versus 3.0 deaths per 1000 men per year in the control group. The results in the other two centres were similar.

Despite the absence of benefit shown in the above general screening trials, it has been suggested that *selective* screening of high risk groups may still assist in reducing mortality. Data from the Surveillance Epidemiology and End Results (SEER) Program [131] shows that men 65 years and older (particularly smokers) are at threefold greater risk of lung cancer than the men 45 to 64 years old that have been targeted in previous studies. Also the trend with age to a larger proportion of squamous cell histology and an increased likelihood of local stage disease could cause the older lung cancer case detected by screening to be more likely to benefit from early surgical intervention than the younger case [132]. This suggestion remains to be proven, however.

Primary prevention

Primary prevention through the avoidance of cigarette smoking offers the most effective prevention strategy (see p. 92). It should also be remembered that primary prevention by cessation of smoking is considered to be many hundred times more efficient than screening for existing disease.

The NCI in the USA and the Finnish National Public Health Institute are currently conducting an innovative collaborative cancer chemoprevention trial. In this study, oral administration of beta-carotene and alphatocopherol are being given to a population of heavy smokers. Incident cancers will be identified and compared with national trends from the Finnish government's health registers [133].

Cost

No details are available specifically on screening the elderly population but screening in general for lung cancer is considered very costly. For example, screening has been estimated to increase the life expectancy of a smoker by 40 days at a cost of $500 000 per person. Further indications of the cost come from the fact that if all the smokers in the USA over the age of 40 years were screened with annual chest X-rays, the annual cost for screening alone (not counting the workups for false positive results) would be approximately $1.5 billion at 1988 prices [121].

In practical terms, some aspects of lung cancer screening would also be difficult to implement in terms of the resources required. An advisory committee to the Director of the Californian State Department of Health estimated that to screen 300 000 workers, exposed at their jobs to lung carcinogens, only twice a year with sputum cytology would require about 550 cytotechnologists plus the full time supervision of 60 pathologists [134].

Endometrial cancer

Importance

Endometrial cancer is the most common of all gynaecological malignancies and the incidence rate appears to be rising. The age-specific incidence peaks at 60 to 64 years at 135 cases per 100 000 women [70]. Although a common disease, relatively few younger women, at least, die from it: it is symptomatic at an early stage, often presenting whilst confined to the uterus and consequently having excellent ten-year survival rates. Overall it accounts for only 1.4 per cent of cancer deaths in women. However, 66 per cent of uterine cancer deaths occur in women 65 years and older [135] and the situation is more grave in this older population. Elderly patients are more likely to present at a later stage of disease [136] and have a much poorer survival with the age-specific death rate increasing to age 70 years [70].

There are many at particular risk of endometrial cancer. This includes those with diabetes, late menses, late onset menopause, infertility, adenomatous hyperplasia of the endometrium and obesity. Also, many postmenopausal women who have taken conjugated oestrogens have up to a nine times higher risk of endometrial cancer [137–139], previous oestrogen use conveying as much risk as current use. However, when progestogens are used in conjunction with oestrogen, they either remove this increased risk or delay its onset [140].

Table 6.6. *Epithelian ovarian cancer:*
five-year survival by stage

Stage	Five-year survival (%)
Ia	69.7
Ib	63.9
Ic	50.3
IIa	51.8
IIb/c	42.4
III	13.3
IV	4.1

Data from Kottmeieir H. Annual Report of the Results of Treatment in Gynaecological Cancer, vol. 18. Stockholm: International Federation of Gynecology and Obstetrics, 1983.

Detection

The few techniques available for diagnosing endometrial cancer in asymptomatic women are far from ideal. The Pap smear will detect only 50 to 60 per cent of uterine cancers [141, 142] and special expertise is required to read these Pap smears accurately. Endometrial biopsy is a relatively uncomfortable and invasive procedure generally considered a poor screening tool. Most interest has centred on cytological uterine sampling, which can be done relatively painlessly in an outpatient setting without general anaesthetic. A further screening technique on which there has been some preliminary work is the use of transvaginal pulsed Doppler ultrasonography with colour flow imaging to detect blood flow as the end point [143].

Effectiveness

There is very limited information about the efficacy of screening for endometrial cancer in asymptomatic populations of any age. It is known that the extensive use of the Pap smear in intensive screening for cervical carcinoma failed to have any concomitant effect (even in elderly people) on mortality from endometrial cancer.

No randomised controlled trials have been aimed specifically at evaluating the effectiveness of preventive screening for endometrial cancer. The one available cohort study of cytological screening did not assess the effect of this screening on stage of distribution in those diagnosed or on patient outcomes [141]. This quite large study performed on more than 25 000 asymptomatic women aged 45 years and over found a prevalence of endometrial cancer of 7 cases per 1000 women. The prevalence in women over 60 years was no different from that in women under 60 years. Twenty per cent of those screened experienced moderate discomfort. No cytology specimen could be obtained in 8 per cent of those studied. The positive predictive value of the test was estimated at only 16.7 to 20 per cent for sensitivity rates of 81 to 100 per cent. Thus after screening, 80 per cent or more of women with abnormal cytology would be free of endometrial disease but would be subjected to at least dilatation and curettage to rule this out.

Cost

No specific details are available for the elderly population.

Ovarian cancer

Importance

The age-specific incidence of ovarian cancer increases with age until it peaks at age 80 years at about 50 cases per 100 000 population, with the age-specific mortality peaking slightly earlier at 75 years when it reaches 43 cases per 100 000 population [70, 144].

Detection

Approximately 45 to 65 per cent of all women newly presenting with ovarian cancer have disease that has already extended out of the pelvis [145, 146] and therefore are likely to have a five-year survival of less than 20 per cent. In contrast, the high mortality associated with extensive tumour must be compared with the good survival achieved by women who present in the earlier stages of the disease (see Table 6.6). Also, increasing age has been shown to correlate significantly with increasing stage at presentation [147].

A number of strategies have therefore been advocated for the detection of the disease in its early stages. The fact that there have been relatively few reports of screening for ovarian cancer is an indication that, until recently, there has been dissatisfaction with the quality of these tests.

Pelvic examination is notoriously unreliable in detecting small adnexal masses [148]. For example, in one study of women of all ages, only six ovarian cancers were discovered during a total of 18 753 pelvic examinations performed in 1319 women over a 15-year period. A further consideration is that nulliparous or arthritic elderly women are the most difficult to examine.

Although cervical Pap smears may detect ovarian cancer (either from metastatic disease or shedding of cells), this cannot be used as a screening instrument because the disease, by this time, is usually in an advanced stage [149, 150].

CA 125 is a newly described high molecular weight glycoprotein antigen expressed by an epithelial ovarian cancer cell line. Serum levels of CA 125 measured by radioimmunoassay are elevated (>35 units/ml) in over 80 per cent of epithelial ovarian cancers [151]. However, it is a relatively non-specific test also being found in a third of patients with pelvic inflammatory disease and 80 per cent of patients with cervical (and other) adenocarcinomas [151]. Some resolution to the problem may come from repeat testing, since many of the elevations not due to ovarian carcinoma will fall to the normal range [151] but sufficient concern still exists that it cannot be used on its own in screening.

Ultrasonography has also been tried as a screening test though it is expensive and cannot distinguish between benign and malignant disease [152]. However, one study from the UK screened 5479 self referred asymptomatic women with a mean age of 52 years [153]. Five patients with primary ovarian cancer were identified. Overall the rate of false positive results was 2.3 per cent.

Because the consequence of a positive screening test is some form of surgical exploration, it is essential that the screening procedure be highly specific for the disease. Consequently some promising (though early) attempts have been made to combine screening tests within an early detection programme to improve the overall quality of the screen. Some figures for combined screening with CA 125, vaginal examination and ultrasonography are shown in Table 6.7 [154]. A further technique being investigated is the use of transvaginal ultrasonography with colour flow imaging [155], which is now being used as a first stage screening procedure in high risk groups, such as asymptomatic women who have had a close relative develop the disease.

Effectiveness

Although the five-year survival for women with ovarian cancer is closely related to the stage at presentation, no trial has yet been performed to assess the impact of early screening on mortality. However, the fact that some studies have found decreased survival for all women over the age of 55 years with

Table 6.7. *Specificity for ovarian cancer in 1010 postmenopausal women of vaginal examination, serum CA 125, and combinations of these tests with ultrasound scanning*

Test	Specificity (%)	95% confidence intervals
CA 125	97.0	95.8– 98.0
Vaginal examination	97.3	96.2– 98.3
Vaginal examination and ultrasound	99.0	98.1– 99.5
CA 125 + ultrasound	99.8	99.3– 99.9
CA 125 + vaginal examination	100.0	99.6–100.0
CA 125 + vaginal examination + ultrasound	100.0	99.6–100.0

Source: Jacobs IJ, Stabile I, Bridges JE et al. Lancet 1988; **1**: 268–71.

early stage disease [145] suggests significant improvements in mortality from early detection may be difficult to achieve.

Cost

No data are available but the use of ultrasonography and CA 125 measurements alone are costly.

Gastric cancer

Importance

Gastric cancer is the fourth-commonest cause of cancer death in the UK [156]. Although the incidence of gastric cancer in the UK is low and has been on the decline for half a century, older generations still experience the risk associated with previous decades [157]. Moreover, overall survival has remained unchanged with very poor five-year survival rates because of the high percentage of late stage disease at presentation. Although there are also a number of factors that predispose to greater risk of this cancer, the atrophic gastritis found in up to 90 per cent of elderly people does not appear to be one of these [158].

Detection

The two commonest screening techniques used have been endoscopy, which is invasive and of limited acceptability, and double contrast barium meal examination, which again is of limited acceptability, and which also carries a radiation hazard, though the potential benefit, at least in Japan, indicates that lives saved considerably outnumber lives lost.

Effectiveness

The overall five-year survival of patients with gastric cancer in the UK remains 10 to 15 per cent. In Japan, aggregate five-year survival following resection is 40 to 50 per cent. This may be accounted for by the massive screening programmes conducted there. Over 30 per cent of all gastric cancers in Japan are classified as 'early' whereas in the UK only 0.3 to 11 per cent are so classified, suggesting that screening leads to early detection and improved survival. Impressive as the Japanese data are, the evidence for the benefit of the Japanese screening rests on case control studies [159] with no prospective randomised studies being available. Screening in Japan was also introduced when both incidence and mortality rates were already falling. Furthermore, experience with multiphasic cancer screening and investigation of patients having symptoms in Italy has shown that the numbers of early gastric cancers detected still remain low, in keeping with reported incidence in Western countries.

More recently however, it has been suggested that *selective* screening by endoscopy of *symptomatic* older patients (for example over 50 years) would yield more gastric cancers than in the other high risk groups outlined above, since mucosal gastric cancers are symptomatic in 50 per cent of cases. This was certainly borne out in an initial screening programme in Birmingham, England, in which endoscopy of all patients over 40 years presenting to their general practitioner with dyspepsia led to a high rate of radical resection and a high proportion of lesions limited to the submucosa (15 per cent), which exceeded that in previous reports [160]. However, the benefits of such screening in terms of mortality rates in larger trials remains to be shown.

Selective screening of other risk groups such as those with pernicious anaemia or those who have had previous benign gastric surgery [161] has not been considered a worthwhile option.

Cost

The low incidence of gastric cancer in the UK is generally considered to preclude widespread screening as a viable economic option. However, few details are available.

Bladder cancer

Importance

Bladder cancer reaches its peak prevalence in the 60 to 70-year-old age group. The average annual incidence rates for bladder cancer per 100 000 for men and women 65 years and older are 185.6 and 44.7 respectively [162]. Bladder cancer is the fifth most common cause of cancer related deaths among men 75 years and older.

The incidence of bladder cancer is higher in industrialised countries and in those who have worked in the rubber and dye industries and have been exposed to carcinogens. Smokers also have a twofold increased risk of bladder cancer in comparison with non-smokers.

Detection

Dipstick urinalysis for haematuria has been recommended as a screening test for bladder cancer. However, because of the relatively low prevalence of this condition, most positive urinalyses are falsely positive. For example, in one study of older men, only 4 to 5 per cent of those testing positive developed cancer or other urological diseases in the first three years after the test [163]. The most optimistic results come from trials of older men [164, 165] which report positive predictive values of around 26 per cent [164].

The method of bladder cancer screening that has been utilised in British industrial screening for many years is that of 6 to 12-monthly urinary cytology estimations. Little is known of the sensitivity and specificity of the test.

Effectiveness

Little is known of the effectiveness of bladder cancer screening even in the relatively high risk population of younger industrial workers exposed to carcinogenic chemicals. Attempts to evaluate it by comparison of survival of screening detected cases with other cases have not shown apparent benefit [166] and no controlled prospective studies have demonstrated that persons with bladder cancer identified through screening have lower mortality than do those detected without screening.

Cost

No information is available on costs specifically relating to the elderly population.

Pancreatic cancer

Importance

During the past 40 years, the adjusted death rate for pancreatic cancer has risen from 3 per 100 000 to more than 10 per 100 000 [167]. The five-year survival rate is one of the lowest of all cancers and 50 per cent of the deaths occur in patients over 65 years of age [168]. Pancreatic cancer is commoner in older smokers [167].

Detection

Ultrasonography is widely accepted as a useful diagnostic investigation for pancreatic cancer in symptomatic persons, but its efficacy in screening asymptomatic populations is not yet proven [169]. Likewise, certain serological markers are elevated in most patients with pancreatic cancer, yet none has achieved sufficient reliability for screening asymptomatic persons. The most accurate tests for diagnosis, such as CT and endoscopic retrograde cholangio-pancreatography (ERCP), are far too costly or invasive for routine screening.

Effectiveness

There is little convincing evidence either from five-year survival rates on the 'natural' history of the disease or from surgical trials [169] that early intervention lowers mortality from pancreatic cancer.

Costs

No detailed information on costs is available.

Skin cancer

Importance

Most skin tumours in elderly people are basal cell and squamous cell carcinomas with the former being about six times more common than the latter. There is a direct correlation of the incidence of basal cell carcinoma with the total lifetime amount of exposure to sunlight with rates as high as 3300 per 100 000 being recorded in those over 75 years old in sunny climates [170].

These tumours are, however, eminently treatable and rarely metastasise. The third common skin tumour is malignant melanoma which is much more serious, being responsible for about 74 per cent of all skin cancer deaths. Although far less common, its incidence in people aged 65 years and over is rising (in one Scottish survey [171] from 12.2 per 100 000 in 1979 to 20.7 per 100 000 in 1989) and a higher proportion present as thick tumours with a poorer prognosis in this age group [171].

Detection

Physical examination of the skin is the principal means of detection but estimates of its sensitivity and specificity vary (33 to 98 per cent and 45 to 95 per cent, respectively) according to the type of cancer being sought [172]. There is also considerable interobserver variation in the interpretation of suspicious lesions, even between experts. Recommendations vary as to whether complete or partial skin examination should be undertaken, as only 20 per cent of melanomas occur on normally exposed body surfaces [172]. The inconvenience, expense, embarrassment and anxiety engendered by the likely high number of false positive findings is not inconsiderable.

Effectiveness

There has been little scientific evaluation of the impact of screening on morbidity and mortality rates for non-melanomatous skin cancers. Also, despite there being strong evidence linking improved survival times with the staging or thickness or malignant melanoma [171, 172], there has been little research on the efficacy of screening and early detection programmes in achieving this aim.

Primary prevention

In view of the role of ultraviolet rays as a risk factor for basal cell and squamous cell carcinomas, there is much advocacy for primary prevention using sunscreen preparations to limit exposure to sunlight. However, there has been little evaluation on the effectiveness of counselling in their use and it is known that, despite awareness of risks, adolescents, at least, fail to use protective measures while suntanning [173].

There are also no studies specifically evaluating the efficacy of primary prevention beginning in old age. Although certain patterns of sunlight exposure have been linked to the occurrence of malignant melanoma, association of this cancer with ultraviolet irradiation (and therefore the role of sunscreen preparations) is much less certain than with non-melanomatous skin cancers.

Despite some early research indicating the possibility of a preventive action on basal cell carcinomas by retinoids and beta carotene, recent prospective trials have failed to show any such benefit when used in populations at high risk of developing such carcinomas [173a, 173b].

Cost

No detailed information is currently available.

Oral cancer

Importance

The age-specific incidence rates for oral cancer (cancers of the lip, tongue, pharynx and other areas of the mouth) increase steadily from middle age until the seventh decade of life [174]. They are more common in men. Alcohol, smoking and the use of 'smokeless tobacco' (chewing tobacco or tobacco used as snuff) are all major risk factors and are thought to account for about 75 per cent of oral cancers in the USA [175]. The majority of deaths from oral cancer occur in persons over 65 years old [176]. For survivors, the psychosocial problems associated with tissue loss and deformity are considerable.

Detection

Studies show that by the time of presentation, 50 per cent of many oral cancers have regional lymph node metastasis with consequent poor prognosis [177]. As elderly people visit their physician more often than they visit their dentist [178], it has therefore been recommended that clinicians should routinely examine for the presence of oral cancer. The principal method of detection of oral cancer is by inspection and palpation of the oral cavity. Protocols for this procedure have been clearly described [179].

Effectiveness

As five-year survival data show significantly improved rates of survival when oral cancers are detected and treated whilst still localised [180], it is possible that early detection programmes might reduce morbidity and mortality.

However, this theoretical benefit of screening has still to be proven in any prospective trial.

Cost

No detailed information is available on the costs of preventing oral cancer in elderly people.

References

1. Silverberg E, Lubera JA. Cancer statistics. Cancer 1988; 11.
2. Office of Population Censuses and Surveys. Cancer Statistics and Registrations, England and Wales, 1984. London: HM Stationery Office, 1988.
3. Marchant, DJ. Epidemiology of breast cancer. Clin Obstet Gynecol 1982; **25**: 387–92.
4. Sondik, E. Annual Cancer Statistics Review 1988. Washington DC: Division of Cancer Prevention and Control, National Cancer Institute, 1990.
5. Adami HO, Malker B, Holmberg L et al. The relation between survival and the age at diagnosis in breast cancer. N Engl J Med 1986; **315**: 559–63.
6. Lynch HT, Guirgis H, Lynch J et al. Genetic factors in breast cancer. In: Lynch HT (ed) Cancer Genetics, pp. 389–423. Springfield IL: CC Thomas, 1976.
7. Vetter NJ. Health promotion and ageing: attitudes of the elderly to health promotion topics. Research Team for Care of the Elderly. University of Wales 1987.
8. UK Trial of Early Detection of Breast Cancer Group. First results on mortality reduction in the UK trial of early detection of breast cancer. Lancet 1988; **2**: 411–16.
9. Dowle, CS, Mitchell A, Elston CW et al. Preliminary results of the Nottingham breast self examination programme. Brit J Surg 1987; **74**: 217–19.
10. Semiglazov VF, Moiseenko VM. Breast self examination for early detection of breast cancer: a USSR/WHO controlled trial in Leningrad. WHO 1986; **65**: 391–96.
11. Roebuck EJ. Mammography in screening for breast cancer. Brit Med J 1986; **292**: 223–6.
12. Miller AB, Baines CJ, To T, Wall C. Canadian National Breast Screening Study: 2. Breast cancer detection and death rates among women aged 50 to 59 years. Can Med Assoc J 1992; **147**: 1477–8.
13. Celentano DD, Shapiro S, Weisman CS. Cancer preventive screening behaviour among elderly women. Prev Med 1982; **11**: 454–63.
14. Gohagan JK, Darby WP, Spitznagel EL et al. Radiogenic breast cancer effects of mammographic screening. J Nat Cancer Inst 1986; **77**: 71–6.
15. Baker, LH. Breast cancer detection demonstration project: five year summary report. Cancer 1982; **32**: 194–225.
16. Cox EB. Breast cancer in the elderly. In: Cohen HJ (ed) Clinics in Geriatric Medicine: Cancer II – Specific Neoplasms, vol. 3, no. 4. Philadelphia, PA: WB Saunders, 1987.
17. Hobbs P, Selwood RA, George WD. Self selection and self referral in breast screening. Clin Oncol 1980; **6**: 143–51.

18. Hobbs P, Kay C, Friedman EHI et al. Response by women aged 65 to 79 to invitation for screening for breast cancer by mammography: a pilot study. Brit Med J 1990; **301**: 1314–16.

19. Eardley A, Elkind A. Breast screening among women aged 65 and over: what do they think of it? J Pub Health Med 1991; **13**: 172–7.

20. Williams EMI, Vessey MP. Randomised trial of two strategies offering women mobile screening for breast cancer. Brit Med J 1989; **299**: 158–9.

21. Herbsman H, Feldman J, Selderna J et al. Survival following breast cancer surgery in the elderly. Cancer 1981; **47**: 2358–63.

22. McCarty KS, Silva JS, Cox EB et al. Relationship of age and menopausal status to estrogen receptor content in primary carcinoma of the breast. Annals Surg 1979; **123**: 1983.

23. Kennedy BJ. Clinical Oncology: focus on the elderly. In: Yancik R, Carbone PP, Patterson WB (eds) Perspectives on Prevention and Treatment of Cancer in the Elderly, pp. 43–50. New York: Raven Press, 1983.

24. Carbone PP, Begg CB, Jensenn L et al. Oncology perspective on breast cancer in the elderly. In: Yancik R, Carbone PP, Patterson WP (eds) Perspectives on Prevention and Treatment of Cancer in the Elderly, pp. 63–72. New York: Raven Press, 1983.

24b. Shapiro S, Venet W, Strax P et al. Periodic screening for breast cancer: the health insurance plan project and its sequelae. Baltimore: Johns Hopkins University Press, 1988.

25. Tabar, L, Faberberg G, Day NE et al. What is the optimum interval between mammographic screening investigations? An analysis based on the latest results of the Swedish two county breast cancer screening trial. Brit J Cancer 1987; **55**: 547–51.

26. Andersson I, Aspergren K, Janzon L et al. Mammographic screening and mortality from breast cancer: the Malmo mammographic screening trial. Brit Med J 1988; **297**: 944–8.

27. Verbeek ALM, Hendriks HJ, Holland R et al. Reduction of breast cancer mortality through mass screening with modern mammography. First results of the Nijmegen project 1975–1981. Lancet 1984; **1**: 1222–4.

28. Palli D, Del Turco MR, Buiatti E et al. A case controlled study of the efficacy of a non-randomised breast cancer screening program in Florence, Italy. Int J Cancer 1986; **38**: 501–4.

29. Collette HJ, Day NE, Rombach JJ et al. Evaluation of screening for breast cancer in a non-randomised study (the DOM project) by means of a case-control study. Lancet 1981; **1**: 1224–6.

30. Eddy DM. Screening for breast cancer. Annals Intern Med 1989; **111**: 389–99.

30a. Mandelblatt JS, Wheat ME, Monane M et al. Breast cancer screening for elderly women with and without comorbid conditions. Annals Intern Med 1992; **116**: 722–30.

30b. Fugh-Berman A, Epstein S. Tamoxifen: disease prevention of disease substitution? Lancet 1992; **340**: 1143–4.

31. Roberts CJ, Farrow SC, Charny MC. How much can the NHS afford to spend to save a life or avoid a severe disability? Lancet 1985; **1**: 89–91.

32. Gravelle HSE, Simpson PR, Chamberlain J. Breast cancer screening and health service costs. J Health Econom 1982; **1**: 185.

33. Holnberg L, Adami HO, Persson I et al. Demands on surgical inpatient services after mass mammographic screening. Brit Med J 1986; **293**: 779–82.

34. Shorthouse AJ. Breast screening and the surgeon. Brit J Hosp Med 1991; **45**: 61.
35. Celentano DD, Shapiro S, Weisman CS. Cancer: preventive screening behaviour among elderly women. Prev Med 1982; **11**: 454–63.
36. Henson D, Tarone R. An epidemiological study of cancer of the cervix, vagina and vulva based on the Third National Cancer Study in the United States. Amer J Obstet Gynecol 1977; **129**: 525–32.
37. Brinton LA, Schairer C, Hasenszel W et al. Smoking and invasive cervical cancer. J Amer Med Assoc 1986; **255**: 3265–9.
38. Siegler E. Cervical carcinoma in the aged. Amer J Obstet Gynecol 1969; **103**: 1093.
39. Mandelblatt J, Gopaul I, Wistreich M. Gynecological care of elderly women. J Amer Med Assoc 1986; **256**: 367–71.
40. Oster S. Cervical vaginal screening in the over 65 female. Mount Sinai J Med 1980; **47**: 192–3.
41. Mandelblatt J, Gopaul I, Weistreich M. Gynaecological care of elderly women: another look at Papanicoulaou smear testing. J Amer Med Assoc 1986; **256**: 367–71.
42. Sala JM, Diaz de Leon AD. Treatment of carcinoma of the cervical stump. Radiology 1963; **81**: 300–6.
43. Benedet JL, Senders BH. Carcinoma in situ of the vagina. Amer J Obstet Gynecol 1984; **148**: 675–700.
44. Eddy DM, Gay JD, Donaldson LD et al. False negative results in cervical cytologic studies. Acta Cytol 1985; **29**: 1043–6.
45. Yobs AR, Plott AE, Hicklin MD et al. Retrospective evaluation of gynecologic cytodiagnosis. ii. Inter-laboratory reproducability as shown in rescreening large consecutive samples of reported cases. Acta Cytol 1987; **31**: L900–10.
46. Roberts ADG, Denholm RB, Cordiner JW. Cervical intra-epithelial neoplasia in post-menopausal women with negative cervical cytology. Brit Med J 1985; **290**: 281.
47. Hudson E. The prevention of cervical cancer: the place of the cytological smear test. Clin Onstet Gynecol 1985; **12**: 33–51.
48. Weintraub NT, Freedman ML. Gynecologic malignancies of the elderly. In: Cohen HJ (ed) Clinics in Geriatric Medicine: Cancer II – specific Neoplasis, vol. 3, pp. 669–94. Philadelphia, PA: WB Saunders, 1987.
49. American Geriatrics Society. Screening for cervical carcinoma in elderly women. J Amer Geriatr Soc 1989; **37**: 885–7.
49a. Mandelblatt J, Traxler M, Lakin P et al. Mammography and Papanicolaou smear use by elderly poor black women. J Amer Geriatr Soc 1992; **40**: 1001–7.
50. Johannesson G, Geirrson G, Day N et al. Screening for cancer of the uterine cervix in Iceland 1965–1978. Acta Obstet Gynecol Scand. 1982; **61**: 199–203.
51. Day NE. Effective cervical cancer screening in Scandinavia. Obstet Gynecol 1984; **63**: 714–18.
52. Hakama M, Chamberlain J, Day NE et al. Evaluation of screening programmes for gynaecological cancer. Brit J Cancer 1985; **52**: 669–73.
53. Ebeling K, Nischan P, Schindler C. Use of oral contraceptives and risk of invasive cervical cancer in previously screened women. Int J Cancer 1987; **39**: 427–30.
54. Duguid HL, Duncan ID, Currie J. Screening for cervical intra-epithelial neoplasia in Dundee and Angus 1962–1981 and its relation with invasive cervical cancer. Lancet 1985; **2**: 1053–6.

55. Dunn JE Jr, Schweitzer V. The relationship of cervical cytology to the incidence of invasive cervical cancer and mortality in Alameda County, California 1960 to 1974. Amer J Obstet Gynecol 1981; **139**: 868–76.

56. Clarke EA, Anderson TW. Does screening by 'Pap' smears help prevent cervical cancer? A case-control study. Lancet 1979; **2**: 1–4.

57. LaVecchia C, Franceschi S, Decarli A et al. 'Pap' smear and the risk of cervical neoplasia: quantitative estimates from a case-control study. Lancet 1984; **ii**: 779–82.

58. Aristizabal N, Cuello C, Correa P et al. The impact of vaginal cytology on cervical cancer risks in Cali, Columbia. Int J Cancer 1984; **34**: 5–9.

59. MacGregor JE. Mortality from carcinoma of cervix uterae in Britain. Lancet 1978; **2**: 774–6.

60. van der Graaf Y, Zielhuis GA, Peer PG, Vooijs PG. The effectiveness of cervical screening: a population-based case-control study. J Clin Epidemiol 1988; **41**: 21–6.

61. Olesen F. A case-control study of cervical cytology before diagnosis of cervical cancer in Denmark. Int J Epidemiol 1988; **17**: 501–8.

62. Shy K, Chu J, Mandelson M et al. Papanicolau smear screening interval and risk of cervical cancer. Obstet Gynecol 1989; **74**: 838–43.

63. IARC Working Group on Evaluation of Cervical Cancer Screening Programmes. Screening for squamous cervical cancer: duration of low risk after negative results of cervical cytology and its implications for screening policies. Brit Med J 1986; **293**: 659–64.

64. Fletcher A. Screening for cancer of the cervix in elderly women. Lancet 1990; **335**: 97–9.

65. Fidler AK, Boyes DA, Worth AJ. Cervical cancer detection in British Columbia. J Obstet Gynec Brit Commonwealth 1968; **78**: 392–404.

66. Stenkvist B, Bergstrom R, Eklund G et al. Papanicolaou smear screening and cervical cancer – what can you expect? J Amer Med Assoc 1984; **252**: 1423–6.

67. Eddy DM. Screening for cervical cancer. Annals Intern Med 1990; **113**: 214–26.

68. Mandelblatt JS, Fahs MC. The cost effectiveness of cervical cancer screening for low-income elderly women. J Amer Med Assoc 1988; **259**: 2409–13.

69. US Department of Health and Human Services Public Health Service, National Institutes of Health, National Cancer Institute. Cancer Statistics Review 1973–1986. Bethesda, MD: NIH Publication No. 89–2789, 1989.

70. Young JL, Percy CL, Asire AJ. Surveillance epidemiology and end results: incidence and mortality data 1973–1977. Bethesda, MD: National Cancer Institute, Monograph 57. DHHS, NIH Pub No. 81–2330, 1981.

71. Seidman H, Mushinski MH, Gelb SK et al. Probabilities of eventually developing or dying of cancer – United States 1985. Cancer 1985; **35**: 36–56.

72. Neilan BA. Colorectal Cancer. In: Cohen HJ (ed) Clinics in Geriatric Medicine: Cancer II – Specific Neoplasms, vol. 3, pp. 625–36. Philadelphia, PA: WB Saunders 1987.

73. Woolf CM. A genetic study of carcinoma of the large intestine. Amer J Human Genet 1958; **10**: 42–7.

74. Talley NJ, Shute CG, Larson DE. Risk for colorectal adenocarcinoma in pernicious anaemia. Annals Intern Med 1989; **111**: 738–42.

75. Grinnel RS, Laing N. Benign and malignant adematous polyps and papillary adenomas of the colon and rectum: an analysis of 1856 tumors in 1335 patients. Surg Gynecol Obstet 1958; **106**: 519–38.

76. Lotfi AM, Spencer RJ, Ilstrup DM et al. Colorectal polyps and the risk of subsequent carcinoma. Mayo Clin Proc 1986; **61**: 337–43.

77. Eide TJ. Risk of colorectal cancer in adenoma-bearing individuals within a defined population. Int J Cancer 1986; **38**: 173–6.

78. Clark JC, Collan Y, Eide TG et al. Prevalence of polyps in an autopsy series from areas with varying incidence of large bowel cancer. Int J Cancer 1985; **36**: 179–86.

79. Stryker SJ, Wolff BJ, Culp CE et al. Natural history of untreated colonic polyps. Gastroenterology 1987; **93**: 1009–13.

80. Atkin WS, Morson BC and Cuzick J. Long term risk of colorectal cancer after excision of rectosigmoid adenomas. N Engl J Med 1992; **326**: 658–62.

80a. Koretz RL. Malignant polyps: are they sheep in wolves' clothing? Annals Intern Med 1993; **118**: 63–8.

81. Frommer DJ, Capparis A, Brown MK. Improved screening for colorectal cancer by immunological detection of occult blood. Brit Med J 1988; **296**: 1092–3.

82. Crowly ML, Freeman LD, Mottet MD et al. Sensitivity of the Guaiac-impregnated cards for the detection of colorectal neoplasia. J Clin Gastroenterol 1983; **5**: 127–30.

83. Knight KK, Fielding JE, Battista RN. Occult blood screening for colorectal cancer. J Amer Med Assoc 1989; **261**: 587–93.

84. Pye G, Ballantyne KC, Armitage MC et al. Influence of non-steroidal anti-inflammatory drugs on the outcome of faecal occult blood tests screening for colorectal cancer. Brit Med J 1987; **294**: 1510–11.

85. Winawer SJ, Andrews M, Flehinger B et al. Progress report on controlled trial of faecal occult blood testing for the detection of colorectal neoplasia. Cancer 1980; **45**: 2959–64.

86. Gilbertsen VA, McHugh RB, Schuman LM et al. The earlier detection of colorectal cancers. A preliminary report of the results of the occult blood study. Cancer 1980; **45**: 2899–901.

87. Kurnick JE, Walley LB, Jacob HH et al. Colorectal cancer detection in a community hospital screening programme. J Amer Med Assoc 1980; **243**: 2056–7.

88. Balock SJ, De Vellis BM, Sandler RS. Participation in fecal ocult blood screening: a critical review. Prev Med 1987; **16**: 9–18.

89. Farrands PA, Hardcastle JD, Chamberlain J. Factors affecting compliance with screening for colorectal cancer. Comm Med 1984; **6**: 12–19.

90. Hobbs FDR, Cherry RC, Fielding JWL et al. Acceptability of opportunistic screening for occult gastrointestinal blood loss. Brit Med J 1992; **304**: 483–6.

91. Siebers MJ. Occult blood testing. Lancet 1986; **2**: 109.

92. Klos SE, Drinka P, Goodwin JS. The utilisation of fecal occult blood testing in the institutionalised elderly. J Amer Geriatr Soc 1991; **39**: 1169–73.

93. Frank JW. Occult blood screening for colorectal carcinoma: the risks. Amer J Prev Med 1981; **1**: 25–32.

94. Report of the US Preventive Services Task Force. Screening For Colorectal Cancer, in: Guide to Clinical Preventive Services, chapter 7. Baltimore, MD: Williams and Wilkins, 1989.

95. Selby JV, Friedman GD, Quesenberry CP et al. A case-control study of screening sigmoidoscopy and mortality from colorectal cancer. N Engl J Med 1992; **326**: 653–7.

96. Friedman GD, Collen MF, Fireman BH. Multifaceted health check up evaluation: a sixteen year follow up. J Chronic Dis 1986; **39**: 453–63.

97. Hardcastle JD, Chamberlain J, Sheffield J et al. Randomised controlled trial of faecal occult blood screening for colorectal cancer. Lancet 1989; **1**: 1160–4.

98. Winawer SJ, Andrews M, Flehinger B et al. Progress report on controlled trial of fecal occult blood testing for the detection of colorectal neoplasia. Cancer 1980; **45**: 2959–64.

99. Hardcastle JD, Armitage NC, Chamberlain J et al. Fecal occult blood screening for colorectal cancer in the general population. Cancer 1986; **58**: 397–403.

100. Kronborg O, Fenger C, Sondergaard O et al. Initial mass screening for colorectal cancer with fecal occult blood tests: a prospective randomised study at Funen in Denmark. Scand J. Gastroenterol 1987; **22**: 677–86.

101. Kewanter J, Bjork S, Haglind E et al. Screening and rescreening for colorectal cancer: a controlled trial of faecal occult blood testing in 27 700 subjects. Cancer 1988; **62**: 645–51.

101a. Simon JB. Colonic polyps, cancer and fecal occult blood. Annals Intern Med 1993; **118**: 71–2.

102. Eddy DM, Nugent FW, Eddy JF et al. Screening for colorectal cancer in a high risk population: Results of a mathematical model. Gastroenterology 1987; **92**: 682–92.

103. Willett W. The search for the causes of breast and colon cancer. Nature 1989; **338**: 389–94.

104. Guillem JG, Matsui MS, O'Brian CA. Nutrition in the prevention of neoplastic disease in the elderly. In: Watkin DM (ed) Clinics in Geriatric Medicine: Nutrition in Older Persons, vol. 3, pp. 373–98. Philadelphia, PA: WB Saunders, 1987.

105. Willett WC, Stampfer MJ, Colditz GA et al. Relation of meat, fat, and fiber intake to the risk of colon cancer in a prospective study among women. N Engl J Med 1990; **323**: 1664–72.

106. Lipkin M. Effect of added dietary calcium and colonic epithelial cell proliferation in subjects at high risk for familial colonic cancer. N Engl J Med 1985; **313**: 1381–4.

107. Thun NJ, Namboodiri MM, Heath CW. Aspirin use in reduced risk of fatal colon cancer. N Engl J Med 1991; **325**: 1593–6.

108. Rosenberg L, Palmer JR, Zauber AG et al. A hypothesis: non-steroidal anti-inflammatory drugs reduce the incidence of large-bowel cancer. J Natl Cancer Inst 1991; **83**: 355–8.

109. Kune GA, Kune S, Watson LF. Colorectal cancer risk, chronic illnesses, operations and medications: case control results from the Melbourne colorectal cancer study. Cancer Res 1988; **48**: 4399–404.

110. Wagner JL, Herdman RC, Wadhwa S. Cost effectiveness of colorectal cancer screening in the elderly. Annals Intern Med 1991; **115**: 807–17.

111. Ransohoff DF, Lang CA. Screening for colorectal cancer. N Engl J Med 1991; **325**: 37–41.

112. Horm JWS, Asire AJ, Young JL et al. (eds). SEER Program: Cancer Incidence and Mortality in the United States, 1973–1981. NIH Publ No. 85–1837. Bethesda, MD: National Cancer Institute, 1984.

113. Gaddipati J, Ahmed T, Friedland M. Prostatic and bladder cancer in the elderly. In: Cohen HJ (ed) Clinics in Geriatric Medicine: Cancer II – Specific Neoplasms, vol. 3, no. 4. Philadelphia, PA: WB Saunders, 1987.

114. Report of the US Preventive Services Task Force. Screening For Prostatic Cancer. Chapter 9, in: Guide to Clinical Preventive Services. Baltimore, MD: Williams and Wilkins, 1989.

114a. Oesterling JE. Prostate-specific antigen. Improving its ability to diagnose early prostate cancer. J Amer Med Assoc 1992; **267**: 2236–7.

114b. Crawford ED, Schutz MJ, Clejan S et al. The effect of digital rectal examination on prostate-specific antigen levels. J Amer Med Assoc 1992; **267**: 2227–8.

115. Chodak GW, Keller P, Schoenberg H. Routine screening for prostate cancer using the digital rectal examination. Prog Clin Biol Res 1988; **269**: 87–98.

116. Littrup PJ, Torp-Pedersen ST et al. Prostate cancer: comparison of transrectal US and digital rectal examination for screening. Radiology 1988; **168**: 389–94.

116a. Johansson JE, Adami HO, Andersson SO et al. High 10 year survival rate in patients with early, untreated prostatic cancer. J Amer Med Assoc 1992; **267**: 2191–6.

116b. Whitmore WF Jr, Warner JA, Thompson IM Jr. Expectant management of localised prostatic cancer. Cancer 1991; **67**: 1091–6.

117. Byar DK, Corle DK. VACURG randomized trial of radical prostatectomy for stages I and II prostate cancer. Veterans Administration Cooperative Urological Research Group. Urol (suppl) 1981; **17**: 7–11.

118. Silverberg E, Lubera J. Cancer statistics 1986. Cancer 1986; **36**: 9–25.

119. Bailar JC, Smith EM. Progress against cancer? N Engl J Med 1986; **314**: 1226–32.

120. Grzybowski S, Coy P. Early diagnosis of carcinoma of the lung. Simultaneous screening with chest X-ray and sputum cytology. Cancer 1970; **25**: 113–20.

121. Eddy DM. Screening for lung cancer. Annals Intern Med 1989; **11**: 232–7.

122. Melamed MR, Flehinger BJ, Zaman MB et al. Preliminary report of the lung cancer detection program in New York. Cancer 1977; **39**: 369–82.

123. Boucot KR, Weiss W. Is curable lung cancer detected by semi-annual screening? J Amer Med Assoc 1973; **224**: 1361–5.

124. Brett GZ. Earlier diagnosis and survival in lung cancer. Brit Med J 1969; **4**: 260–2.

125. Lilienfeld A, Archer PG, Burnett CG et al. An evaluation of radiologic and cytologic screening for the early detection of lung cancer: a cooperative pilot study of the American Cancer Society and the Veterans Administration. Cancer Res 1966; **26**: 2083–121.

126. Berlin NI, Bunchur RC, Fontana RS et al. The National Cancer Institute Cooperative Early lung cancer detection program – results of the initial screen (prevalence). Early lung cancer detection (introduction). Amer Rev Respir Dis 1984; **130**: 545–9.

127. Kubik, A, Polak J. Lung cancer detection: results of a randomised prospective study in Czechoslovakia. Cancer 1986; **57**: 2427–37.

128. Melamed MR, Flehinger BJ, Zaman MB et al. Screening for early lung cancer: results of the Memorial Sloan-Kettering Study in New York. Chest 1984; **86**: 44–53.

129. Tockman MS. Survival and mortality from lung cancer in a screened population. The Johns Hopkins Study. Chest 1986; **89** (suppl): 324S–5S.

130. Saunderson DR. Lung cancer screening: the Mayo Study. Chest 1986; **89** (suppl): 324S.

131. Baranovsky A, Myers M. Cancer incidence and survival in patients 65 years of age and older. Cancer 1986; **36**: 27–34.

132. O'Rourke MA, Crawford J. Lung cancer in the elderly. In: Harvey AJ (ed) Clinics in Geriatric Medicine: Cancer II – Specific Neoplasms, vol. 3, no. 4. Philadelphia, PA: WB Saunders, 1987.

133. Albanes D, Virtamo J, Rautalahti M et al. Pilot study: the US–Finland lung cancer prevention trial. J Nutr Growth Cancer 1986; **3**: 207–14.

134. American Cancer Society. Report on the cancer-related health check up. New York: American Cancer Society, 1980.

135. US Department of Health and Human Services: Vital Statistics of the United States 1978, vol. 2 Mortality, Part A.

136. Berman ML, Ballon SC, Legasse LD et al. Prognosis and treatment of endometrial cancer. Amer J Obstet Gynecol 1980; **136**: 670–88.

137. Shapiro S, Kaufman DW, Sloane D et al. Recent and past use of conjugated estrogens in relation to adenocarcinoma of the endometrium. N Engl J Med 1980; **303**: 485–9.

138. Shapiro S, Kelly JP, Rosenberg L et al. Risk of localised widespread cancer in relation to recent and discontinued use of conjugated estrogens. N Engl J Med 1985; **313**: 969–72.

139. Smith DC, Prentice R, Thompson DJ et al. Association of exogenous estrogen and endometrial carcinoma. N Engl J Med 1975; **293**: 1164–7.

140. Persson I, Adami HO, Bergkvist L et al. Risk of endometrial cancer after treatment with oestrogen alone or in conjunction with progestogens: results of a prospective study. Brit Med J 1989; **298**: 147–51.

141. Kass LG, Schreiber K, Oberlander SG et al. Detection of endometrial carcinoma and hyperplasia in asymptomatic women. Obstet Gynecol 1984; **64**: 1–11.

142. Zucker PJ, Kasdon EJ, Feldstein ML. The validity of Pap smear parameters as predictors of endometrial pathology in menopausal women. Cancer 1985; **56**: 2256–63.

143. Bourne TH, Campbell S, Whitehead MI et al. Detection of endometrial cancer in postmenopausal women by trans-vaginal ultrasonography and colour-flow imaging. Brit Med J 1990; **301**: 369–70.

144. Green MH, Clark JW, Blayney DW. The epidemiology of ovarian cancer. Semin Oncol 1984; **11**: 209–26.

145. Bjorkholm E, Petterson G, Einhorn N et al. Long term follow up and prognostic factors in ovarian carcinoma. Acta Radiol Oncol 1982; **21**: 413–19.

146. Ozols RF, Young RC. Chemotherapy of ovarian cancer. Semin Oncol 1984; **11**: 251–63.

147. Goodwin JS, Samet JM, Key CR et al. Stage at diagnosis of cancer varies with the age of the patient. J Amer Geriatr Soc 1986; **34**: 20–6.

148. Lundberg WI, Wall JE, Mathers JE. Laporoscopy in evaluation of pelvic pain. Obstet Gynecol 1973; **42**: 872–6.

149. Buchsbaum HJ, Lifshitz S. Staging and surgical evaluation of ovarian cancer. Semin Oncol 1984; **11**: 227–37.

150. Smith LI, Ol RH. Detection of malignant ovarian neoplasms. A review of the literature. 1. Detection of the patient at risk: clinical, radiological and cytological detection. Obstet Gynecol Surv 1984; **39**: 313–28.

151. Weintraub NT, Freedman ML. Gynecologic malignancies of the elderly. In: Cohen HJ (ed) Clinics in Geriatric Medicine: Cancer II – Specific Neoplasms, vol. 3, no. 4. Philadelphia, PA: WB Saunders, 1987.

152. Goswany RK, Campbell S, Whitehead MI. Screening for ovarian cancer. Clin Obstet Gynecol 1983; **10**: 621–43.

153. Campbell S, Bhan V, Royston P et al. Trans-abdominal ultrasound screening for early ovarian cancer. Brit Med J 1989; **299**: 1363–7.

154. Oram DH, Jacobs IJ, Brady JL et al. Early diagnosis of ovarian cancer. Brit J Hosp Med 1990; **44**: 320–4.

155. Bourne T, Campbell S, Steer C. Trans-vaginal colour-flow imaging: a possible new screening technique for ovarian cancer. Brit Med J 1989; **299**: 1367–70.

156. Office of Population Censuses and Surveys. Cancer Statistics. London: HMSO, 1986.

157. Correa P. Clinical implications of recent developments in gastric cancer pathology and epidemiology. Semin Oncol 1985; **12**: 2–10.

158. MacDonald JS, Cohn I, Gunderson LL. Cancer of the stomach. In: Cancer: Principles and Practice of Oncology, pp. 659–60. Philadelphia, PA: JB Lippincott, 1985.

159. Hisamichi S, Sugawara N. Mass screening for gastric cancer by x-ray examination. Jpn J Clin Oncol 1984; **14**: 211–23.

160. Hallissey MT, Allum WH, Jeukes AJ et al. Early detection of gastric cancer. Brit Med J 1990; **301**: 513–15.

161. Logan RSA, Langman JS. Screening for gastric cancer after gastric surgery. Lancet 1983; **ii**: 667–70.

162. Gaddipati J, Ahmed T, Friedland M. Prostatic and bladder cancer in the elderly. In: Cohen HJ (ed) Clinics in Geriatric Medicine: Cancer II – Specific Neoplasms, vol. 3, no. 4. Philadelphia, PA: WB Saunders, 1987.

163. Mohr DN, Offord KP, Owen RA et al. Asymptomatic microhaematuria and urologic disease. J Amer Med Assoc 1986; **256**: 224–9.

164. Messing EM, Young TB, Hunt VB et al. The significance of asymptomatic microhaematuria in men 50 or more years old: findings of a home screening study using urinary dipsticks. J Urol 1987; **137**: 919–22.

165. Britton JP, Dowell AC, Whelan P. Dipstick haematuria and bladder cancer in men over 60: results of a community study. Brit Med J 1989; **299**: 1010–12.

166. Cartwright RA, Cadian T, Carland JE et al. The influence of malignant cell cytology screening on the survival of industrial bladder cancer cases. Brit J Epid Comm Health 1981; **35**: 35–8.

167. Gordis L, Gold EB. Epidemiology of pancreatic cancer. World J Surg 1984; **8**: 808–21.

168. American Cancer Society. 1985 Cancer Facts and Figures. New York: American Cancer Society, 1985.

169. Report of the US Preventive Services Task Force. Screening for Pancreatic Cancer. Chapter 14 in: Guide to Clinical Preventive Services. Williams and Wilkins, 1989.

170. Scotto J, Kopf AW, Urbach F. Non-melanoma skin cancer among Caucasians in four areas of the United States. Cancer 1974; **34**: 1333.

171. McHenry PM, Hole DJ, MacKie RM. Melanoma in people aged 65 and over in Scotland, 1979–1989. Brit Med J 1992; **304**: 746–9.

172. Report of the US Preventive Services Task Force. Screening for Skin Cancer. Chapter 11 in: Guide to Clinical Preventive Services. Williams and Wilkins, 1989.

173. Public awareness of the effects of sun on skin. A survey conducted for the American Academy of Dermatology. Princeton NJ: Opinion Research Corporation, 1987.

173a. Robinson JK, Salasche SJ. Isotretinoin does not prevent basal cell carcinoma. Arch Dermatol 1992; **128**: 975–6.

173b. Greenberg ER, Baron JA, Stukel TA. A clinical trial of betacarotene to prevent
      basal cell and squamous cell cancers of the skin. N Engl J Med 1990; **323**:
      789–95.
174. National Cancer Institute, Division of Cancer Prevention and Control. 1987
      Annual Cancer Statistics Review, Bethesda, MD: DHHS, NIH Publication
      No. 88–2789.
175. Blot WJ, McLaughlin JK, Winn DM et al. Smoking and drinking in relation to
      oral and pharyngeal cancer. Cancer Res 1988; **48**: 3282–7.
176. Baden E. Prevention of cancer of the oral cavity and pharynx. Cancer 1987; **37**:
      49–62.
177. Chiodo GT, Eigner T, Rosenstein DI. Oral cancer detection: the importance of
      routine screening for prolongation of survival. Postgrad Med 1986; **80**: 231–6.
178. Vital and Health Statistics, National Center for Health Statistics: Series 3,
      DHHS Publication No. (PHS) 87–1409 and No. 25, and Series 10, No. 165.
      DHHS Publication No. (PHS) 88–1593. Hyattsville, MD, 1986.
179. Fedele DJ, Jones JA, Niessen LC. Oral cancer screening in the elderly. J Amer
      Geriatr Soc 1991; **39**: 920–5.
180. Report of the US Preventive Services Task Force. Screening for Oral Cancer.
      Chapter 15, in: Guide to Clinical Preventive Services, Baltimore, MD:
      Williams and Wilkins, 1989.

7

The prevention of non-cancerous
health problems

Hypertension

Importance

Although some studies have shown a lack of association between hypertension and mortality in elderly people and two [1, 2] have even shown an unexpected survival advantage, the considerable bulk of evidence indicates that hypertension is not a benign accompaniment of ageing. It is associated with greater mortality and morbidity from stroke and cardiovascular disease. Cardiovascular risk gradients actually increase with advancing age (see Fig. 7.1). Diastolic blood pressure is a predictor of risk in its own right but systolic pressure is equally, if not more, predictive of risk for cardiovascular morbidity and mortality and for future stroke events [4].

Prevalence estimates of both diastolic and isolated systolic hypertension in elderly people vary widely, tending to decrease with increasing numbers or occasions on which the blood pressure is measured prior to making the diagnosis. Between ages 60 to 70 years, the prevalence of elevated levels of combined *casual* systolic and diastolic pressure (upon which risk estimates may be based) range between 17 and 24 per cent [5]. However, the prevalence of *sustained* levels for systolic and diastolic hypertension (upon which treatment decisions should be based) is about a third of this. Isolated systolic hypertension ranges between 3 and 13 per cent in an elderly population based on *casual* readings, but in the Systolic Hypertension in the Elderly Program study (see below), just over 1 per cent of all elderly subjects screened fulfilled the entry criteria of *sustained* isolated systolic hypertension recorded as the mean of six measurements at a minimum of three visits.

Detection

The estimation of blood pressure by sphygmomanometry is the usual detection manoeuvre. There are many well-documented sources of error in making these recordings [6] to which pseudohypertension [7] due to a calcified and incompressible brachial artery should be added in the older age group. When considering subsequent treatment, hypertension should be based on repeated estimations, hypertension not being considered present unless there has been more than one elevated reading obtained on each of three separate visits [6].

Effectiveness

There are now numerous well-conducted, controlled trials that show clear benefit for treating hypertension in elderly persons [8–16]. Treatment of diastolic hypertension in elderly people is therefore highly beneficial. Almost all the trials have shown a reduction in the rates of stroke and cardiovascular events. For example, the most recent UK Medical Research Council study reported a 25 per cent reduction in stroke and a 19 per cent reduction in coronary events [11]. Only two studies [10, 12] have shown a beneficial impact on total mortality however and only one [8] a beneficial impact on myocardial infarction.

There is now good evidence from the Systolic Hypertension in the Elderly Program (SHEP) [17] that treatment is beneficial. A further European study of hypertension in elderly people is also underway. In the SHEP study, it was estimated that treatment of 33 elderly patients with isolated systolic hypertension for five years was likely to prevent one stroke or two cardiovascular events.

There has for some time been a suggestion that excessive reduction of diastolic blood pressure in patients with preexisting coronary disease may actually cause coronary events. This hypothesis is refuted by the evidence from the SHEP study in which pretreatment diastolic pressures were low and in which coronary events were still *reduced* at the end of the trial in the treatment group.

Despite numerous trials, the insufficient numbers still allow few firm recommendations to be made for treating hypertension in people over 80 years. Nevertheless, the preponderance of evidence in younger older people indicates that the onus should be to treat rather than not to treat. However, the risk–benefit equation in this very old age group will need to be carefully and individually considered.

In comparison with younger patients, those over 60 years treated for hypertension have the same relative reduction in cardiovascular morbidity and mortality. However, because elderly people have higher rates of cardiovascular events, the same percentage benefit from drug treatment results in a greater absolute reduction in events [4].

The compliance of elderly individuals in some hypertensive trials has been surprisingly high [18]. However, most of these reports have come from specialist centres under highly supervised research conditions, and they may not equate with compliance rates in the service arena of primary care, the arena that would be involved if antihypertensive treatment were adopted on a national scale.

The increased risk of side effects from antihypertensive therapy in elderly patients is well known and must be carefully weighed in the balance before starting therapy. Particular care must be taken to avoid too rapid a reduction in blood pressure [19].

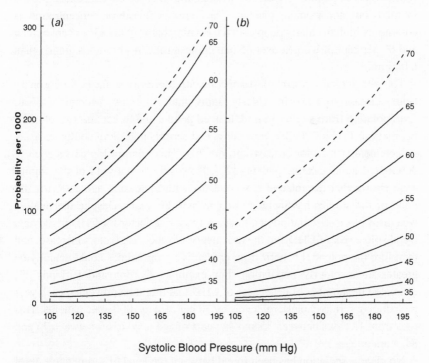

Fig. 7.1. Probability of cardiovascular disease in eight years according to systolic blood pressure at specified ages in (*a*) men and (*b*) women (Framingham Study: 18-year follow up, low risk subjects). Adapted from ref. [3].

Cost

The cost of mounting blood pressure treatment programmes for elderly people is unknown but must be considerable. Weinstein and Stason [20] have estimated that, for the population as a whole, treating hypertension may add more to medical expenditures than it saves in terms of emergency services, hospitalisation and vascular surgery. Programmes for the treatment of moderate to severe hypertension were estimated to be four times as expensive and for treating mild hypertension the costs were considered to be six times as great.

Hyperlipidaemia

Importance

Levels of blood cholesterol increase with age. Mean blood cholesterol concentrations run parallel in men and women until their 60s when concentrations in men, but not women, plateau. The serum cholesterol concentration is commonly high in elderly people; in the Framingham cohort 35 per cent of men and 60 per cent of women over 65 had cholesterol concentrations greater than 6.0 mmol/l.

The role of total serum cholesterol concentration as a risk factor for coronary heart disease (CHD) in elderly individuals is now becoming clear. Extrapolation from studies in middle aged people and direct analysis of older populations (Table 7.1) [21] now show that serum cholesterol continues as an independent risk factor at least into the 70s. This relationship exists even in debilitated nursing home patients [22]. However, virtually all of the studies have shown that the relative risk weakens with increasing age and virtually none of the studies has included people over 80 years. Despite the relative weakness of the association of cholesterol as a risk factor for CHD in old age, the absolute risk of CHD and the prevalence of other risk factors increase, and therefore the potential benefit from preventive programmes could actually be greater in an elderly population. For example, Gordon and Rifkind [23] estimated the number of new cases of CHD that might be prevented each year by reducing serum cholesterol levels by 30 per cent in 1000 male patients. This rose from 12 cases between 35 and 44 years of age to 20 cases between 75 and 84 years of age.

No clear association has been found between the level of serum cholesterol and stroke disease, though this may reflect the lack of inclusion of older people in the studies concerned [21]. Finally, hypocholesterolaemia has been

Table 7.1. *Studies of the relationship between cholesterol and coronary heart disease involving older people*

Study	Number of subjects	Age (years)	Summary of results
Agner and Hansen (1983)	440	70	CHD mortality 37% if cholesterol is in upper quartile, compared with 17% in other quartiles combined
Barrett-Connor et al. (1984)	3187	50–79	*RR* of CHD death = 1.4 for each standard deviation (= 1 mmol litre) increase in cholesterol
Harris et al. (1988)	998	>65	*RR* = 1.5 for all CHD for cholesterol >90th percentile, compared with those having a cholesterol level of < 5.2 mmol litre
Benfante and Reed (1990)	6860	65–74	*RR* = 1.64 for all CHD for upper compared with lower quartiles of cholesterol
Rabin et al. (1990)	2746	60–79	*RR* = 1.5 for fatal CHD for upper compared with all other quartiles of cholesterol

CHD, coronary heart disease; *RR*, relative risk.
References cited: Agner E, Hansen PF. Acta Med Scand 1983; **214**: 3–41.
Barrett-Connor E, Svarez L, Khaw K et al. J. Chron Dis 1984; **37**: 903–8.
Harris T, Cook EF, Kannel WB, Goldman L. J Amer Geriatr Soc 1988; **36**: 1023–8.
Benfante R, Reed D. J Amer Med Assoc 1990; **263**: 393–6.
Rabin SM, Sidney S, Black DM et al. Annals Intern Med 1990; **113**: 916–20.
Source: ref. [21].

found as a risk factor for death in elderly men [24] and in elderly women in nursing homes [25]. Although these low levels of cholesterol have been suggested as a consequence of malignant disease, other nursing home studies suggest the association is most likely to be due to malnutrition and infection [26]. Hypocholesterolaemia has also been suggested as a risk factor for haemorrhagic stroke in the elderly population [27].

Detection

Estimation of serum cholesterol is the most reliable and validated screening test available. Due to substantial physiological fluctuations repeated measurements may give a more reliable estimate of true risk of CHD. Estimation of high density lipoprotein (HDL), considered a protectant factor for ischaemic heart disease and which increases with age [28], or the ratio of HDL to cholesterol, may further refine the extent of risk associated with CHD, but they have not yet been widely used in screening programmes.

Effectiveness

Although randomised trials of cholesterol reduction in asymptomatic younger adults have shown a significant reduction in cardiovascular morbidity and mortality (though no decrease in overall mortality) [29], the impact of such measures on elderly people has not been evaluated. Only one trial of a diet relatively high in polyunsaturated fat has included significant numbers of people over 65 years. The diet resulted in only a very small reduction in serum cholesterol and the reduction in CHD was not significant [30]. It is also likely that the side effects of cholesterol-lowering medications will be greater in elderly people, that there may become a problem of interaction with other drugs, and that antihyperlipidaemic therapy in the majority of trials has been associated with an increase in non-cardiac mortality [31].

Cost

The available evidence suggests that antihyperlipidaemic therapy for asymptomatic elderly individuals would have an extremely high cost for any benefits obtained. Using cholestyramine for antihyperlipaemic therapy, the cost effectiveness in men, starting treatment at age 65 years with a pretreatment cholesterol level of 7.49 mmol/l (290 mg/dl), has been estimated as $993 700 per year of life saved [32].

Stroke

Importance

Bonita [33] provides a detailed account of the epidemiology of stroke. Incidence of stroke (first-ever events), rises exponentially with age being 20 to 32 per 10 000 persons aged 55 to 64 years depending on geographic locality and similarly 184 to 397 per 10 000 persons 85 years and over. After first stroke, the recurrence is about 13 per cent in the first year and about 5 per cent in each year thereafter. The age-specific death rate from stroke doubles each five-year age increment. Stroke disease is the third most common cause of death in western societies; about 88 per cent of deaths attributed to stroke are among people over 65 years.

The burden from stroke has been estimated for a number of settings. Between 15 and 22 per cent of patients remain disabled after stroke depending on whether non-fatal cases that occur outside hospital have been included in the estimate. The cost of stroke care in the USA in 1984 was estimated at

$5 billion per year. In Scotland in 1988, stroke accounted for 4.3 per cent of all NHS resources and 5.5 per cent of hospital resources [34]. Stroke also accounted for 22.5 of family practitioner consultations per 1000 aged 65 to 74 years and 47.4 per 1000 aged 75 years and over [34]. It accounted also for 8.5 per cent of community nursing visits. The costs of stroke to patients and their families is also considerable.

Targeting/detection

A. Targeting of primary preventive measures should be aimed at the following subgroups of elderly people.
1. *Hypertensives*. Hypertension is the most important risk factor for stroke of all ages and may contribute to as many as 70 per cent of all strokes. Details of the association are discussed on p. 77.
2. *Those with atrial fibrillation*. Atrial fibrillation associated with rheumatic heart disease increases the risk of stroke 17 times. Perhaps more important for an elderly population is the risk associated with non-rheumatic atrial fibrillation (NRAF). NRAF is associated with a fivefold increase in the risk of stroke (perhaps even higher if 'silent' cerebral infarcts are included) that increases further with age [35]. It is suggested that NRAF is the single most important characteristic associated with stroke in women over 70 years, cerebral infarction eventually occurring in up to 35 per cent of such people. Further studies suggest the presence of recent congestive heart failure, a history of hypertension or previous thromboembolism and various echocardiographic findings can predict a subset of those with NRAF at high risk of embolism [36, 37].
3. *Smokers*. Recent evidence implicates cigarette smoking as a risk factor for stroke [38] and the relative risk in heavy smokers is twice that in light smokers [39]. One case control study estimated the relative risk to be 5.7 for patients with ischaemic stroke due to extracranial or intracranial vascular disease [40].
4. *Patients with coronary artery disease*. Those with symptomatic coronary artery disease have an ischaemic stroke risk which falls between that subsequent to patients with transient ischaemic attack (TIA) or stroke and the age-matched population.

Targeting elderly people with other risk factors for primary prevention seems less justified. Although the presence of an asymptomatic carotid bruit has generated much interest as a risk factor for stroke in younger age groups, the frequency of occurrence of carotid bruits increase with advancing age and do not greatly increase the risk for subsequent attributable stroke in elderly people [41]. They often disappear without clinical sequelae [42]. Some ethnic groups such as blacks in the USA and Afro-Caribbeans in the UK have high risk of stroke. Although attention to other concomitant risk factors such as hypertension is important, a proportion of the ethnic risk will remain immutable [43]. Diabetes and impaired glucose tolerance are important risk factors for stroke but targeting those suffering from the disorder for primary preventive measures is not recommended because there is no convincing evidence that control of glycaemia alters the risk. Alcohol has been implicated as a risk factor for stroke [44] but studies reporting no or even a decreased risk from ischaemic stroke have also been published [45]. The relationship of stroke to hyperlipidaemia is discussed on p. 80.

B. Detection of TIA or small stroke for secondary preventive measures is essentially by clinical assessment though a minority will require further investigation which may include continuous wave Doppler ultrasound or duplex scanning to assess carotid arterial patency.

Primary prevention

Primary preventive strategies are those applied to the elderly population who have not yet experienced a first stroke episode. They may be considered as follows.

Antihypertensive treatment

The evidence for its efficacy is summarised on p. 78.

Quitting smoking

The evidence for its efficacy is summarised on p. 92.

Aspirin therapy

It is not yet known whether the elderly population in general would benefit from prophylactic aspirin therapy for the primary prevention of stroke. Two clinical trials on the use of low-dose aspirin in relatively healthy persons (most of whom were in middle age) showed no reduction in the rate of stroke [46, 47]. Furthermore, there was some evidence indicating a slightly *increased* risk for disabling haemorrhagic stroke [46]. In a retirement community, aspirin use has also been implicated with an increased risk of kidney cancer and ischaemic heart disease [48]. Current evidence does not therefore support the use of aspirin for stroke prevention in healthy persons.

Prophylactic therapy after myocardial infarction

Although not specifically analysing older populations, the results from large-scale trials in patients with recent or remote myocardial infarction have shown a substantial reduction in the incidence of subsequent stroke amongst patients treated with aspirin [49, 50].

Prophylactic therapy for those with atrial fibrillation

Four randomised trials investigating the use of low-dose warfarin as a measure in people with NRAF have recently been published [51–53]. All four studies showed that low-dose warfarin can substantially reduce stroke (risk reduction rates varying from 42 to 86 per cent) with minimal risk of significant haemorrhage. Withdrawal rates from the warfarin ranged from 10 to 38 per cent. Two of the studies [51, 52] contained large numbers of those with paroxysmal, rather than persistent, atrial fibrillation. Two of these randomised trials [52, 53] also studied the effect of low-dose aspirin therapy. One study (mean age of patients 74 years) showed no benefit. The other showed the primary event rate in the aspirin group to be 3.2 per cent per year compared with 6.3 per cent for the placebo group. No benefit was observed for patients over 75 years however. Possible explanations for these findings are discussed by Chesebro [35].

Carotid endarterectomy

Available evidence from surgical trials on the use of carotid endarterectomy in *asymptomatic* persons with carotid bruits have yet to show conclusive benefit. Indeed the American College of Physicians concludes that the non-selective use of carotid endarterectomy in such patients represents the most inappropriate use of this procedure [54].

Secondary prevention

The following secondary preventive strategies have been employed with variable success.

Antihypertensive treatment

See p. 78.

Aspirin therapy

The results of several large studies and particularly meta-analysis of these trials have shown convincingly that aspirin reduces the risk of subsequent stroke by 20 to 25 per cent after TIA or minor stroke [55]. This effect is seen in both sexes. There is also some evidence indicating that neurological deficits may be less severe in persons receiving aspirin therapy [56]. The same preventive benefits have *not* been shown with aspirin after a major stroke [57].

Most preventive trials have used aspirin in dosages ranging from 900 to 1500 mg per day. However, a British trial showed no difference in benefit between aspirin 1200 mg daily and aspirin 300 mg daily [58]. A recent Dutch trial has further shown that 30 mg of aspirin daily is as effective as 300 mg daily [59]. The most effective dose of aspirin for prevention nevertheless remains controversial.

Other antiplatelet agents

Two large clinical trials [60, 61] have failed to demonstrate that the addition of dipyridamole to aspirin therapy was beneficial in reducing further the incidence of stroke. A relatively new antiplatelet drug Ticlopidine has also been shown to reduce subsequent risk of fatal and non-fatal stroke after recent TIA or minor stroke [62]. However, Ticlopidine is a more expensive therapy than aspirin and it carries a 1 per cent risk of reversible neutropenia. Current evidence suggests it is somewhat more effective than aspirin for stroke prevention [63].

Anticoagulant therapy

Based on clinical trials performed many years ago, there has been a suggestion that anticoagulation with warfarin may reduce the subsequent incidence of ischaemic stroke for at least the first six months after TIA. Three more recent randomised trials from Sweden [64–66] have, however, failed to show any relative benefit of anticoagulation over antiplatelet therapy.

Prophylactic anticoagulation therapy for those with atrial fibrillation

There is very limited evidence on the efficacy of anticoagulation with warfarin in the *secondary* prevention of stroke [67]. One non-randomised comparative trial with small numbers of patients, yet including many elderly individuals, failed to show any significant benefit either in the rate of recurrent stroke or the rate of survival in the anticoagulated group [68].

Carotid endarterectomy

There is now evidence from a North American and from a European trial that carotid endarterectomy is highly beneficial in preventing further stroke in patients with recent hemispheric and retinal transient ischaemic attacks or non-disabling and ipsilateral high grade stenosis (70 to 99 per cent) of the internal carotid artery [69, 70]. However, results were obtained in patients under 80 years of age without widespread cerebrovascular disease. The benefits of intervention would be diminished if performed at a centre with a perioperative risk of major stroke and death exceeding 2.1 per cent and would vanish entirely if the complication rate approached 10 per cent. There is no evidence of benefit when operating for lesser degrees of carotid stenosis.

Extracranial–intracranial arterial bypass

A large prospective randomised trial in the United States, Canada and Japan comparing extracranial–intracranial arterial bypass to standard therapy for the prevention of stroke in symptomatic patients with carotid occlusion or surgically inaccessible stenosis failed to show any benefit overall or in any subgroup [71]. Subsequent concern has been expressed over selection bias for the trial and the results have been reanalysed [72], but the onus still remains with the proponents of the technique to prove its efficacy.

Cost

Little information is available relating specifically to an elderly population, but high costs will be incurred if surgical techniques are increasingly adopted to prevent stroke. For example, in the USA (where 433 carotid endarterectomies per million population are performed, compared with 20 per million in the UK) the total cost of this procedure was $1.2 billion in 1984.

Recently, Gustafsson et al. [72a] studying the total Swedish population with chronic atrial fibrillation found that primary prevention of stroke with anti-coagulants and, if contraindications exist, with aspirin was cost effective, provided that the risk of serious haemorrhagic complications due to anti-coagulants was kept low. The total savings from this regimen was estimated to be Kr175 million per year corresponding to £2 million per million inhabitants each year.

Abdominal aortic aneurysms

Importance

Recent screening studies suggest that asymptomatic small aneurysms are frequent in the elderly population [73]. In men aged 65 to 74 years of age the incidence of abdominal aortic aneurysm of more than 4 cm diameter is 2.3 per cent. The age-specific incidence of rupture of an abdominal aortic aneurysm as a cause of death rises after age 55 years and continues to increase beyond 85 years [74]. It is four times more common in men than in women, being the principal cause of death in 1.7 per cent of men 65 to 74 years of age [73].

Detection

Detection of aneurysms by abdominal palpation is inefficient, particularly in obese patients, yet can be satisfactorily achieved by ultrasonography or computed tomography (CT) scanning. Accurate though the identification and measurement of aneurysmal diameter may be, it still only provides an approximation of the risk of rupture, which is the main problem associated with the condition. Previous data based on patients referred to specialist centres have suggested significant expansion rates for small aneurysms and significant rupture rates for larger aneurysms. Community based studies [75], however, have found considerably lower average rates of expansion and a risk of rupture of only 8 per cent by 10 years. The risk of rupture ranged from 3 per cent at 10 years for aneurysms less than 5 cm in diameter to 25 per cent at 5 years for aneurysms 5 cm or more in diameter [75].

Effectiveness

A number of screening surveys have provided epidemiological information [76, 77], but so far no comprehensive screening programme has yet been mounted to evaluate the benefits of an early detection and treatment programme. One of the proponents of screening, Collin [78], in estimating the impact of a screening programme for men 65 to 74 years in England and Wales, calculated on identifying 585 aneurysms. Death from ruptured aneurysm might be prevented in 185 patients but there would be 30 operative deaths, 20 of which would be in men who would otherwise have died from natural causes. There would therefore be a net saving of 165 lives. However, if all the patients had been allowed to rupture their aneurysms about 25 might be expected to survive; the adjusted number of lives saved by screening therefore drops to 140. No calculation of the morbidity from operation was taken into account in these calculations.

Whilst some indication is available of the number of men willing to undergo ultrasound screening (see above), no information is available on the number of asymptomatic elderly individuals who would subsequently be willing to undergo the sorts of risks of such surgery outlined above, yet the efficacy of the screening programme is ultimately dependent on this.

Cost

Looking at the direct costs of medical care only, Collin [78] estimated a screening programme in England and Wales for men in the age group 65 to 75 years of age would amount to £100 000, the operations would cost £550 000 and the postoperative hospital care £650 000. The total cost per life saved was £9000. Later estimates by the same author suggest a medical cost of £450 per quality adjusted life year [78a].

Ischaemic heart disease

Importance

There is a progressive increase in both the attack rate and case fatality rate of myocardial infarction with increasing age [78b]. By the age of eighty, pathological evidence of moderate to severe coronary atheroma can be found in most persons and evidence of myocardial infarction is present in over 50 per cent of both sexes. Approximately 10 per cent of male and female patients between 70 and 80 years of age have symptomatic angina pectoris [78c]. Ischaemic heart disease (IHD) is the commonest cause of cardiac failure in elderly people. IHD is the leading cause of death in old people in industrialised countries [78d].

Detection/targeting

Detection measures for the primary identification of risk factors for IHD are discussed in the relevant sections of this book.

Confirmation of symptomatic IHD is usually reliably performed through a combination of clinical and electrocardiographic examinations. Identification of presymptomatic IHD by these techniques is much less reliable. Details are provided elsewhere [78e]. In general, screening electrocardiography is not recommended in asymptomatic persons. Yet, it may be prudent to perform screening electrocardiograms in high risk groups (men who have hypertension, a family history of IHD, high blood cholesterol, diabetes mellitus, smoke etc.) and, in view of the marked prevalence of IHD in very old people (those over 75 years) they too may be considered a high risk group. Also, some of the criticism levelled against false positive electrocardiogram results in a younger population such as their disqualifying some people from employment or making them ineligible for insurance, are less relevant in the extremes of old age.

Effectiveness

Primary prevention

The effectiveness of various strategies in the primary prevention of IHD is discussed on the following pages: hypertension, p. 78; hyperlipidaemia, p. 82; quitting smoking, p. 92; exercise, p. 173. The use of low-dose aspirin as a primary preventive care measure against IHD has recently been reviewed [78f]. In the United States Physicians' Aspirin Trial, which enrolled male physicians 40 to 84 years old, after five years of therapy the incidence of myocardial infarction was 44 per cent lower in the aspirin group. The treatment effect was seen only in those aged 50 years or older. A number of criticisms have been levelled at a smaller study with British physicians that showed no significant differences between control and treated groups that may explain the apparent lack of benefit. However, no studies have as yet looked at the primary preventive impact of low-dose aspirin in older women, though a study of its use in younger nurses did show a significant reduction in fatal and non-fatal myocardial infarction.

Secondary prevention

The following goals for preventive care may be considered once symptomatic ischaemic heart disease has become established:

1. Reduction in the incidence and severity of ischaemic events. In trials with both young and old patients, low-dose aspirin has been shown to reduce the incidence of non-fatal myocardial infarction in patients with unstable angina and the reinfarction rate in patients who survive acute myocardial infarction [78f].
2. Reduction in mortality rates. Low-dose aspirin has also been shown to reduce the incidence of cardiac death in patients with unstable angina and to reduce the mortality of acute myocardial infarction [78f]. Likewise, thrombolysis after acute myocardial infarction also effectively reduces mortality. For example in the ISIS–2 trial among patients 80 years of age or older who received streptokinase and aspirin as compared with placebo, one-month mortality was reduced from 37 to 20 per cent [78g].
3. Reduction in other vascular events. Low-dose aspirin reduces the incidence of transient cerebral ischaemic attacks and strokes after myocardial infarction.
4. Reduction in disability and handicap. Exercise rehabilitation programmes for elderly patients recovering from myocardial infarction may improve

exercise capacity and reduce functional and psychological dependence [78h].

5. Reduction in subsequent cardiac failure. Attention is now focussing on the possibility that the use of angiotensin-converting-enzyme (ACE) inhibitors may assist in the prevention of cardiac failure in patients with ischaemic heart disease. Although there are no published studies specifically on elderly patients, an analysis of the results of existing trials [78i], in which some elderly patients were included, suggests that treatment with ACE inhibitors started within 24 hours of acute myocardial infarction is contra-indicated but that, started after a delay of a few days in patients with systolic dysfunction before severe dilatation has occurred, it can result in a signifi-cant reduction in mortality. In a further trial of patients with chronic left ventricular dysfunction but without symptomatic heart failure, the use of ACE inhibitors resulted in only a small survival benefit (about one life saved for every 300 patients treated per year) but did result in a more substantial reduction in incidence of clinical heart failure (about three episodes prevented for every 100 patients treated per year).

Cost

Based on a cost analysis of the literature, Krumholz et al. [78j] have shown that there is a clear-cut favourable benefit-to-risk ratio for thrombolytic treatment in elderly patients with suspected myocardial infarction. The cost per year of life saved for an eighty year old in such circumstances was £21 200.

Although not dealing specifically with elderly patients, cardiac rehabili-tation has also been shown to be a cost effective strategy by lowering the cost of readmission to hospital.

Smoking

Importance

Many elderly people continue to smoke [79]. Figures for the prevalence of this habit found during a British survey are given in Table 7.2. Smoking rates tend to fall in old age and more women than men are not current smokers or have never smoked [80].

All available evidence indicates that smoking is a potentially harmful activity for elderly people. Lacroix and Omenn [81] report at least 11 studies in populations over 60 years where nearly all show an increased risk of death from smoking continuing into old age. Whilst the *relative* risk of total mortality from smoking in elderly people may be rather lower than the relative risk associated with smoking in middle aged subjects, the *attributable* risk actually increases with age.

Smoking has a well-documented correlation with coronary disease, peripheral vascular disease and chronic obstructive lung disease. Smoking makes a major contribution to the incidence of lung, pancreatic, bladder and cervical cancer. It also contributes to stroke disease, osteoporosis, loss of body weight, decreased muscle strength, and accelerated lung ageing. It probably also contributes to hip fracture [82]. Smoking is also associated with an increased risk of functional decline [81]. In addition, demented elderly people who smoke often pose a fire risk to themselves and others.

Targeting

No reliable methods are available for detecting those at future risk of illness and physiological impairment. All elderly smokers, particularly heavy smokers, should therefore be targeted for quitting smoking. Quality of life considerations may need to modify this policy (see Chapter 11).

Effectiveness

Even lifelong smokers can achieve significant gains in life expectancy by quitting smoking on reaching old age. This information is summarised in Fig. 7.2 [83].

Recent evidence has also shown that stopping smoking late in life is associated with a rapid and sustained reduction in mortality from coronary disease [84] and cessation of smoking lessens the risk of death or myocardial reinfarction in older as well as younger persons with existing coronary artery disease [85].

The reduction in the risk of lung cancer from quitting smoking is not merely confined to younger age groups. A case-control study of lung cancer in New Mexico compared patients and control subjects under 65 with those over 65 years. The decline in lung cancer that occurred with smoking cessation was similar for the two groups [86].

Older adults who quit smoking show improved lung function [87] and a reduction in respiratory symptoms [88]. There is also a reduction in associated pneumonia and influenza death rates [89]. Quitting smoking has also been shown, after two years, to result in a significant reduction in risk of stroke [90].

Many methods designed to assist people in quitting smoking have been shown to be effective [91]. These include simple counselling by physicians,

Table 7.2. *Smoking habits according to age and sex*

Smoking habits	Age (years)							
	17–34		35–64		65–74		75–100	
Males								
Present smoker	247	(36)	386	(42)	83	(40)	37	(31)
Previous smoker	106	(16)	313	(34)	101	(48)	69	(58)
Never smoked	324	(48)	219	(24)	26	(12)	12	(10)
Total	677	(100)	918	(100)	210	(100)	118	(100)
Females								
Present smoker	294	(37)	355	(37)	61	(26)	18	(14)
Previous smoker	136	(17)	242	(25)	81	(34)	44	(33)
Never smoked	362	(46)	363	(38)	93	(40)	70	(53)
Total	792	(100)	960	(100)	235	(100)	132	(100)

Values in parentheses are percentages of each age group.
Adapted from ref. [80].

with or without various information aids. Nicotine gum has been shown in a number of randomised controlled trials to enhance quit rates when used in conjunction with these counselling strategies [91].

Of the numerous methods that have been employed to assist individuals to quit smoking, their success rates in elderly compared with younger individuals are virtually unknown, but may well be lower. Seventy per cent of smokers below retirement age want to quit smoking but only 40 per cent of those over 75 years wish to do so. Of this latter age group, 46 per cent consider their smoking not at all harmful to their health [80].

Surveys of patients suggest that many physicians do not routinely counsel smokers to quit. A further strategy to increase quit rates is therefore to improve physician participation in these programmes. Recent evidence suggests that physicians who receive a continuing education programme about how to counsel smokers discuss smoking with more patients who smoke, spend more time counselling them about smoking, give out more self-help booklets and help more patients to quit smoking, as assessed at one-year follow up [92].

Cost

One study found the cost effectiveness of brief counselling advice on stopping smoking, made during routine doctor–patient contact, to be $950 and $1411 per year of life saved for men and women respectively aged 65 to 69 years [93].

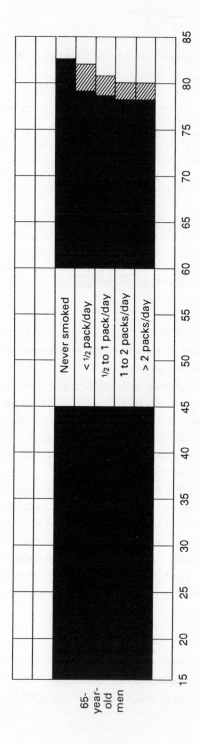

Fig. 7.2. Life expectancy for 65-year-old men who have never smoked compared with life expectancy loss from cigarette smoking. The 65-year-old who has never smoked has a life expectancy to age 82, 17 additional years. The filled bars show the reduced life expectancy as a function of the number of cigarettes smoked. Thus, a man who has smoked more than two packs per day from adolescence has, at age 65, a life expectancy remaining of 13 to 14 years, 3 to 4 years less than if he had never smoked. If he stops smoking at age 65, even though he has smoked since adolescence, he will regain about half of that lost life expectancy (indicated by cross-hatched bars). Adapted from ref. [83].

Anaemia

Importance

Using the WHO criteria of 13 and 12 g/dl to define anaemia in elderly men and women respectively, the frequency of anaemia in several surveys has been found to vary considerably from as high as 41 per cent to as low as 5 per cent [94]. The National Center for Health Statistics in the USA recorded a haemoglobin level less than 12 g/dl in persons over 65 years in 2.3 per cent of men and 5.5 per cent of women [95]. Anaemia by itself does not have a readily apparent morbidity unless the haemoglobin level falls below 10 g/dl. Its importance lies in the symptoms it may produce when severe and, when asymptomatic, its being an indicator of underlying disease. There is controversy as to whether it is associated with an increased susceptibility to infection [96].

Detection/targeting

Haemoglobin and haematocrit determinations are cheap, simple and reliable detection manoeuvres. In view of the lack of morbidity associated with asymptomatic anaemia and the lack of benefit of treatment at this stage (see below), general screening of the elderly population is not recommended. However, significant anaemia mimics the fatigue, low exercise tolerance, impaired cognition and failure to thrive, problems so often attributed to the ageing process or to concomitant chronic illness in the elderly that health professionals should have a high index of suspicion for anaemia and employ opportunistic screening for it when clinically appropriate.

Effectiveness

There is no evidence that treating elderly people who have mild asymptomatic anaemia that has been detected early by screening reduces morbidity or improves wellbeing. On the contrary, there is evidence that iron supplementation in asymptomatic iron deficiency anaemia in younger subjects has no effect on symptoms or psychomotor performance [97]. Recent research also suggests high levels of body iron stores may increase the risk of cancer [98].

Although screening for anaemia may subsequently lead to the identification of underlying cancer, there are no data to suggest this is an effective preventive strategy for malignant disease.

Cost

No detailed information on costs for an elderly population is available.

Open angle glaucoma (OAG)

Importance

Glaucoma is one of the major causes of blindness in the elderly population. The prevalence rate of open angle glaucoma (OAG) requiring treatment because of visual field deficit increases with age to reach 2 to 4 per cent in those over 75 years [99]. Black races are particularly at risk [100], as are those suffering from myopia and a family history of glaucoma.

Detection

The two most used screening procedures are tonometry and ophthalmoscopy. Neither is ideal. Tonometry is based on detecting ocular hypertension (OH), which in many cases is a harbinger of OAG. Yet the specificity of the test is poor, the majority of those with OH never developing OAG. For example, about 10 per cent of patients found to have OH at the time of screening will have glaucoma and only 10 per cent of the remainder will develop glaucoma within ten years [101]. Furthermore, a single measurement of intraocular pressure has limited negative predictive value in ruling out glaucoma and the accuracy and reliability of tonometry is affected by the method chosen (Schiotz, applanation or non-contact), and the experience of the examiner [102].

The other screening test, ophthalmoscopy, has low sensitivity, fundoscopic findings being apparent in only 50 to 60 per cent of cases of glaucoma [103]. It is also not particularly specific, the ophthalmoscopic findings of glaucoma being seen in about 15 per cent of persons lacking the visual field deficits characteristic of OAG [104].

A third screening test, oculokinetic perimetry (OKP) has been advocated for use in geriatric assessment units [104a] but, in a recent study of elderly patients attending a day hospital, only 47 per cent could be screened adequately using this technique [104b].

Effectiveness

The benefits of reducing very high intraocular pressures (e.g. over 35 mmHg) are well accepted but the treatment of mild to moderate ocular hypertension, such as is commonly found in screening, is less certain. The results of five controlled trials have suggested that such treatment may reduce the incidence of OAG [105–109], but there have been serious methodological problems affecting most of them [102] and in only two have the benefits reached statistical significance. Contrarily, numerous other trials have failed to show such benefit [102].

It should be remembered that the majority of those who, on screening, are found to have intraocular hypertension and who are given antiglaucoma treatment would *not* in any case have developed glaucoma, yet may experience significant side effects from almost any of the antiglaucoma drugs or from surgery [110].

Cost

Studies in both the general population and in frail elderly subjects have provided evidence that widespread screening programmes would be a costly health maintenance strategy. In the USA, a screening programme for elderly people was costed at $100 million to $300 million for the first year, rising with the rescreening of the same people every two years [111]. Eddy also calculated that at 1983 prices the cost of screening 100 000 asymptomatic individuals over 40 years with Schiotz tonometry, working up those with ocular hypertension and treating 120 patients with chronic simple glaucoma for 10 years (assuming 75 per cent adherence) would be about £1.5 million or about £13 000 per patient potentially benefited [101].

Bacteriuria

Importance

Bacteriuria is commonly seen in elderly people, the frequency of those afflicted depending on the characteristics of the population studied. Several studies have reported a prevalence of more than 20 per cent in elderly women living in the community [112] and bacteriuria is even more common in institutionalised populations, with levels of over 30 per cent commonly being recorded [112]. For most however, bacteriuria is an asymptomatic relatively benign accompaniment of ageing. There have been several studies that have failed to show an association between bacteriuria and worsened renal function [113–115] and in the study that has linked the two [116], it is far from certain that the association is causal. The same may be said for any association between bacteriuria and hypertension. Also, Dontas [117] and Sourander [115] have shown a relative increase in mortality in elderly persons affected by bacteriuria. Recently, Nicolle et al. [118] suggested that this decreased survival (in persistently bacteriuric institutionalised elderly patients) occurred in those who could be shown to mount a more vigorous local host response as identified by elevated levels of urine antibody to the major outer membrane of *E. coli*. Again however there are studies that have failed to show decreased survival with bacteriuria and it is suggested that bacteriuria merely serves as a marker for senile debility from dementia or stroke disease. It may be these conditions and not the bacteriuria that is responsible for the higher death rate. Although traditional studies from younger (and particularly paraplegic) populations suggest that urinary tract infection is a major cause of septicaemia, a more critical study by Quintiliani [119] found that only 8 per cent of hospital associated cases of septicaemia were definitely related to urinary tract infections and that in the absence of immunosuppression or urethral instrumentation the association is quite rare.

Detection

Culture of one clean-catch sample of urine is a reliable detection manoeuvre and the 'gold standard' for screening. However, Flanagan et al. [120] have evaluated four simple screening tests for bacteriuria in elderly people. They found that a *combination* of visual appearance of the urine and dipstick testing for nitrite and leucocyte esterase gave a sensitivity of 96.1 per cent with a specificity of 50.6 per cent. Employing this strategy might reduce about a third of the number of urine samples requiring to be submitted to the laboratory for processing. The detection of pyuria alone is neither sufficiently sensitive nor specific as a screening measure for bacteriuria, since the incidence of pyuria in those with infection varies between 36 and 79 per cent. Pyuria also occurs in about 15 per cent of elderly people without significant bacterial counts [115].

Effectiveness

If symptoms or obstructive uropathy are present, then bacteriuria should be treated. However, in the absence of these conditions, the benefits of treating asymptomatic bacteriuria are much less certain. Antibiotic therapy can clear the urine of bacteria [122], but the relapse rate is very high. For example, Brocklehurst [123] found 47 per cent of infections recurred within 14 months following a successful course of antibiotic treatment. Therefore, further courses of antibiotics need to be given or long term suppression with low-dose antibiotics implemented. The benefits of such treatment may vary depending on the population treated. Nicolle et al. [124] have shown that in institutional elderly men, mortality and infective morbidity after a treatment strategy aimed at eliminating bacteriuria was the same as in untreated patients. Conversely, Boscia et al. [125], in ambulatory non-hospitalised women, showed that during a six-month follow up after antibiotic treatment for asymptomatic bacteriuria, only 8 per cent of the therapy group developed *symptomatic* bacteriuria compared with 16 per cent of the non-therapy group. Despite this, the principal investigator concluded ' . . . it is not feasible to attempt to eradicate all asymptomatic bacteriuria in elderly persons. The adverse reaction rate to antimicrobial agents is sufficiently high in this population to warrant caution in adopting too vigorous an approach . . . furthermore the cost of screening . . . would be difficult to justify with the current state of knowledge' [126].

Cost

No detailed information on costs is available.

Benign prostatic hypertrophy

Importance

The incidence of benign prostatic hypertrophy (BPH) increases with age, peaking around 65 years of age. Exact rates vary depending on the definition. One recent Scottish survey, defining BPH as enlargement of the prostate gland to greater than 20 g in the presence of symptoms of urinary dysfunction and/or a urinary peak flow rate less than 15 ml/s and without evidence of malignancy, found it to be present in 138 per 1000 men aged 40 to 49 years and 430 per 1000 men aged 60 to 69 years [127].

BPH gives rise to significant morbidity, not only from the distress caused by obstructive symptoms associated with voiding, but from urinary retention, overflow incontinence, infection, renal insufficiency and hypertension. Studies of the natural history of benign prostatic hypertrophy indicate that the mean decrease in maximal flow is about 0.2 ml per second per year [127a] but the rates of occurrence of problems resulting from this are not well defined due to lack of information on the natural history of the disease. However, among men aged sixty or older with prostatic enlargement and obstructive symptoms the twenty-year probability of requiring surgery was found in the Baltimore Longitudinal Study of Aging to be 39 per cent [127b].

Detection

Digital rectal examination provides an unreliable estimate of prostatic size [128]. Furthermore, symptoms of prostatism correlate poorly with prostate size as measured by transrectal ultrasonography [127]. Therefore, early detection measures depend mostly on numerical symptom scoring systems and/or uroflowmetry. Again more information is required on the natural history of BPH before reliable cut-off points can be defined with these techniques for early screening for the disease.

Effectiveness

Transurethral resection of prostatic tissue (TURP) is still the commonest form of treatment and the standard against which other treatment modalities are measured. Nevertheless, TURP provides less effective outcomes when performed in the earlier stages of the disease and carries with it a small mortality and significant morbidity [129, 130]. This, plus the implications of earlier preventive care for surgical resources, therefore indicate that other, non-surgical modalities may be more likely to be the measures employed. Recently, the use of the selective 5-alpha reductase inhibitor drug finasteride in a dose of 5 mg per day was found to result in a significant decrease in symptoms of obstruction, an increase in urinary flow and a decrease in prostatic volume [131].

Cost

No detailed information on costs is available.

The complications of 'silent' gallstones

Importance

Autopsy and ultrasonographic surveys show gallstones to be present in 30 per cent of white women in their 60s and up to 38 per cent of white women in their 80s [132]. Rates for white men are lower. In blacks the prevalence is roughly one-half of that in whites. In American Indians the prevalence is approximately twice that in whites.

Gallstones can be responsible for biliary colic, jaundice and the presentation of non-specific physical and mental debility in elderly patients [133]. Gallstones are also implicated in the aetiology of gallbladder cancer. However, at least 12 cohort and other studies [132] now attest to the essentially benign prognosis of gallstones. For silent stones, the 15-year cumulative probability of developing biliary pain or complications is only 18 per cent [134]. The risk of developing cancer in a gallbladder with stones is also low. Newman and Northup [135] estimate that for a 65-year-old person with a 14.1 year life expectancy, the risk of developing cancer of the gallbladder during this time is 0.44 per cent. They further comment that if a lower incidence of carcinoma (as reported by the US Bureau of Vital Statistics compared with hospital autopsy rates) is used in the calculation, the probability is reduced by half.

Detection

Radiography and ultrasonography have now largely replaced the oral cholecystogram as the screening method of choice for detecting the presence of gallstones.

Effectiveness

Previously, there has been much advocacy for prophylactic cholecystectomy in patients with silent gallstones. Currently however, expectant care is normally considered the optimal course for managing such cases in an elderly population. This recommendation is based on a better understanding of the natural history of the condition and its essential benign nature, plus the results of decision analysis models which have shown that the difference in mean survival between expectant care and intervention with cholecystectomy is less than one month of life and with expectant management being favoured [136]. The effect of newer therapies for gallstones on the optimal strategy for silent gallstones has not been detailed but will probably not detract from a wait-and-see policy.

The expectant management for silent stones should not be confused with symptomatic stones for which operative intervention has traditionally and almost universally been recommended. Even this has been challenged by the results of a recently published decision analysis which suggests that expectant management may still be appropriate for the elderly person who has had only a single episode of colic [137].

Cost

No information is available on the net impact on costs of prophylactic cholecystectomy in elderly people.

Hypothermia

Importance

The increase in mortality that accompanies cold weather is more prominent in the elderly (see Table 7.3) with excess deaths doubling for every nine years of advancing age over 40 years [138]. Hypothermia (core body temperature of less than 35 °C (95 °F)) makes its impact on health in two main ways.

i. Hypothermia makes a direct and immediate contribution to the cause of death. This is fortunately rare, with few cases being reported even in a severe winter [139]. Most occur in lightly clothed elderly people who have developed an intercurrent illness and who have fallen indoors and lain for significant periods of time [140]. Mortality statistics from England and Wales show hypothermia as contributing to the immediate cause of death in only about 300 out of the 40 000 excess deaths that occur every winter. The concern that this may merely reflect failure to detect abnormally low, deep body temperatures has been negated by one study that made accurate estimates of all new patients entering casualty departments and that failed to show that hypothermia was more widespread [141]. Herity et al. [142] have calculated the age- and sex-specific incidence, mortality and case-fatality rates according to the ambient outside temperature. They found the incidence of hypothermia doubled with each fall in temperature of five degrees centigrade and the mortality rate doubled with each fall in temperature of four degrees centigrade. Men had a 30 per cent higher case fatality than women did. Single men and single women were particularly prone to hypothermia and its associated mortality.
ii. Hypothermia results in secondary illness which is the major contributor to the cause of death. This effect is responsible for the bulk of morbidity and mortality from hypothermia. Subclinical hypothermia increases blood pressure and plasma viscosity [143]. Partly as a consequence, and after a time lag of a few days [144], this results in an increased death rate from stroke disease and myocardial infarction. Some idea of this overall excess mortality can be seen from the progressive rise in winter mortality ratio into old age (see Fig. 7.3 [145]).

Detection

Hypothermia often goes unrecognised by medical and nursing staff because of failure to record the core body temperature or because of the lack of availability of low-reading rectal thermometers.

Table 7.3. *Age- and sex-specific incidence, mortality and case fatality rates for hypothermia*

	No. of cases	No. of deaths	Annual incidence (per million)		Annual mortality (per million)		Case fatality rate (%)	
Sex								
Male	639	244	52.8	(48.8– 57.0)	20.2	(17.7– 22.9)	38.2	(34.4–12.1)
Female	653	191	54.5	(50.3– 58.8)	15.9	(13.7– 18.3)	29.3	(25.7–32.9)
Age[a] (years)								
<49	203	27	11.0	(9.5– 12.6)	1.5	(1.0– 2.1)	13.3	(9.0–18.8)
50–69	304	93	75.9	(67.6– 84.9)	23.2	(18.7– 28.4)	30.6	(25.5–36.1)
70+	736	313	447.4	(415.7–480.9)	190.3	(169.8–212.6)	42.5	(38.9–46.2)
Total	1292	435	53.6	(50.7– 56.6)	18.1	(16.4– 19.8)	33.7	(31.1–36.3)

Values in parentheses are 95% confidence index limits.
[a]Details are lacking in 46 cases, including two deaths.
Adapted from ref. [142].

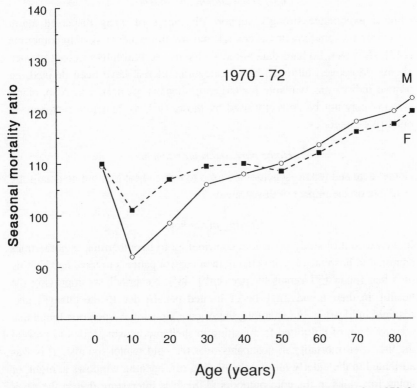

Fig. 7.3. Seasonal mortality ratios by age and sex in England and Wales for 1970–2. M, male; F, female. Adapted from ref. [143]. Original data were from: McDowell M. Population Trends 1981; **26**: 16–19.

None of the detection manoeuvres available is entirely satisfactory. Recording room temperature is a simple procedure that can be carried out by community staff. The correlation between a low environmental temperature and the complications of hypothermia is, however, very poor. Recording core temperature with a low-reading rectal thermometer or by measuring the temperature of freshly passed urine are too aesthetically unpleasing to be employed on a widespread basis, and they record the problem only after it has occurred. A subset of elderly people initially presenting with autonomic disorders are particularly prone to future hypothermia [146] but the time lag is unknown.

Effectiveness

A number of strategies have been proposed to prevent hypothermia.

Dispersed community alarms

Clinical experience strongly supports the value of using dispersed alarm systems to prevent long lies after a fall and any subsequent risk of hypothermia [147]. However, no hard data are available on the preventive impact of such alarms. Moreover, although broad categories of risk have been defined, no refined indices are available for targeting those at greatest risk. Also, alarm systems may not be correctly used by those, such as dementia sufferers, in other risk categories.

Home care and repair schemes

Home 'care and repair' schemes are used to reduce heat loss but no details are available on the impact of this strategy.

Heating in the home

In a case-control study of factors contributing to hypothermia, hypothermics admitted to hospital were less likely than control patients to have had heating on when found (50 versus 89 per cent [148]). Nevertheless, improving the heating in their homes may be of limited benefit due to the changes also required in lifestyle. For example, the Anchor Housing Association found that the provision of unlimited free heating in sheltered housing failed to prevent the increased mortality in occupants over the cold winter months. This was attributed to the elderly turning the heating off, opening windows at night, or going for walks in the cold outdoors [148]. It is interesting that in the case-control study mentioned above, 93 per cent of patients in both the hypothermic and control groups had heating available [140].

The study of ageing in mice has shown that intermittent cold acclimation effectively reduced hypothermia during cold challenge, so there has been the theoretical irony that the more elderly people are encouraged to live in warm environments the less they may be able to acclimatise to cold conditions when encountered. However, work by Collins [149] suggests that old people are not likely to acquire significant acclimatisation to the effects of cold when living in cold indoor surroundings.

Financial supplements for heating

Over a quarter of all people over 75 years state that cost sometimes prevents them from using their heating as much as they would like. The provision of a financial supplement to those at risk of hypothermia with low incomes would therefore seem an appropriate strategy. However, this may be of limited benefit because, in a survey of deaths from hypothermia, lack of use of heating facilities was associated with financial hardship in only 20 per cent [150].

Education of the elderly public

This is a strategy widely employed in most countries that experience cold winters. However, in the UK the impact of distributing by post an information pack *Warmth in Winter* was not found effective for people aged 75 and over. There was no difference in the knowledge and action taken between those who received the pack and those who did not [151]. The work of Tester and Meredith [152] suggests this information might have more impact if given in person to those at risk rather than delivered in an impersonal fashion.

Counselling by general practitioners

This has also been shown to have limited benefit. When those elderly people on a register for being at risk of developing hypothermia were counselled by their doctor and re-evaluated at a later visit, several improvements to heating arrangements were noted, but the median temperature in the bedrooms of houses with no central heating was 10 °C below the WHO recommended temperature. Even with media publicity and visits from carers and a doctor, 17 of the 27 elderly people studied continued to live in an environment in which they were at risk of developing hypothermia [153].

Other strategies

Although the majority of hypothermic patients are found indoors, in the minority occurring outdoors in old age, alcoholism and wandering from dementia have been implicated factors [140]. Strategies to combat alcoholism

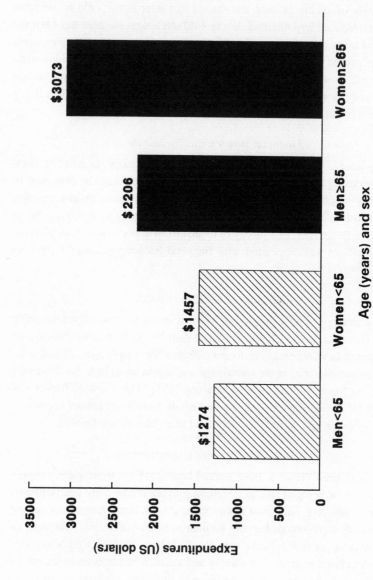

Fig. 7.4. Health care expenditures attributable to non-insulin-dependent diabetes mellitus per case, by age and sex, 1986. Prices are in US dollars. Adapted from ref. [156].

and to improve surveillance of those with restless behaviour may, therefore, have some benefit in preventing hypothermia.

Cost

No detailed costing information is available.

Glucose intolerance

Importance

Diabetes mellitus is an extremely common condition in elderly people. Estimates of its prevalence vary from 18.7 per cent of women 65 to 74 years to 29.9 per cent aged 65 to 84 years [154]. Prevalence rates of those with *diagnosed* diabetes are less, around 9.6 per cent of people over 65 years. Over 98 per cent of diabetes in this age group is of the type II, or non-insulin-dependent diabetes mellitus (NIDDM) variety. It accounts for a considerable mortality, morbidity and health care cost [155]. This has recently been detailed for the US population by Huse et al. [156] and figures relating to the older population are summarised in Fig. 7.4.

Whilst there is undoubtedly a group of individuals who suffer from a clinical diabetic syndrome which includes metabolic and/or pathological lesions, the problem lies in defining inclusion criteria. At present, this depends essentially on the existence of a degree of hyperglycaemia. Yet only a minority of hyperglycaemics can be identified as suffering from true diabetes. A greater proportion will have impaired glucose tolerance: however, of this group only 1.5 to 4 per cent per annum will worsen to develop true diabetes. There is no greater trend for this to occur in older than in younger subjects [157].

Detection

Age has a significant effect on carbohydrate metabolism that must be taken into account when screening. During oral glucose tolerance tests the one-hour value rises by approximately 0.5 mmol/l per decade and the two-hour value by 0.3 mmol/l per decade [158]. Far higher proportions of elderly people will therefore be labelled as diabetic (or having impaired glucose tolerance) than in younger age groups, if traditional criteria are used. The additional risk that this incurs, in terms of eventual tendency to metabolic or pathological complications, is virtually unknown. There is, therefore, a strong likelihood of identifying a larger number of 'false-positive' elderly people with higher than normal glucose levels who may then be subjected to preventive measures despite being at no risk of developing the disease state. Similarly, caution should be exercised in using a random plasma glucose estimation as a screening measurement in older people, because postprandial plasma glucose levels rise by about 0.2 mmol/l per decade [158]. Possibly the most valuable screening tool in the elderly population is the fasting plasma glucose level, which is only minimally raised with age (0.06 mmol/l per decade). A recent evaluation of this strategy has been reported [159].

Effectiveness

There is conflicting evidence on the efficacy of treatment in reducing the progression of younger individuals with impaired glucose tolerance to the definite biochemical or pathological criteria for clinical diabetes [160]. Evidence for or against such prevention is lacking for an elderly population.

There is also some evidence that strenuous efforts to maintain euglycaemia reduce the incidence of microvascular complications. However, this benefit has not been consistently shown under rigorous experimental conditions and the evidence relates almost entirely to younger populations with insulin-dependent diabetes. There is also no convincing evidence that treatment can prevent macrovascular complications and one study using oral hypoglycaemic agents, although surrounded by controversy, showed an *increase* in macro-vascular complications [161].

Against the contested evidence for the benefits of preventive treatment must be weighed a number of significant disadvantages to elderly people. These include the inconvenience of taking medication (which may include insulin injections), a change in long-established lifestyle or dietary habits, undesired levels of monitoring or supervision to ensure safe compliance and an increased risk of hypoglycaemia and other drug side effects.

Cost

No detailed information is available on the costs of screening and preventive care for diabetes mellitus in an elderly population.

Hypothyroidism

Importance

Most studies of community screening of older persons have shown a prevalence of unsuspected hypothyroidism of from 0 to 7 per 1000 men and from 3 to 18 per 1000 women [162]. The prevalence of the condition in a relatively unfit group of elderly patients presenting to their physicians is shown in Table 7.4 [163].

Detection

Detection is relatively simple by assaying the TSH level. However, false positive and negative results are not uncommon in the presence of other concomitant disease [162].

Helfand and Crapo [163] have reviewed the value of various targeting strategies in some detail. They emphasise the distinction between testing an apparently healthy elderly public with tests intended to find early evidence of the disease and testing patients who have come to their physicians for reasons unrelated to the disease in question. They conclude that the former community-type of screening programmes are not indicated. On the one hand, apart from some minor changes in cardiac and cognitive function, treating hypo-thyroidism when it is diagnosed on biochemical parameters alone without clinical features is of questionable benefit [162]. On the other hand, because only a proportion of biochemically diagnosed hypothyroid cases will proceed to clinical disease, many will end up being treated unnecessarily. For example, using diagnostic criteria of a TSH level greater than 10 mU/L and positive antithyroid antibodies, Helfand and Crapo [163] estimated that for every 1000 elderly women that are screened, 60 (at most) would be diagnosed as having subclinical hypothyroidism and 12 of these women would progress to overt disease within five years. Even if follow up and early treatment helped these 12, the other 48 patients would be treated unnecessarily.

Opportunistic testing however, can be justified for patients being admitted to departments of geriatric medicine with vague, chronic unexplained disability, depression or mental impairment. The evidence for this is summarised in Table 7.5 [163]. Opportunistic testing is not indicated in acutely ill elderly patients unless they have signs and symptoms related to thyroid disease.

Table 7.4. *Studies of case-finding or periodic health examination in clinical patients*

Study description	Number of patients (n)	Primary screening test	Test performance		Prevalence (n/1000)			
			Sensitivity[a]	Specificity[b]	Overt hyperthyroid		Overt hypothyroid	
					Men	Women	Men	Women
Health maintenance organisation, Oakland, CA, USA	2704	FT4I	1.0	0.996	0	5	3	6
Private hospital and clinic, MA, USA	5002	TT4	1.0[c]	0.906	0.5	2	5	5
Primary care centre, Sweden	2000	s-TSH	Not given	0.93[d]	1[e]	5	1	12
Outpatient clinic of a large hospital, Sweden	496	FT4	Not given	0.92	NA	6	NA	10
Private practice, CT, USA	1554	History and physical examination	Not given	Not given	0	8	3	5
Primary care centre, Japan	1114	FT4 or TT4	Not given	0.96	4	2	0	5

FT4I, free thyroxine index; TT4, total thyroxine; s-TSH, sensitive thyrotropin; FT4, free thyroxine; NA, not available.

[a] Patients with hyperthyroidism and hypothyroidism are combined to calculate the true positive rate (sensitivity). Most studies use a specially calculated reference range to increase sensitivity.

[b] Falsely elevated and falsely decreased test results are combined to calculate the false positive rate (1 − specificity).

[c] Estimated from initial study of 200 patients.

[d] Estimated after excluding patients receiving thyroxine.

[e] Assumes 1250 women and 750 men in population.

Adapted from ref. [163].

Table 7.5. *Case-finding in patients admitted to geriatric units*

Description of patient conditions	Number of patients (n)	Primary screening test[a]	Response to therapy reported?	Prevalence (n/1000)	
				Overt hyperthyroid	Overt hypothyroid
General disability, failure to thrive, mental slowing	3417	Clinical suspicion	Yes	5	17
Similar to above	490	PII, T3 uptake	Yes	23	20
Apathy, depression, non-specific symptoms, anaemia, arthritis and other medical problems	2000	PBI, FT4I	Yes	NA	21
Geriatric assessment, hip fracture, rehabilitation	229	TT4, FT4I, TT3, TSH	Yes	30	26
Similar to above (one third of patients were transferred from acute care facility for rehabilitation)	307	FT4I	Yes	3	7
Geriatric assessment, some rehabilitation, medical problems	125	TSH, TT4, FT4I, TT3	No	8	94[b]
Geriatric patients	4780	PBI	No	12	6

[a]PBI, protein-bound iodine; T3 uptake, T3 resin uptake; TT4, total thyroxine; FT4I, free thyroxine index; TT3, total triiodothyronine; TSH, thyrotropin; NA, not available.
[b]Includes previously diagnosed and asymptomatic patients with elevated levels of TSH and low levels of FT4I.
Adapted from ref. [163].

Effectiveness

Evidence for the benefit of community screening programmes rests solely in their ability to identify potential cases of clinical hypothyroidism (Table 7.5) [163].

Costs

No detailed analysis of screening or treatment costs is available.

Oral and dental problems

Importance

Numerous surveys of elderly people living in the community [164] and in institutions have shown poor oral health in old age. The most apparent change in the mouth with increasing age is loss of the natural teeth, with high proportions of the elderly population being edentulous. In this group, up to two-thirds require a repair or replacement of their dentures [165]. Nevertheless, the number of elderly people without teeth is lessening significantly, with more today keeping their teeth than ever before [166]. Those elderly people with teeth have a far higher prevalence of root surface caries and periodontal disease than those in younger age groups [167, 168].

Nevertheless, although many of these problems are symptomatic, their importance as ascribed by elderly people themselves, must be viewed in association with the fact that almost three-quarters of elderly people have not seen their dentist in the last year, and half of them not in the last six years [169]. A survey of the literature by Lee [170] found that there was a low level of perceived need among elderly people, regardless of setting.

Detection

The definitive procedure for detection is a specialist dental assessment. Many problems of oral health can, however, be detected by relatively untrained personnel using a structured interview and examination protocol [171].

Effectiveness

An important strategy to maintain oral and dental care for elderly people is to improve geographical and financial access to dental services. Nevertheless, although there is an association between financial status and use of dental services by elderly people [172], lack of attendance cannot be ascribed solely to cost or lack of availability of dentists [173].

There is evidence that primary preventive measures such as long term exposure to a water supply containing optimum levels of fluoride can have a beneficial effect in reducing the prevalence of root surface caries [174]. For many elderly people, secondary preventive measures are the most pertinent. Even in those who have suffered the ravages of periodontal disease there is evidence that the development of new carious lesions can be prevented by intensive individual and professional tooth cleaning [175]. Likewise, various fluoride gels and mouth rinses have been used successfully in the prevention and remineralisation of root surface caries [176].

However, the present cohort of elderly people had reached middle age before the time such preventive dental measures had become accepted care. It is, therefore, not surprising that very few practice preventive behaviour [169]. Nevertheless, elderly people can be made to respond to health education about oral and dental care. In a Canadian health education and screening programme undertaken in an elderly population living in the community, Knazan [177] was able to show statistical improvement in oral health status of the participants, in enhanced awareness of oral health and in greater dental self-care practices at six-month follow up. In general, however, compliance rates in the elderly population for preventive strategies for oral care, and particularly for high intensity strategies or strategies requiring regular professional input, are likely to be low.

Cost

No detailed information is available.

Problems with feet

Importance

In the UK, retired people receive 94 per cent of all chiropody treatment. This is not surprising, since the incidence of foot problems increases with age. A survey from the UK found that, on examination by chiropodists, 64 per cent of a random selection of people 65 years and over had some foot condition, problem or foot deformity. Four per cent of the foot problems were considered of major importance, 22 per cent of moderate and 58 of minor importance [178]. The commonest findings of the chiropodists were corns, callosities, lesser toe deformities, bunions, flat feet and oedema of the feet and ankles. As reported subjectively by the elderly people surveyed, the foot problems ranged from callosities or hard skin, thickened or deformed toenails, corns and aching swollen feet.

By far the commonest problem with foot care is being unable to cut toenails. Community surveys have shown that over 67 per cent of elderly people are unable to do this, many lacking the flexibility to bend down to perform this task.

Although there is a clear association between foot problems and immobility [179], it is far less certain that this association is causal, the possibility being that arthritic or vascular problems are often responsible for both. Although one study found that *serious* foot problems were associated with an increased relative risk of falling of 1.4 [180], similar comments to the above may be made about the causality of this association.

Detection

Ideally, problems are detected by clinical examination and treatment by a qualified chiropodist. However, several other professional groups are involved in foot care of elderly people in the community, but as yet no comparative study of the benefits afforded by them has been undertaken.

Effectiveness

Other than descriptive studies, there has been little scientific evaluation of the benefit of chiropody services to the elderly population. The bulk of lay and clinical experience, however, attests to their benefit in improving both the physical and psychological aspects of foot comfort and hygiene. Several studies also suggest that a foot care programme in frail elderly people, particularly those with diabetes, reduces the amputation rate [181–183]. However, 39 per cent of diabetics are unable to reach their toes and only 14 per cent can respond to plantar lesions [184]. Foot care education programmes unsupported by trained assistance may therefore be ineffective in reducing the morbidity of foot problems in this population.

There is surprisingly little evidence to show that foot care improves the mobility of significant numbers of the elderly population.

Cost

No detailed information is available.

Pressure ulcers

Importance

The risk of pressure ulcers increases with age. In a Scottish population requiring nursing care, the percentage of patients with pressure sores rose from 1.1 per cent in the 20 to 29 year age group to 13.2 per cent in those over 90 years [185]. The prevalence of pressure ulcers is 3 to 11 per cent in acute care hospitals and nursing homes in the USA. Pressure ulcers can result in discomfort, immobility, prolonged institutionalisation, anaemia and septicaemia. Among geriatric patients and nursing home residents, pressure ulcers are associated with a fourfold increase in the risk of death [186]. They also incur significant costs [187].

Detection

Several simple validated rating scales are available for use by nursing staff for assessing the likelihood of developing pressure ulcers [188–191]. An example is shown in Table 7.6.

Effectiveness

The employment of alternating-pressure air mattresses has been shown in controlled trials to prevent and heal pelvic and heel ulcers without the need for repositioning [192–194]. Likewise, the use of air-fluidised beds is associated with a more than fivefold increase in the odds of showing improvement as compared with conventional therapy [195]. One study, using historical controls, suggests that the use of rating scales coupled with such preventive apparatus reduces the incidence of pressure ulcers [190].

Cost

Few details are available, although it has been suggested that making nurses more aware of the need to identify patients at risk of pressure ulcers could save the NHS in the UK £10 million per annum and a further £15 million by implementing up to date preventive measures.

Recently, the US Public Health Service released practice guidelines 'Pressure Ulcers in Adults: Prediction and Prevention' [195a]. An essential component of these is the recommendation that all bedbound or chairbound patients be systematically assessed for pressure ulcer risk. The implementation

Table 7.6. *Waterlow pressure-sore prevention treatment policy*

Build/weight for height •		Skin type visual risk areas •		Sex •		Special risks •	
Average	0	Healthy	0	**Age**		**Tissue malnutrition**	
Above average	1	Tissue paper	1	Male	1	e.g. terminal cachexia	8
Obese	2	Dry	1	Female	2	cardiac failure	5
Below average	3	Oedematous	1	14–49	1	peripheral vascular	
		Clammy (temp↑)	1	50–64	2	disease	5
Continence •		Discoloured	2	65–74	3	anaemia	2
Complete/catheterised	0	Broken/spot	3	75–80	4	smoking	1
Occasionally incontinent	1			81+	5		
Cath/incontinent of faeces	2	**Mobility** •				**Neurological deficit** •	
Doubly incontinent	3	Fully	0	**Appetite** •		e.g. diabetes, M.S., C.V.A.,	
		Restless/fidgety	1	Average	0	motor/sensory,	
		Apathetic	2	Poor	1	paraplegia	4–6
		Restricted	3	N.G. tube/fluids only	2		
		Inert/traction	4	N.B.M./anorexic	3	**Major surgery/trauma** •	
		Chairbound	5			Orthopaedic –	
						below waist, spinal	5
						on table >2 hours	5
						Medication •	
						Steroids, cytotoxics,	
						high dose anti-	
						inflammatory	4

Score:	⩾ 10 at risk	⩾ 15 high risk	⩾ 20 very high risk
		Waterlow score =	

Ring scores in table, add total. Several scores per category can be used.
Cath, catheterised; temp↑, fever; N.G., nasogastric; N.B.M., nil by mouth; M.S., multiple sclerosis; C.V.A., cerebrovascular disease (stroke).
Adapted from ref. [188].

of such a formal preventive policy will not be without cost. However, a recent comparison of patient risk for pressure ulcer development with nursing use of preventive interventions [195b], suggests that such interventions are very commonly employed in long term nursing care facilities, that their use is based on nursing intuition and may not be targeted to those at greatest risk and that savings might be achieved by *not* employing the interventions in those at lower risk after more formal risk assessment has been made. Clearly, further study is needed to define the cost, efficacy and related cost effectiveness of routine pressure ulcer risk assessment.

Overweight

Importance

Overweight is the commonest form of malnutrition in elderly people. A national survey in the USA of over 13 000 people revealed that the percentage that were overweight did not differ significantly between older and younger age groups, but for the age group 60 to 69 years, 24 per cent of men and 30 per cent of women were at least 10 per cent overweight and 11 per cent of men and 15 per cent of women were at least 20 per cent overweight [196]. Even greater degrees of overweight are not uncommon. In a New Zealand community, 14 per cent of women over 70 years were more than 40 per cent above ideal weight [197].

The extent of mortality risk associated with overweight in old age is still the subject of debate. Although recent data from the Framingham study indicates that being overweight at 65 years is significantly related to early subsequent mortality in non-smoking individuals [198], other studies have refuted this association [199]. Several studies, including the recent Framingham report, show that the mortality risk associated with being moderately [196] or morbidly obese [200] (50 to 150 per cent above standard weight) nevertheless lessens with increasing age.

Overweight also carries with it a certain morbidity. It is known to predispose to symptomatic osteoarthritis [201] of the knees and to aggravate knee pain in existing osteoarthritic joints. Overweight is also known to limit exercise toler-ance in those with cardiopulmonary complaints and to aggravate hypertension. It also causes back injuries in the attendants of those who are dependent.

Detection

The commonest detection measure used is an evaluation of body weight and height with subsequent estimation of the body mass index. More precise measures for obesity using skinfold thickness are less often used as a screening measure in clinical practice.

Effectiveness

Weight loss

There is little evidence from controlled trials that weight loss improves longevity, although a mortality risk reduction, from 179 to 109, has been reported in males 30 per cent over ideal weight on their return to standard weight [202].

Recently, weight loss of approximately 5.1 kg in the preceding ten years was found to decrease the odds for developing symptomatic knee osteoarthritis by over 50 per cent [201].

Loss of weight may also lessen pain from established osteoarthritis of the knees. Weight loss modifies risk factors such as hypertension, elevated serum cholesterol and impaired glucose tolerance.

Counselling for weight loss

Although a variety of weight reducing regimens are available, it is usually the most conservative, such as nutritional and exercise counselling, that are most applicable to elderly individuals. The success of these strategies in this older population is unknown, though in younger age groups outcomes are highly variable [203].

Cost

No information is available.

Subnutrition

Importance

The importance of subnutrition in elderly people is difficult to quantify due to the variable definitions attributed to its various facets. There is no doubt that high percentages of the frail elderly population have serum or tissue levels of nutrients (or of substances affected by nutrients) that fall well below norms for the young and/or for fit age-matched controls. In many cases, however, those suboptimal levels are due to concomitant illness and are unresponsive to dietary manipulation.

Many elderly people also have nutrient intakes well below those in younger subjects and/or below 'recommended dietary intakes' [204]. However, interpretation is difficult because of the extensive controversy surrounding the appropriate definition for these recommendations [205].

Morbid illness caused by an identifiable deficiency state is actually quite unusual in elderly people living in the community. Studies in the UK 20 years ago showed only 2 per cent of those surveyed were suffering from serious subnutrition [206]. Similar surveys in the USA have mirrored these findings [207]. These percentages should now be lower, due to the improved living conditions and wellbeing of the elderly population.

Deficient intake of nutrients, particularly of the vitamin B complex and iron, have been found in the institutionalised elderly, but is largely confined to those with feeding dependency [208].

Detection

The availability of a suitable screening instrument for the presence of subnutrition is complicated by the ill-precision in defining subnutrition. Nevertheless, a simple measure for assessing the risk of poor nutrition has been developed and validated for use with elderly people living in the community [209]. High scorers displayed a consistent pattern of higher rates of known nutrition-related problems and their sequelae than did low scorers. In view of the low prevalence of subnutrition in the community, routine screening of the older population with this instrument is not recommended. In selected cases, however, its use may assist in the diagnosis of subnutrition when used in conjunction with routine clinical assessment.

In frail elderly people in institutions, various biochemical profiles have been used to detect subnutrition. However, the problem is largely confined to those with feeding dependency, and monitoring for inability to perform this activity, coupled with serial weight measurements, may achieve similar results.

Effectiveness

A number of preventive strategies have been implemented with variable success.

Dietary supplementation

There is little evidence to support widespread dietary supplementation for elderly people. There is evidence that numerous specific supplementary strategies are probably *not* of benefit. These include: increased protein intake to improve plasma albumin and transferrin levels in institutionalised patients [210]; zinc supplementation to improve wound healing in pressure sores [211]; vitamin D supplementation to institutionalised patients to improve muscle function and activities of daily living [212]; iron supplementation in non-anaemic subjects to improve haemoglobin levels and wellbeing [97]; vitamin C supplementation to prevent osteoporosis and reduce mortality rates [213]; long term anabolic steroid supplementation to increase weight or activity levels [214]; potassium supplements in normokalaemic individuals to improve muscle strength [215]; and vitamin B supplements to improve the skin and mucosal changes [216].

Indiscriminate dietary supplementation is also not without risk as has been shown by the association between iron supplementation and the risk of cancer in men [98].

Meal service programmes

Meal services in elderly peoples' homes in the UK consist of the Home Help and Meals on Wheels programmes. There is substantial experience to support their importance to the frail elderly who are dependent on others to make their meals. Nevertheless, it is estimated that four full meals need to be provided each week if an adequate nutrient intake is to be achieved [217] and this is in excess of the usual quota provided. The necessary relocation of resources may be ensured by case-managed community care programmes but this has still to be validated.

Food stamps

In the USA, the Food Stamp Program provides a monthly financial supplement to households headed by older persons. However, it has had only a limited impact on their food expenditures and nutrient intake, as participants substitute income otherwise spent on food for housing, heating and other essentials [218].

Cost

No information is available.

Influenza

Importance

Influenza gives rise to a substantial burden of illness in elderly people, causing excess physician contacts, hospitalisations and deaths. The incidence of influenza A in this population is around two per cent per year, but varies considerably [219]. The associated death rate in an average year has been calculated to be 45 per 100 000 of the elderly population per year [220]. During an epidemic year, and for patients 65 years or older, additional general practice contacts for acute respiratory disease are estimated at 6000 per 100 000, additional hospitalisations from influenza for those with high risk conditions at 640 per 100 000 and excess deaths at 100 per 100 000 [220]. Schoenbaum [221] has estimated that, for all ages in the USA, the direct costs of influenza exceed $1 billion per year and may reach $3 billion to $5 billion.

Targeting

This primary preventive measure should be targeted at the elderly living in the community, particularly those with chronic cardiovascular, pulmonary, renal, metabolic, neurological or neoplastic disease. It may similarly be targeted at those in institutional care.

However, vaccination coverage is low in the UK, currently being around 20 per cent. In a postal questionnaire to all consultant geriatricians in Great Britain and Northern Ireland less than one in five offered influenza vaccine to patients in continuing care wards [222]. This is partly because of scepticism about the vaccine's efficacy and partly because of the implicit adoption of limited treatment plans for very frail aged persons.

It is important to consider ethical constraints when contemplating vaccination of frail patients. In particular, those in institutional care should be carefully selected, omitting those on limited treatment plans in whom the prolongation of life would merely prolong suffering. Care should be taken to identify the elderly person's wishes and to communicate with their family on this matter.

Effectiveness

Flu vaccination

There are several reports on the effectiveness of flu vaccination in ambulatory elderly populations [223–226]. When the vaccine contains antigens similar to the currently circulating influenza A and B viruses, it results in a risk reduction for clinical episodes of flu of up to 67 per cent, a reduction of hospitalisation rates of up to 72 per cent, and of death rates of 81 to 100 per cent. A number of recent studies have also shown flu vaccination to be effective in reducing the impact of influenza in nursing homes [227–229]. Vaccination reduces the flu attack rate, reduces the severity of disease and prevents deaths.

Despite these excellent results, it is recognised that the antibody response is less in older populations [230], and booster vaccination one month after the first and double dose vaccinations have been recommended. These are not routinely necessary.

The vaccine may safely be given concomitantly with pneumococcal vaccination [231]. Concern about side effects often deters people from being vaccinated, but one randomised double-blind crossover trial found no significant differences between the administration of trivalent split-antigen influenza vaccine and a saline placebo with respect to the proportion of subjects reporting disability or symptoms [232]. Subunit vaccines cause little alteration in respiratory status in asthmatics and may be preferentially used, but a comparison of the side effects of subunit and split vaccines showed little difference [233].

Improving vaccination coverage

A number of interventions have been tried and shown to be effective in improving influenza vaccine coverage. Two randomised controlled trials have reported a more than doubling of coverage among elderly family practice patients with the use of mailed reminders [234, 235]. Benefits have also been shown from telephone reminders [236], from delegating responsibility for immunisation to nurses in a medical outpatient department [237] and from computer-generated nurse/physician reminders to offer influenza vaccine to elderly patients [238].

Amantadine

An alternative strategy to vaccination is the administration of amantadine, which is 70 to 90 per cent effective in preventing illness caused by naturally occurring strains of influenza A. It does not prevent influenza B infection. Amantadine administration may be a useful strategy for outbreaks of presumed influenza A in institutions, for short term prophylaxis for those at risk who have not been vaccinated or who were vaccinated late. Amantadine has been shown to be effective in a number of trials, not only in preventing the disease but in reducing the duration of fever once the disease has been contracted [239]. Nevertheless, quite high rates of side effects have been reported in nursing home residents using this technique. Stange et al. [240] found that severe adverse reactions were associated with risk factors such as physical disability and having a greater number of concomitant diagnoses. Recently, rimantadine, an amantadine analogue, has been shown to be slightly less effective (efficiency rates of 85 and 91 per cent, respectively) but to have fewer side effects (4 versus 13 per cent withdrew from the trial because of them [241]).

Cost

The net cost of the US influenza vaccination programme for the elderly population has been estimated to be $310 per life year gained at 70 per cent vaccine efficacy and $600 per life year gained at 50 per cent vaccine efficacy [242]. More recent analyses have estimated the programme to result in net savings in medical costs [243]. Helliwell [244] estimated the Ontario vaccination programme for those 65 or older to yield a net economic benefit of $3.86 per vaccination. More recently, a cost–benefit analysis of four alternative strategies for the prevention of influenza in nursing homes was published by the Division of Immunization at the Centers for Disease Control in the USA. All four approaches (which consisted of various combinations of vaccination and/or amantadine therapy) were found to be cost effective.

The sequelae of Herpes zoster

Importance

Herpes zoster is a serious and common infectious disease of elderly people. Its incidence increases from two to three cases per 1000 in early adult life to seven per 100 in the seventh and eighth decades and 10.1 per 1000 in those 80 years and over [245]. The likelihood of developing one of the major complications, post-herpetic neuralgia, increases with age, from 16 per cent in those under to 47 per cent in those over 60 years of age [246]. In one study no fewer than three-quarters of all patients over 70 had post-herpetic neuralgia [247]. The severity and duration of post-herpetic neuralgia also increase with age.

Detection

The disease is easily detectable in its early stages by clinical examination.

Effectiveness

Primary prevention

Primary prevention consists of the isolation of patients with zoster infection to prevent spread to others. Institutionalised elderly people, many of whom have declining cell-mediated immunity from concomitant disease or extreme age are particularly at risk [248].

Acyclovir

There have been four placebo controlled, randomised double blind trials of acyclovir [249–253] which provide good evidence that early treatment modifies the rash, toxaemia and acute pain. It also lessens the common ocular complications [253]. Acyclovir has also been shown to reduce the number of patients in whom pain persists as post-herpetic neuralgia, where post-herpetic neuralgia is defined as localised pain persisting after healing of the rash [252] (see Fig. 7.5). A lessening of post-herpetic neuralgia has also been reported in a randomised trial of Levodopa [254]; although this drug is without effect on the acute illness, its use led to a reduction in the proportion of patients developing post-herpetic neuralgia.

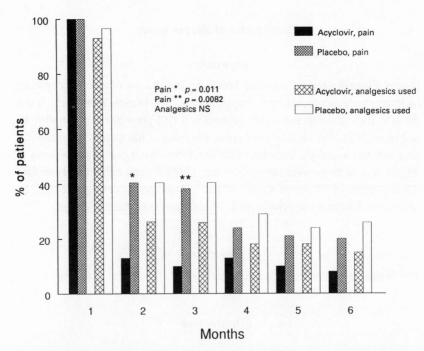

Fig. 7.5. Effects of acyclovir on post-herpetic neuralgia. The percentage of patients reporting pain and analgesic use during each month for six months. The data compare patients treated with acyclovir and those receiving a placebo. Analgesics NS, analgesics made no statistically significant difference to the pain. Adapted from ref. [252].

Cost

Costs associated with the control of both varicella and zoster infections in hospitals following guidelines laid down by the Centers for Disease Control in the USA have been reported to vary between $10 000 and $43 292 per annum [255]. The cost of adopting less stringent procedures against zoster infection only is unknown.

Pneumonia

Importance

Pneumonia is a major illness in the elderly population. Although the exact yearly incidence of community acquired pneumonia in the non-institutionalised is unknown it has been estimated to be between 25 and 44 per 1000 population [256]. In contrast, elderly residents of chronic-care institutions have a reported incidence of 68 to 114 cases of pneumonia per 1000 population per year [257]. At any one time, as many as 2.1 per cent of US nursing home residents may have lower respiratory tract infection [258].

When no other condition co-exists, the mortality from the disease is 9 per 100 000 but this rises to 979 per 100 000 with the co-existence of other illness [256].

Targeting

In the USA, pneumococcal vaccination is recommended for all healthy adults aged 65 or more and for adults with chronic cardiovascular or pulmonary disease, renal failure, cirrhosis, alcoholism, diabetes mellitus, asplenia and sickle cell disease.

In spite of these recommendations, coverage with pneumococcal vaccination in the UK is extremely low, and in the USA influenza coverage is still four times that for pneumococcal vaccine coverage, even though there is Medicare reimbursement for the latter.

There are ethical constraints on the extent to which this preventive measure should be employed in frail patients. In particular, those in institutional care should be carefully selected, omitting those on limited treatment plans in whom the prolongation of life would merely prolong suffering. Care should be taken to identify the elderly person's wishes and to communicate with his or her family on this matter.

Effectiveness

Pneumococcal vaccination

Although a number of non-controlled studies of pneumococcal vaccine suggest its protection to be about 60 to 70 per cent [259–263], lingering doubts about its effectiveness remain. Two prospective randomised placebo-controlled studies undertaken between 1973 and 1979, one on ambulatory patients over 45 years of age and the other on chronic hospitalised patients, failed to show any discernible clinical benefit from the vaccine [264]. There was no reduction in 'respiratory events', clinical pneumonia, X-ray evidence of pneumonia, prevalence of vaccine pneumococci in the sputum, or deaths. Similarly, two further recent trials have shown only limited efficacy [265, 266]. One by the American Veterans' Administration vaccinated 2295 patients according to the national recommendations, but found no significant reduction of pneumococcal respiratory infections [266]. Another study has shown no clear benefit for patients with Hodgkin's disease, myeloma, renal failure or alcoholism, although the numbers studied were few [267].

Pneumococcal vaccine may be safely and effectively administered simultaneously with influenza vaccine. The duration of immunity following pneumococcal vaccination is unknown but is certainly five to eight years and possibly much longer. At present revaccination is not recommended because of the higher risk of reactions.

Improving vaccination coverage

Attempts to improve coverage have included the suggestion that the vaccine be given to high risk patients on discharge from hospital. By this means, 51 to 78 per cent of eligible patients have been immunised before discharge [268, 269]. As many of the elderly people who are being treated as outpatients have conditions that double or treble their risks of pneumococcal disease, coverage can be improved by vaccination when they are attending medical outpatient clinics [270]. However, the vaccine should not be administered during an acute illness.

Cost

Cost effectiveness analysis of the pneumococcal vaccine originally suggested an expenditure of $1000 per quality adjusted life year gained when vaccinating a population 65 years and older [271]. However, large numbers of uncertain variables and a wide range of results in the sensitivity analysis were notable features of the study, and revised estimates on the cost benefits of pneumococcal vaccination have been less favourable, suggesting that for every $6000 (1983 prices) spent on vaccinating 65-year-old Americans, one extra year of healthy life is gained [272].

Tuberculosis

Importance

In the USA, the incidence rate for tuberculosis in 1984–5 was estimated as 21.5 cases per 100000 persons over 65 years living in the community. Of all newly diagnosed cases, 28.6 per cent occur in this age group [273]. However, the death rate attributed to this disease is only 1.3 per 100000 of the population.

The tuberculosis case rate among elderly people residing in chronic care facilities may be up to ten times higher than that for those who live in their own homes [274]. The importance of this problem has been magnified by several reports in the scientific literature of an inordinately high prevalence of tuberculosis in a minority of nursing homes in the State of Arkansas in the USA [275]. The reasons for this high prevalence (approximately 1000 cases per 100000 residents) were not detailed, but may be explained by the low immunity of the indigenous population to tuberculosis as well as the heterogeneity of nursing homes populations in the USA that include young persons, those with immunosuppression (such as AIDS patients), intravenous drug users and ethnic groups at high risk of harbouring active tuberculosis. The relevance of this experience to other settings, particularly that in the UK, is therefore in doubt.

Detection

The tuberculin skin test is the usual screening strategy. Ideally it should be done by the Mantoux test (5 units of tuberculin purified protein derivative injected intradermally). The alternative multiple puncture tests have comparatively poor sensitivity and specificity [276]. However, the Mantoux test is still less than satisfactory as a screening instrument in an older population. Up to 20 per cent of an urban population can show a positive result indicating previous but inactive infection. False negative results can occur from anergy due to severe illness and from a waning of the efficiency of the immune system with age, which in elderly people dictates the need for a two-stage procedure, the second Mantoux test becoming positive because the first has boosted the aged person's immune system [276a].

In the Arkansas nursing homes study, the value of tuberculin skin testing as a screening procedure was shown in that over 60 per cent of the clinical cases of tuberculosis arose in the 15 to 20 per cent of persons showing a significant (10 mm or more) reaction to tuberculin on admission. If left untreated, individuals in this group were 150 times more likely that non-reactors to develop clinical tuberculosis [275]. It should be remembered, however, that the predictive value of the positive tuberculin test in these nursing home residents may be significantly exaggerated above the norm; the rate of tuberculosis was inordinately high, being 5 to 30 times greater than case rates for persons of comparable age in the general population.

Effectiveness

Chemoprophylaxis against tuberculosis in compliant individuals has an efficacy greater than 90 per cent. The most commonly used drug for this purpose is isoniazid. However, it has an increased incidence of side effects, particularly hepatotoxicity, in elderly patients. It is thus uncertain whether the benefits of such chemoprophylaxis outweigh the risks. One study concluded that benefits outweigh risks until the patient exceeds 45 years old [277]. Another analysis for elderly tuberculin skin reactors concluded that isoniazid would neither improve nor worsen five-year survival but would decrease the risk of developing active disease [278].

Experience from the Arkansas nursing homes mentioned above has shown that isoniazid as preventive therapy provides protection to 98.4 per cent of elderly residents who are recent tuberculin skin test converters. Furthermore, the ratio of benefit (reduction of risk for clinical tuberculosis) to risk (for non-fatal isoniazid-related hepatitis) was clearly favourable in persons who had definite conversions (1.6 for women and 3.4 for men), although the ratio was less favourable for persons who had positive tuberculin reactions of unknown duration and for persons with minor increases in size of tuberculin reaction [279].

Cost

No details are available relating to costs in an elderly population.

Tetanus

Importance

Because a large number of elderly people are not immunised against tetanus [280], its incidence [281] and its case-fatality rate [282, 283] increase in this older population and a large proportion of tetanus deaths may be accounted for by elderly people [284]. It is nevertheless a relatively rare disease. In the highest risk group, men 65 to 74 years, the annual risk is less than 1 in 180 000.

Targeting/detection

Tetanus toxoid administered on a routine basis at the time of wounding is probably an ineffective strategy for an elderly population. Interest has therefore centred on improving primary immunisation for this age group: however, no profiles exist to identify those elderly people most at risk, though over half of the cases follow gardening injuries. In younger age groups, agricultural workers are particularly susceptible.

Effectiveness

There is good evidence from a randomised controlled trial of maternal immunisation against tetanus [285] and a series of non-experimental studies involving injured troops [286] that active immunisation against tetanus is an effective strategy. Although no studies relate specifically to old people, there is no reason to believe the procedure significantly less effective in this population.

Some measure of the perceived importance of tetanus immunisation by the older population, and therefore their compliance with it as an effective preventive strategy, can be gained from the results of Dixon and Bibby's [287] study from family practice in the UK. In this study, only 177 of 412 elderly respondents who had not received a tetanus injection in the past five years intended to make an appointment for vaccination and one month later only 37 had done so.

Cost

The mounting of a nationwide tetanus immunisation programme for the elderly would be extremely costly for the benefits obtained. Hutchison [288], analysing the cost effectiveness of a programme of mailed reminders from family physicians to increase primary tetanus immunisation among elderly Canadians, considered that this would produce small health benefits at very high cost. The most favourable cost-effectiveness ratios per case of tetanus averted, per life saved and per life-year gained were $840 000 to $2 970 000 and $520 000 (Canadian 1986 prices), respectively.

Iatrogenic insult from hospitalisation

Importance

The hospitalisation process itself and the accompanying medical care encompass many iatrogenic risks for elderly people. The iatrogenic morbidity from individual procedures, drugs, and nosocomial infections have been well described. Overall, Reichel [289] found 193 adverse effects and 44 cases of intercurrent illness during the admission of 500 elderly consecutive patients to an acute care hospital. Jahnigen [290] showed a complication rate of 17 per cent in medical patients under 65 years of age, and of 42 per cent in surgical patients under 65 years of age. The corresponding figures for those over 65 years were 40 and 43 per cent respectively. Psychological decline is also common. Gillick [291] found depressed psychological functioning associated with hospitalisation in 40.5 per cent of those over age 70 in hospital. The functional problems of impaired mobility, falls and incontinence are poorly dealt with in the traditional acute hospital environment and may even be worsened by the high levels of formal and informal restraint of elderly patients. In one survey of such a setting, body or arm restraints were being used to manage almost 20 per cent of surveyed patients over 70 years of age and psychotropic medications and sedatives were being prescribed (often for restraint purposes) to 43 per cent [292]. The hospitalisation process may also induce stressed family carers to relinquish their long term support.

Targeting/identification

Strategies to minimise the iatrogenic insult experienced during hospitalisation should be targeted mostly at people over 75 years of age because the latter have either a very high percentage of concomitant functional disability with their acute illness or a marked decrease in homeostatic reserve.

Specialised geriatric evaluation and management (GEM) units (see below) are effective only when they are targeted at specific groups of frail elderly patients. As yet, the criteria for inclusion in GEM programmes is a subject of debate [293], but most are based on a combination of patient age, degree of functional impairment, particular diagnostic conditions and psychosocial variables.

Effectiveness

No strategies have yet been described that would help health care providers to appreciate the iatrogenic consequences of their own actions. However, clinical experience strongly suggests that, in the generalised acute hospital environment, improved outcomes may be achieved by the promotion of early rehabilitation, the adoption of stronger case management throughout the numerous consults in the acute care hospital and, for the most frail, by adopting the principle of minimal interference in the medical workup [294] with each move being based on the logical utility of the test or procedure in terms of its contribution towards diagnosis, prognosis and management rather than aiming for a 'complete workup' [295].

Furthermore, several randomised controlled trials now attest to the improved outcomes from hospital care in specialised units for the elderly [296]. Benefit has been shown in survival, in functional status, in decreased use of medications and in lesser need for long term institutional care.

Because of the magnitude and adverse consequences of the use of restraints in hospitals, several guidelines for their application have been produced and numerous alternatives to restraint use have been recommended. These have been well reviewed by Evans et al. [297] and include companionship and supervision, changing bothersome treatment to alternative forms, environmental manipulation, psychosocial interventions, physical and diversionary activities and staff re-education and support. For wanderers, various types of 'creative control' have been suggested instead of physical restraint. Regrettably, there has been little scientific evaluation of the efficacy of these alternatives.

Cost

No details are available, but the potential cost savings from avoiding unnecessary or inappropriate biotechnical care could be significant.

Motoring accidents

Importance

In recent years there has been a marked growth in the proportion of elderly drivers in western countries. In the USA, drivers 65 to 69 years, 70 to 74 years and over 75 years represent, respectively, 4.4, 3.1 and 2.0 per cent of the driving population [298]. Although these elderly drivers limit their driving and avoid potentially dangerous conditions [299] such as night driving, the rate of crashes, the severity of injuries and the mortality rates by distance driven rise dramatically after age 60 and particularly after 75 years of age [298, 300] (see Fig. 7.6). Age-associated deterioration in psychomotor skills, perceptual abilities and information processing have been implicated [301]. Perhaps more important is the impact of age-associated illness such as dementia: elderly drivers suffering from this condition have been reported as having nearly five times as many crashes as age-matched controls [302].

Targeting

Three targeting strategies are currently employed in different countries. In the UK, reliance is placed on a self declaration of health and illness by the elderly person after 70 years. It is likely that there is marked under-reporting of problems with this strategy because elderly people in general may not be aware of age-related impairments or illness and, in any case, tend to underestimate driving dangers while overestimating their own driving skills [301]. Drivers with dementia, in particular, continue to drive despite a striking deterioration in driving performance and usually withdrawal from driving is initiated by a family member or physician rather than by the elderly driver [303].

Another strategy is to require a 'medical' assessment of fitness to drive beyond a certain arbitrary age threshold. In the presence of a clear-cut illness, a decision about future driving ability can be fairly easily taken. For the majority of elderly drivers, however, it can be extremely difficult if the problem is related only to normal ageing processes or to a less clear-cut illness such as insidious dementia. The problem here is that there is insufficient information to establish a normative data bank in elderly drivers and, in the absence of marked psychomotor deficits, the relationship between psychomotor/perceptual/cognitive performance detected on examination and road driving behaviour is unclear [301]. Additional helpful aids to such a 'fitness' examination have included assessment of activities of daily living [303] and traffic sign recognition testing [304]. Nevertheless, their routine use in targeting drivers at risk of crashing is still to be proven.

The third, and possibly most recommended strategy [301] is that of direct assessment of driving ability on the road. Ideally it should be a normal road test, preferably near the elderly driver's home and incorporating various levels of difficulty.

A major deterrent to the adoption of any of the above measures is the lack of acceptability to the elderly public. In the UK, 77 per cent of elderly drivers regard the car as essential or very important to their way of life and 42 per cent think that driving is a right as opposed to 27 per cent who think it is a privilege [305]. One British survey in particular showed resistance among drivers to the concept of regular medical checks to retain a driving licence [305].

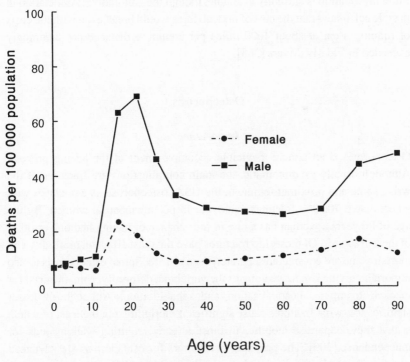

Fig. 7.6. Deaths per 100 000 population from motor vehicle traffic crashes by age and sex, 1977–79. Adapted from ref. [298].

Effectiveness

No detailed information is available on the efficacy of any of the above strategies in reducing trauma from motoring accidents nor has any cross-national comparison been made between the self report system, the requirement of a certificate of health from a doctor at an arbitrary age threshold, and regular driving retesting after such an age threshold. However, from the available evidence, regular driving retesting would seem the most appropriate option [301, 306]. It is, therefore, suggested that a biannual road test become mandatory after age 75 years though there is no evidence to gauge the impact of its introduction. The importance of losing the civil liberty to drive must also be considered. For the time being at least, many countries will need to rely on the use of seat belts as a highly effective strategy for reducing both the morbidity and mortality from accidents [307].

Cost

Little information is currently available, though the Automobile Association in the UK calculated that the cost of taxicab fares would break even with the costs of running a car at about 4000 miles per annum, a distance not commonly exceeded by elderly drivers [308].

Osteoporosis

Importance

Osteoporosis is an almost inevitable accompaniment of the ageing process. Although usually asymptomatic, the main complications are fractures of the wrist, spine and proximal femur. In the USA, osteoporosis is associated with an estimated 700 000 fractures each year in postmenopausal women. By the age of 80 years a woman has a one in four chance of having had one or other of these fractures. Of these, hip fractures have the most effect on morbidity and mortality and are considered separately (see p. 138). Spinal osteoporosis is also important, giving rise to wedging of the vertebrae, deformity, pain, the need for medical treatment, hospitalisation and rehabilitation. Although of lesser significance, wrist fractures cause significant morbidity, not the least of which is that they jeopardise mobility in those already requiring walking aids for independence [309]. The principal risk factors for osteoporosis are advanced age, female gender, Caucasian race, slender build and bilateral oophorectomy before the menopause [310].

Detection

Various screening tools of varying levels of sophistication have been used to measure bone mineral density. Their respective merits are discussed elsewhere [310]. The problem is that, irrespective of their efficacy in so doing, bone mineral density measurements are a relative poor discriminator between those who will remain asymptomatic and those who will go on to develop a fracture. A recent comprehensive review of the evidence found the difference in bone density between patients with hip fracture and controls was only about half of one standard deviation. This was too small for an effective screening test [311] (see Fig. 7.7). Another radiological screening technique used, the Singh index (which measures the extent of bony trabeculae in the femoral neck), has problems of interobserver variation and has been shown a poor discriminator of fracture risk for those over 75 years of age [311].

Effectiveness

Most research on the prevention of osteoporosis has focussed on relatively young, perimenopausal women. This creates difficulties when attempting to extrapolate results to an elderly population with established osteoporosis in which the underlying mechanism for osteoporosis may be quite different

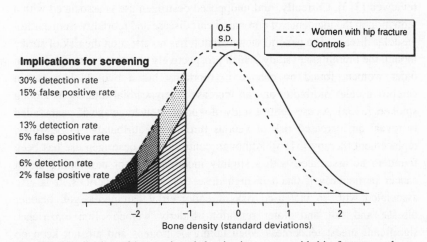

Fig. 7.7. Distribution of bone mineral density in women with hip fracture and age-matched controls. Implied vertical axis is proportion of cases and controls within a marginal unit of bone density. Expected screening performance of measurement is shown by three examples. S.D. standard deviation. Adapted from ref. [311].

[312]. Nevertheless, an increasing number of studies are now including older subjects which allows the following tentative conclusions to be drawn:

Hormone replacement therapy

Randomised trials have shown that oestrogen replacement substantially or totally prevents bone loss in the immediate perimenopausal years, whereas there is a fairly rapid rate of bone loss in untreated controls. However, bone subsequently adjusts to oestrogen deficiency, and in contrast, in elderly post-menopausal women with established osteoporosis, the rate of loss of bone is quite small. In randomised controlled trials among this group of women, oestrogen therapy has still been shown to increase the spinal and femoral trochanteric bone density [312a, 312b] although there is no convincing evidence that oestrogen benefits women over the age of 75 years [312b]. Although there is an epidemiological association between risk of fracture and current oestrogen use, evidence to support oestrogen use as a preventive measure for fractures is still scant. In the randomised controlled trial by Lufkin et al. [312a] in women with established osteoporosis (median age approximately 65 years), vertebral fracture rates were reduced but the results may have been confounded by the small sample size. The epidemiological association between oestrogen and hip fracture in the elderly population is discussed below.

The side effects of hormone replacement therapy are well researched and reviewed [313]. Currently, oral unopposed oestrogen use is associated with a reduction in the incidence of coronary heart disease and mortality from cardio-vascular disease. The general view is that it has no effect on the risk of stroke though the Framingham study, which prospectively examined oestrogen use in older women, found no change in mortality but a twofold increase in cerebrovascular morbidity and an increase in myocardial infarctions among smokers [313a]. A case-control study of women of average age 65 years failed to reveal an increased risk of venous thrombosis attributable to oestrogen replacement therapy [313b]. Although controversial, oestrogen use has been found to be associated with a slightly increased risk of developing breast cancer particularly if taken in high doses for very long periods. It is also associated with an increased risk of endometrial carcinoma, gall bladder disease and salt and water retention. Elderly women often experience significant breast tenderness when taking oestrogens and are not keen on coping with vaginal bleeding again after its absence for many years. However, for most women with an intact uterus, combined preparations with progestogens are nowadays mostly prescribed. Though this confers a degree of protection against endometrial cancer and can avoid the vaginal bleeding, it lessens the beneficial effect the oestrogen has on cardiovascular end points. Newer methods of oestrogen administration such as vaginally or by dermal patch make the side effects of hormone replacement therapy even more difficult to estimate.

Calcium, vitamin D and calcitriol

There is evidence from a number of randomised trials that pharmaceutical preparations of calcium (often administered with a small dose of vitamin D to assist absorption) have a definite but modest (less than half that produced by oestrogen replacement) effect on reducing the rate of vertebral bone loss though in some of these studies there was less benefit to the spine than to the femur or forearm [311].

Recently, interest has focussed on the use of 1,25-dihydroxyvitamin D3 (calcitriol), which not only increases the gastrointestinal absorption of calcium but, in vitro at least, promotes bone mineralisation. Although numbers in previous studies were too small to allow its impact on fracture incidence to be evaluated, Tilyard et al. [313c] have now shown in a larger study of postmenopausal women (mean age 63 years) that continuous treatment with calcitriol for three years is safe and that it significantly reduced vertebral fracture incidence compared with a control group who received calcium supplementation alone in the second (9.3 versus 25.0 fractures per 100 patient-years) and third (9.9 versus 31.5 fractures per 100 patient-years) years of treatment. The benefit was only evident in those women with five or fewer vertebral fractures at baseline.

Other therapies

Sodium fluoride is known to stimulate bone formation, but its use is disfavoured because of concerns about its toxicity, its predominant effect on the axial skeleton and controversy about the quality and strength of the new bone produced. Two recent randomised controlled trials have shown that, for younger elderly women at least, cyclical etidronate appears to achieve a gain in vertebral bone mass and reduction in vertebral fracture rate [314, 315]. The implications of such long term therapy on a widespread scale have not yet been evaluated.

Exercise

In elderly people over 70 years of age two trials of exercise programming now show that bone mineral density can be increased, though this increase in bone mass is proportionately small [316, 317].

Quitting smoking

Although lower bone density and increased fracture rates have been shown to develop in older smokers compared with age matched controls, results from other trials have been conflicting and information on the risk of fracture according to the duration of abstinence among former smokers is not available [81].

Cost

Although no information is available specifically on elderly people, Weinstein [318], in a study of postmenopausal women, compared the risks of endometrial cancer, uterine bleeding and gallbladder disease against the benefits associated with the prevention of osteoporosis and consequent fractures. He found the net effects on life expectancy were probably small in either direction, although they were likely to be positive in women with existing osteoporosis or prior hysterectomy. Treatment appeared to be particularly cost effective in menopausal women with prior hysterectomy. For osteoporotic women aged 55 to 70 years the cost per quality adjusted life year gained was calculated as $5460 to $15 100 depending on whether an annual endometrial biopsy was included in the programme.

It has also been estimated that to treat all women over age 50 years in Britain with calcium supplements, the annual cost would be over £500 million or about 15 per cent of the total National Health Service drug expenditure [311].

Hip fracture

Importance

Hip fracture is a major health problem in elderly women. Its incidence is 6.1 per 1000 at 75 to 79 years rising exponentially to 48.6 at 90 years [319]. There has also been a rising age-specific incidence in previous decades. About 30 per cent of elderly women with hip fracture die within one year [320] and of the survivors (even with walking aids) only 37 per cent of women in one series had regained their prefracture level of mobility [320]. A significant proportion of survivors require to spend substantial periods of time living in residential homes or nursing homes. In the UK, 20 per cent of NHS orthopaedic beds are occupied by patients with hip fracture. The estimated annual cost of hip fracture in the USA in 1983 was $7.3 billion [321].

Table 7.7. *Age-adjusted relative risk of hip fracture in elderly women,
estimated from various trials*

Factor	Duration	Relative risk (95% CI)
Active exercise	More than 1 hour/day	0.6 (0.4–0.8)
	0.5 to 1 hour/day	0.7 (0.5–1.0)
	Less than 0.5 hour/day	1.0
Oestrogen use	In previous 2 years	0.3
	More than 2 years ago	0.7
	Never	1.0
Oestrogen use	In previous year	0.8 (0.5–1.1)
	2–14 years previously	0.9 (0.6–1.2)
	More than 14 years ago	1.2 (0.9–1.5)
	Never	1.0
Current cigarette use		1.1
Current cigarette use		1.2 (0.8–1.6)
Current cigarette use	Never	1.0
	1–10 cigarettes/day	1.3 (0.7–2.2)
	More than 10 cigarettes/day	2.1 (1.5–3.0)
Current cigarette use		5.6 (1.8–17.7)
Visual impairment	20/30 to 20/80 vision	1.5 (1.0–2.5)
	20/100 or worse vision	2.2 (1.2–3.8)

CI, confidence interval.
Adapted from Reid J, Kennie DC. Care Elderly 1992; **4**: 213.

Targeting

Preventive measures may be applied globally or by targeting recurrent fallers
or those with prior fracture.

Effectiveness

Most strategies for the primary prevention of hip fracture have focussed on
reducing the degree of risk associated with osteoporosis. Recent research on
elderly patients with hip fractures, however, has led to an appreciation that,
while osteoporosis does play a part, the main determinant appears to be
postural instability and the resultant fall [322, 323]. Other strategies have
therefore been aimed at prevention of falls and increased exercise. These
are discussed in detail in the appropriate sections. However, some idea of
the potential effectiveness of possible interventions can be gained by
comparing the age-adjusted fracture risk ratios shown in Table 7.7. Tertiary
prevention, i.e. reducing resultant disability after fracture is dealt with on
page 182.

Table 7.8. Studies of relative risk of hip fracture in women who had or had not ever received hormone replacement therapy

Study centre	Age range (mean) (years)	No. of cases who had/had not received hormone replacement therapy	No. of controls who had/had not received hormone replacement therapy	Relative risk (95% confidence interval)
Case-control studies				
Seattle	50–75	52/108	293/274	0.4 (0.3 to 0.6)[a,b]
Oregon	52–80 (70)	49/199	121/215	0.7 (0.5 to 1.1)
Los Angeles	<80 (72)	35/46	85/80	0.7 (0.4 to 1.2)[b]
Connecticut	45–74 (67)	14/80	213/579	0.5 (0.2 to 0.9)[a]
Southampton (UK)	50–99 (78)	6/234	23/457	0.5 (0.2 to 1.3)
New Haven	<80 (70)	3/68	12/59	0.2 (0.1 to 0.7)[b]
Prospective studies				
Los Angeles	(76)[c]	163/166		1.0 (0.8 to 1.3)
Framingham	64–96 (75)	28/135		0.6 (0.4 to 0.9)[a]

[a] Adjusted for the effect of other risk factors.
[b] Calculated by Law [311] from published data.
[c] Median age.
Adapted from ref. [311].

Hormone replacement therapy

Observational studies (summarised in Table 7.8) have, with one exception, shown that oestrogen protects against hip fracture, with a median reduction in incidence of 50 per cent in women who had at some time received post-menopausal oestrogen therapy [311]. However, further data (Table 7.8) strongly indicate that, whilst current use reduces hip fracture risk, this protection is substantially lost within a few years after stopping hormone replacement therapy. Law et al. [311] suggest that even if oestrogen were taken to the age of 70 there would be little protectant effect in women over the age of 75, in whom over 80 per cent of hip fractures occur.

Hormone replacement therapy is likely to have an appreciable effect on the frequency of hip fractures only if it is continued indefinitely after the menopause. This leads to difficult decisions when balancing the benefits to elderly people of hip fracture reduction against the side effects of oestrogen.

Calcium supplementation

Several observational studies on dietary calcium and hip fracture have shown quite discrepant results with no clear protectant effect yet being proven [311]. However, in a recent French prospective randomised controlled trial of healthy ambulatory women of mean age 84 years, the group supplemented with tricalcium phosphate (containing 1.2 g of elemental calcium) and 20 µg (800 IU) of vitamin D3 each day for 18 months had a 43 per cent lower rate of hip fracture ($P = 0.04$) than the control group [311a].

Exercise

There is evidence from six observational studies (most of which contained aged subjects) that exercise has a substantial impact on reducing the risk of hip fracture [311] (see Table 7.9). It is therefore appropriate to recommend exercise programmes as a valuable preventive strategy for osteoporosis and hip fracture.

Cost

Available information on the costs of preventing osteoporosis and falls and on promoting exercise programmes for the elderly population are discussed on pp. 138, 187 and 174 respectively.

Table 7.9. *Results of studies of effect of regular exercise on risk of hip fracture*

Study centre	Extent of habitual exercise	Relative risk (95% confidence interval)
Case-control studies		
Los Angeles	Frequency of active outdoor games:	
	Low	1.0
	Medium	0.5[a]
	High	0.3
Hong Kong	Habitual walking uphill:	
	<Once/day	1.0
	>Once/day	0.6 (0.5–0.9)[a]
Southampton	Physical activity:	
	<2 hours/week	1.0
	3–4 hours/week	0.6 (0.4–0.9)[a]
	>5 hours/week	0.4 (0.3–0.7)
	Previous occupation:	
	Sedentary	1.0
	Intermediate	0.3 (0.2–0.6)[a]
	Weight bearing	0.3 (0.2–0.5)
Oxford	Past activity:	
	Very inactive	1.0
	Moderately inactive	0.7 (0.4–1.2)
	Active	0.5 (0.3–0.8)
Prospective studies		
Los Angeles	Active exercise:	
	<½ hour/day	1.0
	½–1 hour/day	0.7 (0.6–0.9)[a]
	>1 hour/day	0.6 (0.5–0.7)
Britain (DHSS)	Outdoor activity:	
	Low	1.0
	Moderate	1.1 (0.3–4.3)[a]
	High	0.3 (0.04–1.4)

[a] Adjusted for the effect of other risk factors.
Adapted from ref. [311].

Depressive illness

Importance

The extent of depression in the elderly population depends on the criteria upon which it is diagnosed. Blazer [324] discusses the details of this in relation to its epidemiology. Approximately 2 to 3 per cent have a major depressive illness, whilst another 15 per cent suffer only from dysphoric symptoms. It causes much morbidity and reduces quality of life. It can lead to suicide and, because depressed elderly persons frequently present with physical symptoms, unrecognised depression can lead to iatrogenic morbidity due to unnecessary diagnostic testing and treatment [325]. Depression also prolongs hospital stay, consumes community services and results in long term institutionalisation. Those with dysphoric symptoms have implications for resource consumption that are similar to those with severe illness [326].

Detection

Primary care physicians often overlook the diagnosis of depression [327]. The detection rate of functional psychiatric disease in elderly people living in the community has been shown to be improved by the incorporation of a structured questionnaire into the interview technique [328]. Several rating scales are also available specifically for the detection of depressive illness in older people. Although most have reasonable clinical utility, none is entirely satisfactory [329]. Nevertheless, there is considerable day to day fluctuation in the reporting of mood (see below) that may give falsely high estimates of the worth of a screening test. Using particularly rigorous criteria to take account of this and other factors, Koenig et al. [329a] have recently found that among those screened with a positive test, the likelihood of a major depressive disorder was 27% and 28% using the Geriatric Depression Scale (GDS) and the Brief Carroll Depression Rating Scale (BCDRS) respectively. These estimates were considerably below those reported in earlier studies.

Effectiveness

Numerous effective therapies are available, though remissions are obtained in only a quarter to a half of cases [330]. Although some evidence from studies in younger depressives suggests that formal screening leads to earlier diagnosis [325], there is no information available on whether this leads to improved patient outcomes. There is also no information on whether treating elderly dysphorics prevents progression to major depressive illness as the natural history of the former condition is poorly known, though one short-term follow-up study reported that over half of the patients screened as positive for depression showed spontaneous improvement [330a].

Cost

No detailed information on costs is available.

Alcohol dependence

Importance

About 5 to 12 per cent of men and 1 to 2 per cent of women in their 60s are problem drinkers [331]. They often first present to the medical system with subtle symptoms, confusional states, the consequences of accidents and adverse or synergistic effects of the alcohol with their medication [332], and gastrointestinal emergency problems [332a].

Alcohol is also important in about a third of suicides by elderly people [333]. Elderly problem drinkers consume considerable community resources and institutional places.

Detection

Compared with their younger counterparts, elderly alcoholics may be drinking relatively little [334], they may be drinking daily rather than 'binge drinking' [334] and they are more likely to try to hide their drinking habits [334]. For this reason, opportunistic screening with a brief instrument may be valuable for use with elderly patients on admission for hospital care. Willenbring et al. [335] have confirmed that the MAST and UMAST alcohol screening tests, often used with younger alcoholics for this purpose, also have excellent sensitivity and specificity in the elderly population. More recently, the use of a shorter instrument, the CAGE Questionnaire has also been found to discriminate successfully between elderly people with a history of drinking problems and those without such a history [335a].

Effectiveness

There is little evidence that early intervention in asymptomatic persons is of benefit. However, if formal screening in selected individuals leads to earlier diagnosis of *symptomatic* individuals, these people can then be provided with counselling from which some benefit may accrue. However, most alcohol treatment studies have included only a few elderly patients, so scientific evidence is limited. Nevertheless, those elderly alcoholics who began abusing alcohol earlier in life (about two-thirds of the total) appear to do better in treatment programmes than do younger alcoholics, being more responsive and enthusiastic [336]. The remainder often respond to intervention strategies aimed at strengthening coping mechanisms, providing home support and providing socialisation and interaction with peers.

A further goal of screening might be to increase the clinician's awareness that alcohol dependency exists to better diagnose or treat other concomitant health problems; however, no information is available on the benefit of screening in this regard.

Cost

No detailed information is available on costs specific to the elderly population.

Retirement stress

Importance

Retirement is an almost inevitable accompaniment of the ageing process. It has been estimated as the tenth most stressful event occurring over the life cycle [337]. However, despite mortality rates in industrial societies increasing sharply after the age of retirement [338], research has failed to demonstrate that retirement is responsible for this adverse outcome.

Detection

Over 70 per cent of persons adjust well to retirement. Of the 30 per cent minority who have difficulties, 7 per cent relate to missing their job and 23 per cent to other problems surrounding the retirement process [339]. There are no reliable methods for identifying these high risk minority groups.

Effectiveness

The case for the benefit of preretirement counselling has been the subject of little rigorous scientific research. However, some studies have shown that the more satisfied retirees start thinking and planning for retirement at an earlier age [340]. Planning for retirement may also improve adjustment and a positive orientation towards leisure [341]. In part, the success of preretirement counselling depends on the nature of its goals. It is argued that an emphasis on preventing deterioration in physical health may be inappropriate and that more success may accompany efforts to minimise the psychosocial problems of retirement and to enable and empower retirees to make the most of what may be another third of their lifespan.

Cost

No information is available.

Bereavement

Importance

Among those 75 years and over, 30 per cent of men and 64 per cent of women have lost a spouse [342]. Although most elderly people cope well with bereavement, it may cause significant morbidity in terms of prolonged sorrow, depression, attention-seeking behaviour and physical ill-health. Numerous studies also show an association between conjugal bereavement and increased risk of death. This risk seems greatest in the first six months of bereavement for widowers and in the second year for widows [343].

Targeting

No criteria are available to identify those bereaved most at risk of morbid complications. The minority of elderly people with prolonged or abnormal grieving patterns can be detected by sensitive interviewing techniques used by health and social work providers.

Efficacy

Bereavement counselling provided by professional services or by professionally supported voluntary and self-help groups has been shown to improve wellbeing, reduce drug consumption and reduce symptoms that lead to consultations with doctors [344]. The impact of bereavement counselling in reducing mortality is unknown.

Cost

No detailed information on costs is available.

Problems from medication

Importance

There is well-documented evidence that health problems from the medication taken by elderly people arise in a number of ways: from faulty prescriber rationale; from faulty prescribing technique; from altered pharmacokinetics; from altered pharmacodynamics; from a variety of drug interactions; and from the elderly person complying poorly with his or her medication regimen or by taking additional over-the-counter drugs. It will be apparent that many of these health problems due to drugs are, therefore, of iatrogenic origin. In the community, 87 per cent of elderly people over 75 years are responsible for their own medicines and studies have shown that 25 to 59 per cent of them make errors in their medication [345].

Targeting/detection

The risk to elderly people of taking medication is considered to be global, though the very old, those with renal impairment, those with concomitant disease states and those with dementia are known to be at particular risk. Routine review of all medication is widely recommended at each consultation as well as chart review during hospital rounds. Compulsory review of medication every few months for those in continuing institutional care is mandated by law in the USA.

As most clinicians' estimates of the patients' medication is inaccurate [346], detection of drug problems (or potential drug problems) at the above reviews may be significantly enhanced by ensuring that elderly people always bring their medication with them to every consultation.

Effectiveness

Although still strongly recommended clinically, there has been little attempt to evaluate the worth of the above medication reviews. Indeed, in an analysis of the literature on iatrogenic illness (most of which focussed on adverse drug reactions), Fletcher and Fletcher [347] concluded that the main preventive strategy is exhortation and that there is little scientific evidence bearing on the effectiveness of this or other strategies. However, the following measures are also advocated.

Improving prescriber rationale and technique

Advocated guidelines, legislated regulations for the use of certain medications, the development of local drug formularies, the promotion of generic prescribing and supervision by clinical pharmacy services are all commonly used, though relatively unevaluated, techniques of improving prescriber rationale and prescribing habits.

Minimising the use of drugs

The taking of multiple drugs increases the risk of side effects, adverse drug reactions and malcompliance. Drug usage should therefore be minimised by:

- prescribing less by:
  employing more stringent criteria starting therapy,
  employing alternative management strategies (e.g. therapy),
  employing counselling and other forms of support.
- reducing medication once started; several studies now show that, after careful review, digoxin [348] and diuretic therapy can be safely discontinued in a high proportion of cases. Reduction prescribing can also be applied to the use of hypnotics. One study of institutionalised patients showed substitution with a placebo as an effective means of weaning many elderly people off sleeping tablets [349].
- avoiding an overall increase in medication after hospital discharge [350].
- an educational programme in geriatric psychopharmacology for health care providers which in a recent controlled trial of US nursing homes was shown to reduce the use of psychoactive drugs by 27 per cent in the experimental group compared with 8 per cent in the control group [350a].

Reducing adverse drug reactions

This may be achieved by:

- minimising the use of drugs; the incidence of adverse drug reactions rises exponentially with the number of drugs taken by a patient so that minimising the use of drugs is potentially a major deterrent (see above);
- education of medical staff; one educational programme has shown a reduction in digitalis intoxication on a medical inpatient service [351]. Sophisticated aide memoires are also available to remind and educate physicians about potential drug–drug interactions;
- supervision by clinical pharmacists; a comprehensive review of 305 articles on the value and acceptance of clinical pharmacology published between 1974 and 1984 is provided by Hatoum et al. [352].

Improving patient compliance

Counselling, with an illustrative card of instructions, has been shown to reduce medication errors [352, 353] and detailed protocols of how best to achieve this have been outlined. Reducing the number of dosage schedules per day has also been shown to be effective [354]. It is generally believed that compliance may be improved by the better labelling of bottles and the avoidance of childproof containers that are difficult to open [355, 356]. Specialised delivery systems may also be of value in certain patients [357].

Cost

No detailed information on costs is available.

An 'unhealthy lifestyle'

Importance

In younger adults there is some evidence of a statistical correlation between certain health practices and lower mortality rates from all causes. These practices include never smoking, regular physical activity, moderate alcohol consumption, average weight status and sleeping seven to eight hours a night. This has led to the concept of 'healthy' and 'unhealthy' lifestyles in this age group.

Evidence that such apparently 'unhealthy lifestyles' really impact on the health of elderly people is much less apparent. In one study, none of the personal health practices mentioned related significantly to mortality in elderly men and only 'never having smoked' correlated with lower mortality in women [358]. A later study also failed to show an association between lifestyle practices and the onset of disabilities [359].

Targeting

No subgroups of elderly people have been identified as being at particular risk.

Effectiveness

General exhortation of the elderly population to adopt 'healthy lifestyle' practices therefore seems unwarranted. Nevertheless, advice to quit smoking still appears justifiable and the limited information from the above studies on activity levels and benefits must be seen against a background of increasing scientific evidence on the benefits of exercise in older people.

Costs

No information is available, but the non-financial costs (inconvenience, reduced life-satisfaction, etc.) to individuals of changing their ingrained lifestyle patterns must be considerable.

The ageing processes

Importance

In recent years increasing effort has been made to retard or to counteract the effects of the ageing processes in order to extend the human lifespan, to prevent the functional decline with age and/or to prevent the adverse bodily changes with age.

Lifespan is the maximal obtainable age by a human being. Currently documented lifespan is 115 years [360]. The importance attached to longevity by society and particularly by the elderly is unknown, its value being closely interwoven with perceived wellbeing and quality of life. If the consumption of anti-ageing cures is any indication, some people at least wish the choice of extending lifespan as much as possible. The value attributed to the functional and compositional changes with age as a health problem is essentially unknown. Society, and elderly individuals in particular, have not been canvassed for their opinion and it is still extremely difficult to distinguish between the consequences of ageing, the consequences of inactivity and the consequences of concomitant disease.

Targeting

Little information is available about the targeting and timing of applying anti-ageing strategies. There are also significant moral, ethical, political and financial implications in selecting suitable individuals for these strategies, particularly if there is a likelihood of perpetuating or increasing an ill or dependent subpopulation within society.

Effectiveness

Schneider and Reed [361] have reviewed the scientific base for several anti-ageing cures. There are no life-prolonging measures of immediate application to the human population. The restriction of caloric consumption used to extend life in rodents results in the retardation of growth and does not seem immediately applicable to elderly people. Moreover, the mechanism by which this is achieved is unknown and there are contradictory studies regarding the relationship between human body weight and longevity. Although exercise programmes are promoted to increase longevity, there is no consistent relationship between a history of athletic competition and longevity. Exercise begun late in the life of experimental rats has not shown a consistent effect on survival.

The following have all shown variable effects on lifespan in experimental animals: dietary compounds; vitamin E and superoxide dismutase (which act as antioxidants); meclofenoxate (which decreases the accumulation of the age pigment lipofuscin); Levodopa (to combat the age-associated decrease in the amounts of brain aminergic neurotransmitters); hypophysectomy (to eliminate the life-shortening effect of certain as yet unidentified hormones); various immunological interventions (to prevent age-associated loss of immune responsiveness); Gerovital H3 (an anti-age treatment developed in Romania); and dihydroepiandrosterone (to counteract the dramatic decline in this hormone with age). None, however, seems to have an immediate application to the human population.

Apart from life-extension measures, anti-ageing strategies, as exemplified by the following three areas of study, are also being considered as ways to prevent or restore the adverse bodily changes that occur with increasing age. The administration of human growth hormone to elderly men has been shown in one pilot study to increase lean body mass, decrease adipose-tissue mass and increase skin thickness [362]. The practical benefits of such compositional changes have not yet been identified, however, nor have details of the risk–benefit equation for widespread growth hormone administration been elucidated. There has also been considerable research into drugs that might prevent age changes in human articular cartilage and postpone the onset of osteoarthritis. Although some encouraging results have been shown in in vitro and animal studies, the implications for humans are as yet unknown [363]. A third example of an attempt to prevent bodily changes that occur with age is the use of tretinoin to delay the photo-ageing of skin. However, although some interesting results are being reported, there is as yet no convincing evidence that the clinical effect on wrinkles is anything other than that produced by the oedema of mild inflammation [364].

Costs

No detailed information is available on the cost implications of anti-ageing strategies. Estimates will vary depending on the relative fitness (and need for support) of the surviving population and on whether its members were physically and mentally able to compete on the job market or would require to be pensioned.

References

1. Langer RD, Ganiats TG, Barrett-Connor E. Paradoxical survival of elderly men with high blood pressure. Brit Med J 1989; **298**: 1356–8.
2. Mattilea K, Haavisto M, Rajala S et al. Blood pressure and five year survival in the very old. Brit Med J 1988; **296**: 887–9.
3. Kannel WB. Blood pressure and the development of cardiovascular disease in the aged. In: Caird FI, Kennedy R (eds) Cardiology of Old Age. New York: Plenum Press, 1976.
4. Appelgate WB. Hypertension in elderly patients. Ann Intern Med 1989; **110**: 901–15.
5. Bulpitt CJ. Definition, prevalence and incidence of hypertension in the elderly. In: Amery A, Staessen J (eds) Hypertension in the Elderly. Vol. 12 of Handbook of Hypertension. Amsterdam: Elsevier, 1989.
6. Report of the US Preventive Services Task Force. Screening for Hypertension. Chapter 3, in: Guide to Clinical Preventive Services. Williams and Wilkins 1989.
7. Spence JD, Sibbald WJ, Cape RD. Pseudohypertension in the elderly. Clin Sci Mol Med Suppl 1978; **55**: 399S–402S.
8. Amery A, Birkenhager W, Brixko P et al. A mortality and morbidity results from the European Working Party on high blood pressure in the elderly trial. Lancet 1985; **2**: 1349–54.
9. Management Committee. Treatment of mild hypertension in the elderly. A study initiated and administered by the National Heart Foundation of Australia. Med J Aust 1981; **2**: 398–402.
10. Hypertension Detection and Follow Up Program Cooperative Group. Five year findings of the Hypertension Detection and Follow up Programs. J Amer Med Assoc 1979; **242**: 2562.
11. MRC Working Party. Medical Research Council trial of treatment of hypertension in older adults: principal results. Brit Med J 1992; **304**: 405–12.
12. Dahlof B, Lindholm LH, Hansson L et al. Morbidity and mortality in the Swedish Trial in Old Patients with Hypertension (STOP-Hypertension). Lancet 1991; **338**: 1281–5.
13. Kuramoto K, Katsushita S, Kuwajima I et al. Prospective study on the treatment of mild hypertension in the aged. Jap Heart J 1981; **22**: 75–85.
14. Veterans Administration Cooperative Study Group on Antihypertensive Agents. Effects of treatment on morbidity in hypertension. III. Influence of age, diastolic pressure and prior cardiovascular disease. Circulation 1972; **45**: 991–1004.
15. Coope J, Warrender TS. Randomized trial of treatment of hypertension in elderly patients in primary care. Brit Med J 1986; **293**: 1145–51.
16. Sprackling ME, Mitchell JRA, Short AH. Blood pressure reduction in the elderly: a randomised controlled trial of methyldopa. Brit Med J 1981; **283**: 1151–3.
17. SHEP Cooperative Research Group. Prevention of stroke by anti-hypertensive drug treatment in older persons with isolated systolic hypertension. Final results of the systolic hypertension in the elderly program (SHEP). J Amer Med Assoc 1991; **265**: 3255–64.
18. Morisky DE, Levine DM, Green LW, Smith CR. Health education program effects on the management of hypertension in the elderly. Arch Intern Med 1982; **142**: 1835–8.

19. Jackson G, Piersianowski TA, Mahon W et al. Inappropriate anti-hypertensive therapy in the elderly. Lancet 1976; **2**: 1317–18.
20. Weinstein MC, Stason WB. Hypertension: The Policy Perspective. Harvard University Press, 1976.
21. Cohen DL. Serum cholesterol and older people. Brit J Hosp Med 1991; **46**: 323–5.
22. Aronow WS, Starling L, Etienne F et al. Risk factors for coronary artery disease in persons older than 62 years in a long term health care facility. Amer J Cardiol 1986; **57**: L518–L520.
23. Gordon DJ, Rifkind BM, Treating high blood cholesterol in the older patient. Amer J Cardiol 1989; **63**: 48H–52H.
24. Rudman E, Mattson DE, Feller AG et al. A mortality risk index for men in a Veterans' Administration extended care facility. J Parenter Enteral Nutr 1979; **13**: 189–95.
25. Forette B, Tortrat D, Wolmark Y. Cholesterol as a risk factor in mortality in elderly women. Lancet 1989; **1**: 868–70.
26. Verdery RB, Goldberg AP. Hypocholesterolaemia as a predictor of death: prospective study of 224 nursing home residents. J Gerontol 1991; **46**: M84–M90.
27. Iso H, Jacobs DR, Wentworth D et al. Serum cholesterol levels in six year mortality from stroke in 350,997 men screened for the Multiple Risk Factor Intervention Trial. N Engl J Med 1989; **320**: 904–10.
28. Penke MA, Grundy SM. Hypercholesterolaemia in elderly persons: resolving the treatment dilemma. Annals Intern Med 1990; **112**: 780–92.
29. Muldoon MF, Manuck SB, Matthews KA. Lowering cholesterol concentrations and mortality: a qualitative review of primary prevention trials. Br Med J 1990; **301**: 309–14.
30. Deyton S, Pearce ML, Hashimoto F et al. A controlled clinical trial of a diet high in unsaturated fat. Circulation 1969; **40** (Suppl 2): 1–63.
31. Oliver MF. Might treatment of hypercholesterolaemia increase non-cardiac mortality? Lancet 1991; **337**: 1529–31.
32. Oster G, Epstein AM. Cost-effectiveness of anti-hyperlipemic therapy in the prevention of coronary heart disease. J Amer Med Assoc 1987; **258**: 2381–7.
33. Bonita R. Epidemiology of stroke. Lancet 1992; **339**: 342–4.
34. Carstairs V. Resource consumption and the cost to the community. In: Gillingham FJ, Mawdsley C, Williams AE (eds) Stroke. Churchill Livingstone, 1976.
35. Chesebro JH, Fuster V, Halperin JL. Atrial fibrillation – risk marker for stroke. N Engl J Med 1990; **323**: 1556–8.
36. Stroke Prevention in Atrial Fibrillation Investigators. Predictors of thrombo-embolism in atrial fibrillation: i. Clinical features of patients at risk. Annals Intern Med 1992; **116**: 1–5.
37. Stroke Prevention in Atrial Fibrillation Investigators. Predictors of thrombo-embolism in atrial fibrillation: ii. Echocardiographic features of patients at risk. Annals Intern Med 1992; **116**: 6–12.
38. Shinton R, Beavers G. Smoking and stroke: an overview. Br Med J 1989; **298**: 789–93.
39. Wolf PA, D'Agostino RB, Kannel WB et al. Cigarette smoking as a risk factor for stroke. J Amer Med Assoc 1988; **259**: 1025–9.
40. Donnan GA, Adena MA, O'Malley HM. Smoking as a risk factor for cerebral ischaemia. Lancet 1989; 16 September, 643–7.

41. Ruiswck JV, Noble H, Sigmann P. The natural history of carotid bruits in elderly persons. Annals Intern Med 1990; **112**: 340–3.

42. Chambers BR, Norris DW. Outcome in patients with asymptomatic neck bruits. N Engl J Med 1986; **315**: 860–5.

43. Kittner SJ, White LR, Losonczy KG et al. Black–white differences in stroke incidence in a national sample. J Amer Med Assoc 1990; **264**: 1267–70.

44. Gill JS, Zezulka AV, Shipley MJ et al. Stroke and alcohol consumption. N Engl J Med 1986; **315**: 1041–6.

45. Stampfer MJ, Colditz GA, Willett WC et al. A prospective study of moderate alcohol consumption and the risk of coronary disease and stroke in women. N Engl J Med 1988; **319**: 267–73.

46. Steering Committee of the Physicians Health Study Research Group. Preliminary Report: findings from the Aspirin component of the ongoing physicians health study. N Engl J Med 1988; **318**: 262–4.

47. Peto R, Gray R, Collins R et al. Randomised trial of prophylactic daily aspirin in British male doctors. Brit Med J 1988; **296**: 313–16.

48. Paganini-Hill, A, Chao A, Ross RK, Henderson BE. Aspirin use and chronic diseases: a cohort study of the elderly. Brit Med J 1989; **299**: 1247–50.

49. ISIS-2 Collaborative Group. Randomized trial of intravenous streptokinase, oral aspirin, both or neither among 17,187 cases of suspected acute myocardial infarction: ISIS-2. Lancet 1988; **2**: 349–60.

50. Antiplatelet Trialists' Collaboration. Secondary prevention of vascular disease by prolonged antiplatelet treatment. Brit Med J 1988; **296**: 320–31.

51. The Boston Area Anticoagulation Trial for Atrial Fibrillation Investigators. The effect of low-dose warfarin on the risk of stroke in patients with non-rheumatic atril fibrillation. N Engl J Med 1990; **323**: 1505–11.

51a. Connolly SJ, Laupacis A, Gent M et al. Canadian atrial fibrillation anticoagulation (CAFA) study. J Amer Coll Cardiol 1991; **18**: 349–55.

52. Stroke Prevention in Atrial Fibrillation Investigators. Stroke prevention in atrial fibrillation study: final results. Circulation 1991; **84**: 527–39.

53. Peterson P, Boysen G, Godtfredsen J et al. Placebo controlled, randomised trial of warfarin and aspirin for prevention of thromboembolic complications in chronic atrial fibrillation: The Copenhagen AFASAK study. Lancet 1989; **1**: 175–9.

54. American College of Physicians. Indications for carotid endarterectomy. Annals Intern Med 1989; **111**: 675–7.

55. Antiplatelet Trialists' Collaboration. Secondary prevention of vascular disease by prolonged antiplatelet treatment. Brit Med J 1988; **296**: 320–31.

56. Grotta JC, Lemak NA, Gary H et al. Does platelet antiaggregant therapy lessen the severity of stroke? Neurology 1985; **35**: 632–6.

57. Swedish Cooperative Study Group. High-dose acetyl salicylic acid after cerebral infarction. Stroke 1987; **18**: 325–34.

58. UK-TIA Study Group. United Kingdom transient ischaemic attack (UK-TIA) aspirin trial: interim results. Brit Med J (Clin Res) 1988; **296**: 316–20.

59. The Dutch TIA Study Group. The Dutch TIA Trial: protective effects of low-dose aspirin and atenolol in patients with transient ischaemic attack or nondisabling stroke. Stroke 1988; **19**: 512–17.

60. Bousser MG, Eschwege E, Haguenau M et al. 'AICLA' controlled trial of aspirin and dipyridamole in the secondary prevention of atherothrombotic cerebral ischaemia. Stroke 1983; **14**: 5–14.

61. American–Canadian Cooperative Study Group. Persantin aspirin trial in cerebral ischaemia. Part II. Endpoint results. Stroke 1985; **16**: 406–15.

62. Gent M, Easton JD, Hachinski VC et al. The Canadian American Ticlopidine Study (CATS) in thrombo-embolic stroke. Lancet 1989; **1**: 1215–20.

63. Hass WK, Easton D, Adams HP et al. A randomised trial comparing Ticlopidine hydrochloride with aspirin for the prevention of stroke in high risk patients. N Engl J Med 1989; **321**: 501–7.

64. Olssen JE, Brechter C, Backlund H et al. Anticoagulant vs. antiplatelet therapy against cerebral infarction in transient ischaemic attacks. Stroke 1980; **11**: 4–9.

65. Buren A, Ygge J. Treatment program and comparison between anticoagulants and platelet aggregation inhibitors after transient ischemic attack. Stroke 1981; **12**: 578–80.

66. Garde A, Samuelsson K, Fahlgran H et al. Treatment after transient ischemic attacks: a comparison between anticoagulant drug and inhibition of platelet aggregation. Stroke 1983; **14**: 677–81.

67. Cerebral Embolism Study Group. Immediate anti-coagulation of embolic stroke: a randomised trial. Stroke 1983; **14**: 668–76.

68. Lodder J, Dennis MS, Raak LV et al. Cooperative study on the value of long term anti-coagulation in patients with stroke and non-rheumatic atrial fibrillation. Brit Med J 1988; **296**: 1435–8.

69. North American Symptomatic Carotid Endarterectomy Trial Collaborators. Beneficial effect of carotid endarterectomy in symptomatic patients with high grade carotid stenosis. N Engl J Med 1991; **325**: 445–53.

70. European Carotid Surgery Trialists' Collaborative Group. MRC European Carotid Surgery Trial: interim results for symptomatic patients with severe (70–99%) or with mild (0–29%) carotid stenosis. Lancet 1991; **337**: 1235–43.

71. EC/IC Bypass Study Group. Failure of extracranial–intracranial arterial bypass to reduce the risk of ischaemic stroke. N Engl J Med 1985; **313**: 1191–200.

72. Dudley, HAS. Extra-intracranial bypass one, clinical trials, nil. Brit Med J 1987; **294**: 1501–2.

72a. Gustafsson C, Asplund K, Britton M et al. Cost effectiveness of primary stroke prevention in atrial fibrillation: Swedish national perspective. Brit Med J 1992; **305**: 1457–60.

73. Office of Population Censuses and Surveys. Mortality Statistics Cause, Series DH2 No. 11, London: HMSO, 1984.

74. Office of Population Censuses and Surveys. Mortality Statistics Cause: Review of the Registrar General on Deaths by Cause, Sex and Age in England and Wales 1983, Series DH2 No. 10, London: HMSO, 1983.

75. Nevitt MP, Ballard DJ, Hallett JW. Prognosis of abdominal aortic aneurysms: a population-based study. N Engl J Med 1989; **321**: 1009–14.

76. Scott RAP, Ashton HA, Kay BN. Routine ultrasound screening in the management of abdominal aortic aneurysm. Brit Med J 1988; **296**: 1709–10.

77. Collin J, Walton J, Araujo L, Lindsell D. Oxford Screening Programme for abdominal aortic aneurysm in men aged 65 to 74 years. Lancet 1988; **2**: 613–15.

78. Collin J. Screening for abdominal aortic aneurysms. Brit J Surg 1985; **72**: 851–2.

78a. Collin J. The value of screening for abdominal aortic aneurysm by ultrasound. In: Greenhalgh RM, Marrick JS (eds) The Cause and Management of Aneurysms. London: Saunders, 1990.

78b. Goldberg RJ, Gore JM, Gurwitz JH et al. The impact of age on the incidence and prognosis of initial acute myocardial infarction: The Worcester Heart Attack Study. Amer Heart J 1989; **117**: 543.

78c. Lernfelt B, Landahl S, Svanborg A. Coronary heart disease at 70, 75 and 79 years of age: a longitudinal study with special references to sex differences and mortality. Age Ageing 1990; **19**: 297–303.

78d. Stott DJ, Williams BO. Ischaemic heart disease in elderly patients. Reviews Clin Gerontol 1992; **2**: 227–35.

78e. Report of the US Preventive Services Task Force. Screening for asymptomatic coronary artery disease. Chapter 1, in: Guide to Clinical Preventive Services. Baltimore, MD: Williams and Wilkins, 1989.

78f. Dalen JE, Goldberg RJ. Prophylactic aspirin and the elderly population. In: Omenn GS (ed) Clinics in Geriatric Medicine: Health Promotion and Disease Prevention, vol. 8. Philadelphia, PA: WB Saunders, 1992.

78g. ISIS-2 (Second International Study of Infarct Survival) Collaborative Group. Randomised trial of intravenous streptokinase, oral aspirin, both, or neither among 17,187 cases of suspected acute myocardial infarction: ISIS-2. Lancet 1988; **2**: 349–60.

78h. Siddiqui MA. Cardiac rehabilitation and elderly patients. Age Ageing 1991; **21**: 157–9.

78i. Cohn JN. The prevention of heart failure – a new agenda. N Engl J Med 1992; **327**: 725–7.

78j. Krumholz HN, Pasternak RC, Weinstein MC et al. Cost effectiveness of thrombolytic therapy with streptokinase in elderly patients with suspected acute myocardial infarction. N Engl J Med 1992; **327**: 7–13.

79. US Department of Health and Human Services national Center for Health Statistics: Health of the United States 1983. DHHS, Publication No. (PHS) 94–1232, 1984.

80. Vetter NJ, Charny M, Farrow S, Lewis PA. The Cardiff Health Survey. The relationship between smoking habits and beliefs in the elderly. Pub Health 1988; **102**: 359–64.

81. LaCroix AZ, Omenn GS. Older adults and smoking. In: Omenn GS (ed) Clinics in Geriatric Medicine: Health Promotion and Disease Prevention, vol. 8, pp. 69–78. Philadelphia, PA: WB Saunders, 1992.

82. Wienpahl J, LaCroix A, White L et al. Body mass index, alcohol use and smoking in relation to hip fracture in older populations (abstract). Amer J. Epidemiol 1990; **132**: 753.

83. Sachs DPL. Cigarette smoking – health effects and cessation strategies. In: Mahler DA (ed) Clinics in Geriatric Medicine: Respiratory Diseases, vol. 2, pp. 337–62. Philadelphia, PA: WB Saunders, 1986.

84. Jajich CL, Ostfeld AM, Freeman DH. Smoking and coronary heart disease mortality in the elderly. J Amer Med Assoc 1984; **252**: 2831–4.

85. Hermanson B, Omenn GS, Kronmal RA et al. Beneficial six-year outcome of smoking cessation in older men and women with coronary artery disease. N Engl J Med 1988; **319**: 1365–9.

86. Pathak DR, Samet JM, Humble CG et al. Determinants of lung cancer risk in cigarette smokers in New Mexico. J Natl Cancer Inst 1986; **76**: 597–604.

87. Cook NR, Evans DA, Scherr PA et al. Peak expiratory flow rate in an elderly population. Amer J Epidemiol 1989; **130**: 66.

88. Colsher PL, Wallace RB. Demographic and health characteristics of elderly smokers: results from Established Populations for Epidemiologic Studies of the Elderly. Amer J. Prev Med 1990; **6**: 61–70.

89. LaCroix, AZ, Lipson S, Miles TP et al. Prospective study of pneumonia hospitalizations and mortality in US older people: the role of chronic conditions, health behaviours and nutritional status. Pub Health Rep 1989; **104**: 350.

90. Wolf PA, D'Agostino RB, Kannel WB et al. Cigarette smoking as a risk factor for stroke. J Amer Geriatr Soc 1988; **259**: 1025–9.

91. Report of the US Preventive Services Task Force. Counseling to Prevent Tobacco Use. In: Guide to Clinical Preventive Services, pp. 281–95. Baltimore, MD: Williams and Wilkins, 1989.

92. Cummings SR, Coates TJ, Richard RJ et al. Training physicians in counseling about smoking cessation. Annals Intern Med 1989; **110**: 640–7.

93. Cummings SR, Rubin SM, Oster G. The cost-effectiveness of counseling smokers to quit. J Amer Med Assoc 1989; **261**: 75–9.

94. Banerjee AK. The Haemopoeitic System. In: Pathy MSJ (ed) Principles and Practice of Geriatric Medicine, pp. 343–416. Chichester: John Wylie and Sons Limited, 1985.

95. National Center for Health Statistics. Hematological and nutritional biochemistry reference data for persons six months–74 years of age: United States 1976–80. Vital and Health Statistics Series 11 No. 232. Washington, DC: Government Printing Office, 1982 (Publication No. DHHS (PHS) 83–1682).

96. Lukens JN. Iron deficiency and infection. Amer J Dis Child 1975; **129**: 160–2.

97. Elwood PC, Hughes D. A clinical trial of iron therapy on psychomotor function in anaemic women. Brit Med J 1973; 254–5.

98. Stevens RG, Jones Y, Micozzi MS, Taylor PR. Body iron stores and the risk of cancer. N Engl J Med 1988; **319**: 1047–52.

99. Podgor MJ, Leske MC, Ederer F. Incidence estimates for lens changes, macular changes, open-angled claucoma and diabetic retinopathy. Amer J Epidemiol 1983; **118**: 206–12.

100. Tielsch JM, Sommer A, Katz J et al. Racial variations in the prevalence of primary open-angle glaucoma. J Amer Med Assoc 1991; **266**: 369–74.

101. Eddy DM, Sanders LE, Eddy F. The value of screening for glaucoma with tonometry. Surv Ophthalmol 1983; **28**: 194–205.

102. Report of the US Preventive Services Task Force. Glaucoma. In: Guide to Clinical Preventive Services, Chapter 32. Williams and Wilkins, 1989.

103. Shutt HKR, Boyd TAS, Salter AB. The relationship of visual fields, optic disc appearances and age in non-glaucomatous and glaucomatous eyes. Can J Ophthalmol 1967; **2**: 83–90.

104. Wood CM, Bosanquet RC. Limitations of direct ophthalmoscopy in screening for glaucoma. Brit Med J 1987; **294**: 1587–8.

104a. Bruce DW, Damato E, Williams BO et al. Screening for glaucoma in geriatric practice using oculokinetic perimetry. J Clin Exper Gerontol 1991; **12**: 13–24.

104b. Machado J, Woodhouse K. Is oculokinetic perimetry (OKP) a useful glaucoma screening test in a day hospital setting? Paper presented at British Geriatrics Society, Scientific Meeting, London, 1992.

105. Kitazawa Y. Prophylactic therapy of occular hypertension: a prospective study. Trans Ophthal Soc NZ 1981; **33**: 30–2.

106. Shin DH, Colker AE, Kass MA et al. Long term Epinephrine therapy on occular hypertension. Arch Ophthalmol 1976; **94**: 2059–60.

107. Krug JH, Hertzmark E, Remis LL et al. Long term study of Timolol vs no treatment in the management of glaucoma suspects (abstract). Invest Ophthalmol Vis Sci (Suppl) 1987; **28**: 148.

108. Becker V, Morton RW. Tropical Epinephrine in glaucoma suspects. Amer J Ophthalmol 1966; **62**: 272–7.

109. Hoff M, Parkinson JM, Cass MA et al. Long term trial of unilateral Timolol treatment in occular hypertensive subjects (abstract). Invest Ophthalmol Vis Sci (Suppl) 1988; **29**: 16.

110. Everitt DE, Avorn J. Systemic effects of medications used to treat glaucoma. Annals Intern Med 1990; **111**: 120–5.

111. Power EJ, Wagner JL, Duffy BM. Screening for open-angle glaucoma in the elderly – assessment. Washington, DC: Health Program Office of Technology, Congress of the United States, 1988.

112. Brocklehurst JC. The Urinary Tract. In: Rossman I (ed) Clinical Geriatrics, pp. 317–30. Philadelphia, PA: JB Lippincott, 1979.

113. Carty M, Brocklehurst JC, Carty J. Bacteriuria and its correlates in old age. Gerontology 1981; **27**: 72–5.

114. Akhtar, HR, Andrews GR, Caird FI. Urinary tract infection in the elderly – a population study. Age Ageing 1972; **1**: 48–54.

115. Sourander LB. Urinary tract infection in the aged: an epidemiological study. Annals Med Intern Fenn 1966; **55** (Suppl 45): 1–55.

116. Dontas AS, Papanayitou PC, Marketas SG. The effect of bacteriuria on renal functional patterns in old age. Clin Sci 1968; **34**: 73–81.

117. Dontas AS, Kasviki-Charvati B, Papanayitou PC. Bacteriuria and survival in old age. N Engl J Med 1981; **304**: L939–43.

118. Nicolle LE, Brunka J, Murray D, Harding GKM. Asymptomatic bacteriuria, urinary antibody, and survival in the institutionalized elderly. J Amer Geriatr Soc 1992; **40**: 607–13.

119. Quintiliani R, Cunha BA, Klimek J, Maderazo EG. Bacteremia after manipulation of the urinary tract: the importance of pre-existing urinary tract disease and compromised host defences. Post-Grad Med J 1978; **54**: 668–71.

120. Flanagan PG, Davies EA, Rooney PG, Stout RW. Evaluation of four screening tests for bacteriuria in elderly people. Lancet 1989; **1**: 1117–19.

122. Lacey RW, Simpson MHC, Lord VL et al. Comparison of single-dose Trimethoprim with a 5 day course for treatment of urinary tract infections in the elderly. Age Ageing 1981; **10**: 179–85.

123. Brocklehurst JC, Bee P, Jones D, Palmer MK. Bacteriuria in geriatric hospital patients: its correlates and management. Age Ageing 1977; **6**: 240–5.

124. Nicolle LE, Bjornson J, Harding GKM, MacDonell JA. Bacteriuria in elderly institutionalised men. N Engl J Med 1983; **309**: 1420–5.

125. Boscia JA, Cobasa WD, Knight RA et al. Therapy v. no therapy for bacteriuria in elderly ambulatory non-hospitalised women. J Amer Med Assoc 1987; **257**: 1067.

126. Boscia JA, Kaye D. Asymptomatic Bacteriuria in the Elderly. In: Kaye D, Posner JD (eds) Clinics in Geriatric Medicine: Common Clinical Challenges in Geriatrics, vol. 4, no. 1. Philadelphia, PA: WB Saunders, 1988.

127. Garraway WM, Collins GN, Lee RJ. High prevalence of benign prostatic hypertrophy in the community. Lancet 1991; **2**: 469–71.

127a. Drach GW, Layton TN, Binard WJ. Male peak urinary flow rate: relationships to volume voided and age. J Urol 1979; **122**: 210–14.

127b. Arrighi HM, Metter EJ, Guess HA, Fozzard JL. Natural history of benign prostatic hyperplasia and risk of prostatectomy. Urology 1991 Supplement; **38**: 4–8.

128. Mayhoff HH, Hald T. Are doctors able to assess prostatic size? Scand J Urol Nephrol 1978; **12**: 219–21.

129. Roos NP, Ramsay EW. A population-based study of prostatectomy outcomes associated with differing surgical approaches. J Urol 1987; **137**: 1184–8.

130. Wennberg JE, Murray AG, Hanley D et al. An assessment of prostatectomy for benign urinary tract obstruction; geographic variations and the evaluation of medical care outcomes. J Amer Med Assoc 1988; **259**: 3027–30.

131. Gormley GJ, Stoner E, Burkewitz RC et al. The effect of finasteride in men with benign prostatic hyperplasia. N Engl J Med 1992; **327**: 1185–91.

132. Krasman ML, Gracie WA, Strasius SR. Biliary tract disease in the aged. In: Sklar M (ed) Clinics in Geriatric Medicine: Gastroenterologic Problems, vol. 2, no. 2. WB Saunders, 1991.

133. Cobden I, Lendrum R, Venables CW et al. Gallstones presenting as mental and physical debility in the elderly. Lancet 1984; **1**: 1062.

134. Gracie WA, Ransohoff DF. The natural history of silent gallstones: the innocent gallstone is not a myth. N Engl J Med 1982; **307**: 798.

135. Newman HF, Northup JD. Gallbladder carcinoma in cholelithiasis. Geriatrics 1964; June: 453–5.

136. Ransohoff DF, Gracie WA, Wolfenson L et al. Prophylactic cholecystectomy or expectant management for silent gallstones: a decision analysis to assess survival. Annals Intern Med 1983; **99**: 199.

137. Ransohoff DF, Gracie WA. Management of patients with symptomatic gallstones: a quantitative analysis. Amer J Med 1990; **88**: 154.

138. General Registrars Office. Deaths in London from the cold weather. Weekly Return No. 51, vol. 35. London: HMSO, 1974.

139. Collins KJ. Hypothermia, the facts. Oxford: Oxford University Press, 1983.

140. Woodhouse P, Keatinge WR, Coleshaw SRK. Factors associated with hypothermia in patients admitted to a group of inner city hospitals. Lancet 1989; **2**: 1201–5.

141. Goldman A, Exton-Smith AN, Francis G, O'Brien A. A pilot study of low-body temperatures in old people admitted to hospital. J Roy Coll Phys 1977; **11**: 291.

142. Herity B, Daly L, Bourke GJ, Horgan JM. Hypothermia and mortality and morbidity. An epidemiological analysis. J Epidem Comm Health 1991; **45**: 19–23.

143. Collins KJ. Effects of cold on old people. Brit J Hosp Med 1987; **38**: 506–14.

144. Bull, GM, Morton J. Relationships of temperature with death rates from all causes and from certain respiratory and arteriosclerotic diseases in different age groups. Age Ageing 1975; **4**: 232–46.

145. McDowell M. Long-term trends in seasonal mortality. Population Trends 1981; **26**: 16.

146. MacMillan AL, Corbett JL, Johnson RH et al. Temperature regulation in survivors of accidental hypothermia of the elderly. Lancet 1967; **2**: 1650–9.

147. McWhirter M. A dispersed alarm system for the elderly and its relevance to local General Practitioners. J Roy Coll Gen Pract 1987; **37**: 244–7.

148. Keatinge WR. Seasonal mortality among elderly people with unrestricted home heating. Brit Med J 1986; **293**: 732–3.

149. Collins, KJ, Easton JC, Bellfield-Smith H et al. Effects of age on body temperature and blood pressure in cold environments. Clinical Sci 1985; **69**: 465–70.

150. Slater DN. Death from hypothermia: are current views on causative factors well-founded? Brit Med J 1988; **296**: 1643–4.

151. Salvage AV. Warmth in winter: evaluation of an information pack for elderly people. Research Team for Care of the Elderly. University of Wales. College of Medicine, Cardiff, December 1988.

152. Tester S, Meredith B. Ill-informed? a study of information and support for elderly people in the inner city. London: Policy Studies Institute, 1987.

153. Otty CJ, Roland MO. Hypothermia in the elderly: scope for prevention. Brit Med J 1987; **295**: 419–20.

154. Harris MI. Epidemiology of diabetes mellitus among the elderly in the United States. In: Froom J (ed) Clinics in Geriatric Medicine: Diabetes Mellitus in the Elderly, vol. 6, no. 4. WB Saunders, 1990.

155. Weinberger M, Cowper PA, Kirkman MS, Vinicor F. Economic impact of diabetes mellitus in the elderly. In: Froom J (ed) Clinics in Geriatric Medicine: Diabetes in the Elderly, vol. 6, no. 4. WB Saunders 1990.

156. Huse DM, Oster G, Killen AR et al. The economic costs of non-insulin dependent diabetes mellitus. J Amer Med Assoc 1989; **262**: 2708–13.

157. Keen H, Fuller JH. The epidemiology of diabetes. In: Exton Smith AN, Caird FI (eds) Metabolic and Nutritional Disorders in the Elderly. Bristol: John Wright and Sons Limited, 1980.

158. Wright AD, Kilvert A. Diabetes mellitus. In: Isaacs B (ed) Recent Advances in Geriatric Medicine 3. Edinburgh: Churchill Livingstone, 1985.

159. Blunt BA, Barrett-Connor E, Wingard DL. Evaluation of fasting plasma glucose as screening test for NIDDM in older adults. Rancho Bernardo Study. Diabetes Care 1991; **14**: 989–93.

160. Report of the US Preventive Services Task Force. Screening for Diabetes Mellitus. In: Guide To Clinical Preventive Services, pp. 95–103. Baltimore, MD: Williams and Wilkins, 1989.

161. University Group Diabetes Program. A study of the effects of hypoglycemic agents on vascular complications in persons with adult-onset diabetes (ii) Mortality results. Diabetes 1970; **19** (Suppl No. 2): 7–830.

162. Report of the US Preventive Services Task Force. Screening For Thyroid Disease. Chapter 17, in: Guide To Clinical Preventive Services. Baltimore, MD: Williams and Wilkins, 1989.

163. Helfand M, Crapo LM. Screening for thyroid disease. Annals Intern Med 1990; **112**: 840–9.

164. National Survey of Oral Health in US Employed Adults and Seniors, Oral health of United States Adults 1985–1986. Bethesda, MD: National Institute of Dental Research; National Institutes of Health Publication 87–2868, 1987.

165. Macpherson AS. 'A Smile For All Seasons'. Dental Health Promotion For Seniors: A Strategy for 1986. Toronto: Department of Public Health, 1986.

166. Niessen LC, Douglass CW. Preventive Actions for Enhancing Oral Health. In: Omenn GS (ed) Clinics in Geriatric Medicine: Health Promotion and Disease Prevention, vol. 8, no. 1. Philadelphia, PA: WB Saunders, 1992.

167. Vehkalahti MM, Rajala M, Tuomien R et al. Prevalence of root caries in an adult Finnish population. Commun Dent Oral Epidemiol 1983; **11**: 188–90.

168. Fejerskov O, Nyvad V. Pathology and treatment of dental caries in the aging individual. In: Hom-Pedersen P, Loe H (eds) Geriatric Dentistry, pp. 238–62. Copenhagen: Munksgaard, 1986.

169. The City of Toronto Community Health Survey: a description of the health status of Toronto residents. City of Toronto Community Health Department, 1983.

170. Lee J. Oral health: a gerontologic perspective. Burnaby, British Columbia: Simon Fraser University, 1984.

171. Gordon SR, Jahnigen DW. Oral assessment of dentulous elderly patients. J Amer Geriatr Soc 1986; **34**: 276–81.

172. Birch S. Hypothesis: charges to patients impair the quality of dental care for elderly people. Age Ageing 1989; **18**: 1136–40.

173. Rise J. Distributive effects of dental programs for old age pensioners in Norway. Community Dent Oral Epidemiol, 1985; **13**: 14–18.

174. Brustman BA. Impact of exposure to Fluoride-adequate water on root surface caries in the elderly. Gerodontics 1986; **2**: 203–7.

175. Lindhe, J, Nyman S. The effect of plaque control and surgical pocket elimination on the establishment and maintenance of periodontal health. A longitudinal study of periodontal therapy in cases of advanced disease. J Clin Period 1975; **2**: 67–79.

176. Johansen E, Papas A, Fong W, Olsen TO. Remineralisation of carious lesions in elderly patients. Gerodontics 1987; **3**: 47–50.

177. Knazan YL. Personal communication. Faculty of Dentistry, University of Manitoba, 1986.

178. Cartwright A, Henderson G. More trouble with feet: a survey of the foot problems and chiropody needs of the elderly. London: HMSO, 1986.

179. Vetter NJ, Jones DA, Victor CR. Chiropody services for the over 70s in two General Practices. Chiropodist 1985; 315–23.

180. Tinetti ME, Speechley M, Ginter SF. Risk factors for falls among elderly persons in the community. N Engl J Med 1988; **319**: 1701–7.

181. Lippman HI, Perotto A, Farrar R. The neuropathic foot of the diabetic. Bull NY Acad Med 1976; **52**: 1159–78.

182. Edmonds ME, Blundell MP, Morris M, Watkins PJ. Reduction in the number of major and minor limb amputations: impact of a combined new diabetic foot clinic (abstract). Diabetologia 1984; **272**: 130.

183. Assal JP. Self management of diabetes: a therapeutic success or a teaching failure. Diabetic Med 1976; **52**: 1159–78.

184. Thompson FJ and Masson EA. Can elderly diabetic patients cooperate with routine foot care? Age Ageing 1992; **21**: 333–7.

185. Clark MO, Barbanel JC, Jordan MM, Nicol SM. Pressure sores. Nursing Times 1978; **74**: 363–6.

186. Allman RM. Pressure ulcers among the elderly. N Engl J Med 1989; **320**: 850–3.

187. Dinsdale SM. Decubitus ulcers: role of pressure and friction in causation. Arch Phys Med Rehabil 1974; **55**: 147–52.

188. Pritchard V. Calculating the risk. Nursing Times 1986; **82**: 59–61.

189. Waterlow JW. Risk assessment guard. Nursing times 1985; **81**: 51–5.

190. Andersen KE, Jensen O, Kvorning SA, Bach E. Prevention of pressure sores by identifying patients at risk. Brit Med J 1982; **284**: 1370–1.

191. Exton-Smith AM, Norton D, Mclaren R. An investigation of Geriatric Nursing Problems in Hospital. Edinburgh: Churchill Livingstone, 1975.

192. Bliss MR, McLaren R, Exton-Smith AN. Preventing pressure sores in hospital: controlled trial of a large-celled ripple mattress. Brit Med J 1967; **1**: 394–7.

193. Exton-Smith AN, Overstall PW, Wedgewood J, Wallace G. Use of the 'Airwave System' to prevent pressure sores in hospital. Lancet 1982; **1**: 1288–90.

194. Andersen KE, Jensen O, Kvorning SA, Bach E. Decubitus prophylaxis: prospective trial of the efficiency of alternating pressure air-mattresses and water mattresses. Acta Derm Venereol (Stockh) 1982; **63**: 227–30.

195. Allman RM, Walker JM, Hart MK et al. Air-fluidized beds or conventional therapy for pressure sores. Annals Intern Med 1987; **107**: 641–8.

195a. Panel for the Prediction and Prevention of Pressure Ulcers in Adults. Pressure Ulcers in Adults: Prediction and Prevention. Clinical Practice Guideline, Number 3. AHCPR Publication No. 92–0047, Rockville, MD: Agency for Health Care Policy and Research, Public Health Service, US Department of Health and Human Services, May 1992.

195b. Makellis GC, Frantz RA, Arteaga M et al. A comparison of patient risk for pressure ulcer developments with nursing use of preventive interventions. J Amer Geriatr Soc 1992; **40**: 1250–4.

196. Society of Actuaries. Build Study, 1979. Chicago: Society of Actuaries, 1980.

197. Benson-Cooper D, Bird D, Laing JK et al. Obesity in a New Zealand community. NZ Med J 1975; **82**: 115.

198. Harris T, Cook EF, Garrison R et al. Body mass index and mortality among non-smoking older persons. The Framingham Heart Study. J Amer Med Assoc 1988; **1259**: 1520–4.

199. Mattila K, Haavisto M, Rajala S. Body mass index and mortality in the elderly. Brit Med J 1986; **292**: 867–8.

200. Drenick EJ, Bale GS, Seltzer F, Johnson DG. Excessive mortality and causes of death in morbidly obese men. J Amer Med Assoc 1980; **243**: 443.

201. Felson DT, Zhang Y, Anthony JM et al. Weight loss reduces the risk for symptomatic knee osteoarthritis in women. Annals Intern Med 1992; **116**: 535–9.

202. Blackburn H, Parlin RW. Antecedents of disease. Insurance mortality experience. Annals NY Acad Sci 1966; **134**: 965.

203. Report of the US Preventive Services Task Force. Screening for Obesity. Chapter 18, in: Guide to Clinical Preventive Services. Williams and Wilkins, 1989.

204. US Department of Agriculture, Agriculture Research Service (by Consumer and Food Economics Division). Consumption of Households in the United States, Spring 1965. Household Food Consumption Survey 1965–1966. Report No. 1, Washington, DC: Government Printing Office, 1968.

205. Schneider EL, Vining EM, Hardy EC et al. Recommended dietary allowance and the health of the elderly. N Engl J Med 1986; **314**: 157–60.

206. Maclennan WJ. Sub-nutrition in the elderly. Brit Med J 1986; **293**: 1189–90.

207. Barrows CH, Roeder LM. Nutrition. In: Finch CE, Hayflick L (eds) Handbook of the Biology of Aging. New York: Van Nostrand Reinhold, 1977.

208. Maclennan WJ, Martin P, Mason BJ. Causes for reduced dietary intake in a long stay hospital. Age Ageing 1975; **4**: 175–80.

209. Wolinsky, FD, Prendergast JM, Miller DK et al. A preliminary validation of a nutritional risk measure for the elderly. Amer J Prev Med 1985; **1**: 53–9.

210. Banerjee AK, Brocklehurst JC, Wainwright H, Swindell R. Nutritional status of long stay geriatric inpatients: the effects of a food supplement (Complan). Age Ageing 1978: **7**: 237–42.

211. Carruthers R. Oral zinc in cutaneous healing. Drugs 1973; **6**: 161–4.

212. Corless D, Dawson E, Fraser F et al. Do vitamin D supplements improve physical capabilities of elderly hospital patients? Age Ageing 1985; **14**: 76.

213. Wilson TS, Datta SB, Murrell JS, Andrews CT. Relation of vitamin C levels to mortality in a geriatric hospital: a study of the effects of vitamin C administration. Age Ageing 1973; **2**: 163–71.

214. Lye MD, Ritch AES. Long-term anabolic therapy in the elderly. Age Ageing 1977; **6**: 221–7.

215. Burr ML, St Leger AS, Westlake A, Davies HEF. Dietary potassium deficiency in the elderly: a controlled trial. Age Ageing 1975; **4**: 148.

216. MacLeod RDM. Abnormal tongue appearances and vitamin status of the elderly – a double-blind trial. Age Ageing 1972; **1**: 99–102.

217. Exton-Smith AN. Nutritional status: diagnosis and prevention of malnutrition. In: Exton-Smith AN, Caird FI (eds) Metabolic and Nutritional Disorders of the Elderly, pp. 66–76. Bristol: John Wright and Sons, 1980.

218. US Department of Agriculture. Food and Nutritional Service. Blanchard L, Butler JS, Doyle P et al (eds) Food stamp SSI/Elderly Cash Out Demonstration Evaluation. Princeton Mathematica Policy Research Inc., 1982.

219. Smith JWG. Vaccination strategy in influenza. In: Selby P (ed) Virus Vaccines and Strategy, pp. 271–94. New York: Academic Press, 1976.

220. Barker WH, Mulloly JP. Impact of epidemic type A influenza on a defined adult population. Amer J Epidemiol 1980; **112**: 793–813.

221. Schoenbaum SC. Economic impact of influenza: the individual's perspective. Amer J Med 1987; **82** (Suppl 6A): 26–30.

222. Lennox IM, Macphee GJA, McAlpine CH et al. Use of influenza vaccine in long-stay geriatric units. Age Ageing 1990; 19: 169–72.

223. Mostow SR, Schoenbaum SC, Dowdle WR. Studies with activated influenza vaccines purified by zonal centrifugation. i. Adverse reactions in serological responses. WHO Bull 1969: **41**: 525–30.

224. Stewart-Harris CH, Andrews BE, Belyavin G et al. Clinical trials of oil–adjuvent influenza vaccines 1960–1963. Brit Med J 1964; **2**: 267–71.

225. Barker WH, Mulloly JP. Influenza vaccination in elderly persons: reduction in pneumonia and influenza hospitalisation and deaths. J Amer Med Assoc 1980; **244**: 2547–9.

226. Barker WH, Mulloly JP. Effectiveness of inactivated influenza vaccine among non-institutionalised elderly persons. In: Kendal AP, Patriarca PA (eds) Options for Influenza Control: Proceedings of a Viratek UCLA Symposium, pp. 169–82. New York: Viratek.

227. Strassburg MA, Greenland S, Sorvillo FJ et al. Influenza in the elderly: report of an outbreak and a review of vaccine effectiveness reports. Vaccine 1987: **4**: 38.

228. Gross PA, Quinnan GV, Rodstein M et al. Association of influenza immunization with reduction in mortality in an elderly population. A prospective study. Arch Intern Med 1988; **48**: 562.

229. Saah AJ, Neufeld R, Rodstein M et al. Influenza vaccine and pneumonia mortality in a nursing home population. Arch Intern Med 1986; **146**: 2353.

230. Ruben FL. Prevention of influenza in the elderly. J Amer Geriatr Soc 1982; **30**: 577–80.

231. DeStefano F, Goodman RA, Noble GR. Simultaneous administration of influenza and pneumococcal vaccines. J Amer Med Assoc 1982; **247**: 2551–4.
232. Ryan MP, MacLeod AF. A comparison of adverse effects of two influenza vaccines and the influence on subsequent uptake. J Roy Coll Gen Practit 1984; **34**: 442–4.
233. Albazazz MK, Harvey JE, Grilli EA et al. Subunit influenza vaccination in adults with asthma: effect on clinical state, airway reactivity, and antibody response. Brit Med J 1987; **294**: 1196–7.
234. McDowell I et al. Comparison of three methods of recalling patients for influenza vaccination. Can Med Assoc J 1986; **135**: 991–7.
235. Larson EB et al. Do post-card reminders improve influenza vaccination compliance? A prospective trial of different post-card 'cues'. Medcare 1982; **20**: 639–48.
236. McDowell I et al. Comparison of three methods of recalling patients for influenza vaccination. Can Med Assoc J 1986; **135**: 991–7.
237. Hoey JR et al. Expanding the nurse's role to improve preventive services in an out-patient clinic. Can Med Assoc J 1982; **127**: 27–8.
238. Hutchison B. Effectiveness of computer generated nurse/physician reminders as a means of increasing influenza vaccine coverage in the elderly. Unpublished data. Department of Family Medicine McMaster University, Ontario, 1986.
239. Little JW, Hall WJ, Douglas RG. Amantidine effect on peripheral airway abnormalities in influenza. Annals Intern Med 1976; **85**: 177–80.
240. Stange KC, Little DW, Blatnik B. Adverse reactions to amantadine prophylaxis of influenza in a retirement home. J Amer Geriatr Soc 1991; **39**: 700–5.
241. Dolin R, Reichman RC, Madore HP. A controlled trial of Amantidine and Rimantidine in the prophylaxis of influenza A vaccine. N Engl J Med 1982; **307**: 580-4.
242. Klarman HE, Guzick D. Economics of influenza. In: Selby P (ed) Influenza: Virus, Vaccines and Strategy. New York: Academic Press, 1976.
243. Riddiough MA et al. Influenza vaccination: cost-effectiveness and public policy. J Amer Med Assoc 1983; **249**: 3189–95.
244. Helliwell BE, Drummond M. The costs and benefits of preventing influenza in Ontario's elderly. Unpublished Manuscript, Department of Clinical Epidemiology and Biostatistics, McMaster University, Ontario 1984.
245. Jolleys J. Treatment of shingles and post-herpetic neuralgia. Brit Med J 1989; **298**: 1537–8.
246. Russell K, Portenoy RK, Duma C, Folley KM. Acute herpetic and post-herpetic neuralgia: clinical review on current management. Annals Neurol 1986; **20**: 651–61.
247. Demorgas JM, Kierland RR. The outcome of patients with herpes zoster. Arch Dermatol 1957; **75**: 193–6.
248. Weller TH, Varicella and herper zoster: changing concepts of the natural history, control and importance of a not-so-benign virus. N Engl J Med 1983; **309**: 1362–8.
249. McKendrick MW, McGill JI, White JE et al. Oral Acyclovir in acute herpes zoster. Brit Med J 1986; **293**: 1529–32.
250. Wood MJ, Ogan PH, McKendrick MW et al. Efficacy of oral Acyclovir treatment of acute herpes zoster. Amer J Med 1988; **85**: 79–83.
251. Huff JC, Bean B, Balfour HH et al. Therapy of Herpes zoster with oral Acyclovir. Amer J Med 1988; **85**: 84–9.

252. Morton P, Thomson AN. Oral Acyclovir in the treatment of herpes zoster in General Practice. NZ Med J 1989; **102**: 93–5.
253. Cobo M. Reduction in the occular complications of herpes zoster ophthalmicus by oral Acyclovir. Amer J Med 1988; **85**: 90–3.
254. Kernbaum S, Hauchecorne J. Administration of levadopa for relief of herpes zoster pain. J Amer Med Assoc 1981; **246**: 132–4.
255. Weber DJ, Rutala WA, Parham C. Impact on costs of varicella prevention in a university hospital. Amer J. Public Health 1988; **78**: 19–23.
256. Schneider EL. Infectious diseases in the elderly. Annals Intern Med 1983; **98**: 395–400.
257. Bentley DW. Pneumococcal vaccine in institutionalised elderly. Review of past and recent studies. Rev Infect Dis 1981; **3**: S61–S70.
258. Garibaldi RA, Brodine S, Matsumiya S. Infections among patients in nursing homes. Policies, prevalence and problems. N Engl J Med 1981; **305**: 731–5.
259. Farr BM, Cobb DK, Johnston BC et al. Case-controlled study of pneumococcal vaccine (pv) efficacy in preventing pneumococcal bacteriaemia (pb) (abstract). 29th Inter-Science Conference on Anti-microbial Agents and Chemotherapy 1989, p. 174.
260. Shapiro ED, Berg AT, Austrian R et al. The protective efficacy of polyvalent pneumococcal polysaccharide vaccine. N Engl J Med 1991; **325**: 1453.
261. Sims RV, Steinman WC, McConvill JH et al. The clinical effectiveness of pneumococcal vaccine in the elderly. Annals Intern Med 1988; **108**: 653–7.
262. Broome CV, Facklam RR, Fraser DW. Pneumococcal disease after pneumococcal vaccination: an alternative method to estimate the efficacy of pneumococcal vaccine. N Engl J Med 1980; **303**: 549.
263. Shapiro ED, Clemens JD. A controlled evaluation of the protective efficacy of pneumococcal vaccine for patients at high risk of serious pneumococcal infections. Annals Intern Med 1984; **101**: 325.
264. Hirschmann JV, Lipsky BA. Pneumococcal vaccine in the United States – a critical analysis. J Amer Med Assoc 1981; **246**: 1428–32.
265. Bolan G, Broome CV, Fackle M et al. Pneumococcal vaccine efficacy in selected populations in the United States. Annals Intern Med 1986; **104**: 1–6.
266. Simberkoff MS, Cross AP, Al-Ibrahim M et al. Efficacy of pneumococcal vaccine in high-risk patients: results of a Veterans' Administration Co-operative study. N Engl J Med 1986; **315**: 1318.
267. Forrester HL, Jahnigen DW, LaForce FM. Inefficacy of pneumococcal vaccine in a high risk population. Amer J Med 1987; **83**: 425.
268. Fedson DS. Improving the use of pneumococcal vaccine through a strategy of hospital-based immunisation. A review of its rationale and implication. J Amer Geriatr Soc 1985; **33**: 142–50.
269. Klein RS, Adochi N. An effective hospital-based pneumococcal immunisation program. Arch Intern Med 1986; **146**: 327–9.
270. Siebers MJ, Hunt VV. Increasing the immunococcal vaccination rate of elderly patients in a general internal medicine clinic. J Amer Geriatric Soc 1985; **33**: 175–8.
271. Willems JS, Sanders CR, Riddiough et al. Cost-effectiveness of vaccination against pneumococcal pneumonia. N Engl J Med 1980; **303**: 553–9.
272. Sisk JE, Riegelman RK. Cost-effectiveness of vaccination against pneumococcal pneumonia: an update. Annals Intern Med 1986; **104**: 79–86.
273. Blagg N. Tuberculosis. In: Gleckman RA, Gantz NM (eds) Infections in the Elderly. Boston, MA: Littlebrown and Company, 1983.

274. Yoshikawa TT. Tuberculosis in aging adults. J Amer Geriatr Soc 1992; **40**: 178–87.
275. Stead WW, To T. The significance of Tuberculin skin testing in elderly patients. Annals Intern Med 1987; **107**: 837–42.
276. Report of the US Preventive Services Task Force. Screening for Tuberculosis. Chapter 21, in: Guide to Clinical Preventive Services. Baltimore, MD: Williams and Wilkins, 1989.
276a. Pattee JJ, Burton JR, Ryan JJ et al. The American Geriatrics Society statement on two-step PPD testing for nursing home patients on admission. J Amer Geriatr Soc 1988; **36**: 77–8.
277. Comstock GW, Edwards PQ. The competing risks of tuberculosis and hepatitis for adult tuberculin reactors. Amer Rev Resp Dis 1975; **111**: 573–7.
278. Tsevat J, Taylor WC, Wong JB et al. Isoniazid for the tuberculin reactor: take it or leave it. Amer Rev Resp Dis 1988; **137**: 215–20.
279. Stead WW, To T, Harrison RW et al. Benefit risk considerations in preventive treatment for tuberculosis in elderly persons. Annals Intern Med 1987; **107**: 843–5.
280. Grabenstein JD, Smith LJ, Carter DW et al. Comprehensive immunisation delivery in conjunction with influenza vaccination. Arch Intern Med 1986; **146**: 1189–92.
281. Centers for Disease Control. Tetanus reported cases by age group. United States 1980 and 1981. Morbid Mortal Weekly Rev 1982; **30**: 87–8.
282. Centers for Disease Control. Leads from the MMWR: Tetanus United States 1982–1984. J Amer Med Assoc 1985; **254**: 2877–8.
283. National Communicable Disease Center Tetanus Surveillance Report No. 4, 1970–1971. Atlanta: Centers for Disease Control.
284. Varughese DVM. Surveillance summary, tetanus in Canada – 1921–1978. Can Dis Wkly Rep 1986; 113–18.
285. Newell KW, Duenas-Lehmann A, Leblanc DR et al. The use of toxoid for the prevention of tetanus neonatorum: final report of a double-blind controlled field trial. Bull WHO 1966; **35**: 863–71.
286. Boyd JSK. Tetanus in the African and European theatres of war 1939–1945. Lancet 1946; **1**: 113–19.
287. Dixon AM, Bibby JA. Tetanus immunization state in a General Practice population. Brit Med J 1988; **297**: 598.
288. Hutchison B. Cost-effectiveness of a program to increase primary tetanus immunization among elderly Canadians. Thesis, Department of Family Medicine, McMaster University, Ontario, Canada.
289. Reichel W. Complications in the care of 500 elderly hospitalised patients. J Amer Geriatr Soc 1965; **13**: 973–81.
290. Jahnigan D, Hannon S, Laxson L, LaForce FM. Iatrogenic disease in hospitalised elderly veterans. J Amer Geriatr Soc 1982; **30**: 387–90.
291. Gillick MR et al. Adverse consequences of hospitalisation in the elderly. Soc Sci Med 1982; **16**: 1033.
292. Warshaw GA, Moore J, Friedman SW et al. Functional disability in the hospitalised elderly. J Amer Med Assoc 1982; **248**: 847.
293. Winograd CH. Targeting strategies: an overview of criteria and outcomes. J Amer Geriatr Soc 1991; **39**: 25S–35S.
294. Segal D. The principles of minimal interference in the management of the elderly patient. J Chron Dis 1964; **17**: 299–300.
295. Hardison JE. To be complete. N Engl J Med 1979; **300**: 193–6.

296. Rubenstein LZ, Stuck AE, Siu AL, Wieland D. Impact of geriatric evaluation in management programs on defined outcomes: overview of the evidence. J Amer Geriatr Soc 1991; **39**: 8S–16S.
297. Evans LK, Strumpf NE. Tying down the elderly: a review of the literature on physical restraint. J Amer Geriatr Soc 1989; **37**: 65–74.
298. Malfetti J. Drivers Fifty Five Plus. Falls Church Virginia: AAA Foundation for Traffic Safety, 1985.
299. Retchin SR, Cox J, Fox M, Irwin L. Performance-based measurements among elderly drivers and non-drivers. J Amer Geriatr Soc 1988; **36**: 813–19.
300. Evans L. Older driver involvement in fatal and severe traffic crashes. J Gerontol 1988; **43**: S186–S193.
301. O'Neill D. Physicians, elderly drivers and dementia. Lancet 1992; **339**: 41–3.
302. Friedland RP, Koss E, Kumar A et al. Motor vehicle crashes and dementia of the Alzheimer type. Annals Neurol 1988; **24**: 782–6.
303. O'Neill D, Neubauer K, Boyle M et al. Dementia and driving. J Roy Soc Med 1992; **85**: 199–202.
304. Carr D, Madden D, Cohen HJ, Jackson TW. The use of traffic identification signs of identify drivers with dementia. J Amer Geriatric Soc 1991; **39A**: 62.
305. Automobile Association Foundation for road safety research. Motoring and the older driver. Basingstoke, Hants: Automobile Association, 1988.
306. Drachmann DA. Who may drive? Who may not? Who shall decide? Annals Neurol 1988; **24**: 787–8.
307. Simson JNL. Seat belts six years on. J Roy Soc Med 1989; **82**: 125–6.
308. MCAP/AA Working Group. Helping the older driver. Basingstone, Hants: The Medical Commission on Accident Prevention and the Automobile Association, 1990.
309. Nankhonya JM, Turnbull CJ, Newton JT. Social and functional impact of minor fractures in elderly people. Brit Med J 1992; **303**: 1514–15.
310. Report of the US Preventive Services Task Force. Screening for Post-Menopausal Osteoporosis. Chapter 40, in: Guide to Clinical Preventive Services. Baltimore, MD: Williams and Wilkins, 1989.
311. Law MR, Wald NJ, Meade TW. Strategies for prevention of osteoporosis and hip fracture. Brit Med J 1991; **303**: 453–9.
311a. Chapuy MC, Arlot ME, Duboeuf F et al. Vitamin D3 and calcium to prevent hip fractures in elderly women. N Engl J Med 1992; **327**: 1637–42.
312. Riggs BL, Melton LJ. Involutional osteoporosis. N Engl J Med 1986; **314**: 1676–85.
312a. Lufkin EG, Wahner HW, O'Fallon WM et al. Treatment of postmenopausal osteoporosis by transdermal oestrogen administration. Annals Intern Med 1992; **117**: 1–9.
312b. Quigley ME, Martin PL, Burnier AM, Brooks P. Estrogen therapy arrests bone in elderly women. Amer J Obstet Gynecol 1987; **156**: 1516–23.
313. Goddard MK. Hormone replacement therapy and breast cancer, endometrial cancer and cardiovascular disease: risks and benefits. Brit J Gen Pract 1992; **42**: 120–5.
313a. Wilson PWF, Garrison RJ and Castelli WP. Postmenopausal estrogen use, cigarette smoking and cardiovascular morbidity in women over 50. New Engl J Med 1985; **313**: 1038–43.
313b. Devor M, Barrett-Connor E, Renwall M et al. Estrogen replacement therapy and the risk of venous thrombosis. Amer J Med 1992; **92**: 275–82.

313c. Tilyard MW, Spears GFS, Thomson J, Dovey S. Treatment of postmenopausal osteoporosis with calcitriol or calcium. N Engl J Med 1992; **326**: 357–61.

314. Watts NB, Harris ST, Genant HK et al. Intermittent cyclical etidronate treatment of post-menopausal osteoporosis. N Engl J Med 1990; **323**: 73–9.

315. Storm T, Thamsborg G, Steiniche T, et al. Effect of intermittent Etidronate therapy on bone mass and fracture rate in women with postmenopausal osteoporosis. N Engl J Med 1990; **322**: 1265–71.

316. Smith E, Reddan W, Smith P. Physical activity and calcium modalities for bone mineral increase in aged women. Med Sci Sports Exer 1981; **13**: 60–4.

317. Rundgren A, Aniansson A, Ljungbrg P et al. Effects of a training program for elderly people on mineral content of the heel bone. Arch Gerontol Geriatr 1984; **3**: 243–8.

318. Weinstein MC. Estrogen use in post-menopausal women: cost, risks and benefit. N Engl J Med 1980; **303**: 308.

319. Knowelden J, Buhr AJ, Dunbar O. Incidence of fractures in persons over 35 years of age: a report to the M.R.C. Working Party on Fractures in the Elderly. Brit J Prev Soc Med 1964; **18**: 130–41.

320. Reid J, Kennie DC. Geriatric rehabilitative care after fractures of the proximal femur: one year follow up of a randomised clinical trial. Brit Med J 1989; **299**: 25–6.

321. Holbrook TL, Grazier K, Kelsey JL et al. The Frequency of Occurrence, Impact on Cost of Selected Musculo-skeletal Conditions in the United States. Chicago: American Academy Orthopedic Surgeons, 1984.

322. Aitken JM. Relevance of osteoporosis in women with fracture of the femoral neck. Brit Med J 1984; **288**: 597–600.

323. Cooper C, Barket DJP, Morris J, Briggs RSJ. Osteoporosis, falls and age in fractures of the proximal femur. Brit Med J 1987; **295**: 13–15.

324. Blazer DG, Williams CD. Epidemiology of dysphoria and depression in an elderly population. Amer J Psychiatr 1980; **137**: 439–44.

325. Report of the US Preventive Services Task Force. Depression. Chapter 44, in: Guide to Clinical Preventive Services. Baltimore, MD: Williams and Wilkins 1989.

326. Bergmann K. Recent Developments in Psychogeriatrics. London: RMPA Publications, 1971.

327. Prestidge BR, Lake CR. Prevalence and recognition of depression among primary care out patients. J Fam Pract 1987; **25**: 67–72.

328. McNab A, Philip AE. Screening an elderly population for psychological well-being. Health Bull (Scot) 1980; **38**: 160.

329. Weiss IK, Nagel CL, Aaronson MK. Applicability of depression scales to the old person. J Amer Geriatr Soc 1986; **34**: 215–18.

329a. Koenig HG, Meador KG, Cohen HJ, Blazer DG. Screening for depression in hospitalized elderly medical patients: taking a closer look. J Amer Geriatr Soc 1992; **40**: 1013–17.

330. Post F. The management and nature of depressive illnesses in later life. Brit J Psych 1972; **121**: 393–409.

330a. McCrea D, Kaufman B, Marchevsky D, Arnold E. Screening for depression in elderly attending a hospital clinic. Paper presented at British Geriatrics Society, Scientific Meeting, London, 1992.

331. Atkinson RM. Substance use and abuse in late life. In: Atkinson RM (ed) Alcohol and Drug Abuse in Old Age, pp. 1–21. Washington, DC: American Psychiatric Press 1984.

332. Dunne FJ, Schipperheijn JAM. Alcohol in the elderly. Brit Med J 1989; **289**: 1660–1.
332a. Adams WL, Magruder-Habib K, Trued S, Brooke HL. Alcohol abuse in elderly emergency department patients. J Amer Geriat Soc 1992; **40**: 1236–40.
333. American Medical Association. Manual on Alcoholism. 3rd edit. Chicago: American Medical Association, 1977.
334. Horton AM. Alcohol in the elderly. Md Med J 1986; **35**: 916–18.
335. Willenbring ML, Christensen K, Spring WD et al. Alcoholism screening in the elderly. J Amer Geriatr Soc 1987; **35**: 864–9.
335a. Buchsbaum DG, Buchanan RF, Welsh J et al. Screening for drinking disorders in the elderly using the CAGE Questionnaire. J Amer Geriatr Soc 1992; **40**: 662–5.
336. Post F. Functional Disorders II. Treatment and its relationship to causation and outcome. In: Levy R, Post F (eds) The Psychiatry of Late Life, pp. 197–221. Oxford: Blackwell Scientific Publications, 1982.
337. Holmes TH, Rahe RH. The social readjustment rating scale. J Psychosom Res 1967; **11**: 213.
338. Haynes SG, McMichael AJ, Tyroler HA. Survival after early and normal retirement. J Gerontol 1978; **33**: 269.
339. Howard JH, Marshall J, Rechnitzer PA et al. Adapting to retirement. J Amer Geriatr Soc 1982; **30**: 488.
340. Draper JE. Work Attitudes and Retirement Adjustment. Madison, WI: University of Wisconsin Bureau of Business Research and Service, 1967.
341. McPherson B, Guppy N. Pre-retirement lifestyle and the degree of planning for retirement. J Gerontol 1979; **34**: 254.
342. Office of Population Censuses and Surveys. Social Trends No. 16, London: HMSO, 1968.
343. McAvoy BR. Death after bereavement. Brit Med J 1986; **293**:835.
344. Parkes CM. Bereavement counselling: does it work? Brit Med J 1980; **281**: 3–6.
345. Vestal RE. Drug use in the elderly: a review of problems and special considerations. Drugs 1978; **16**: 358–82.
346. Price D et al. Doctors unawareness of the drugs their patients are taking: a major cause of overprescribing? Brit Med J 1986; **292**: 99–100.
347. Fletcher RH, Fletcher SW. Iatrogenic illness and the elderly. In: Petersen MD, White DL (eds) Health Care of the Elderly – An Information Sourcebook, pp. 451–7. Newbury Park, CA; Sage Publications, 1989.
348. Dall JLC. Maintenance digoxin in elderly patients. Brit Med J 1970; **2**: 705–6.
349. Bayer AJ, Pathy MSJ. Requests for hypnotic drugs and placebo response in elderly hospital inpatients. Postgrad Med J 1986; **6**: 317–20.
350. Beers MH, Dang J, Hasegawa J et al. Influence of hospitalization on drug therapy in the elderly. J Amer Geriatr Soc 1989; **37**: 679–83.
350a. Avorn J, Soumerai SB, Everitt DE et al. Reducing the use of psychoactive drugs in nursing homes. N Engl J Med 1992; **327**: 168–73.
351. Ogilvie RI, Ruedy J. An educational program in digitalis therapy. J Amer Med Assoc 1972; **222**: 50–5.
352. Hatoum HT, Catizone C, Hutchinson RA, Purohit A. An eleven-year review of the pharmacy literature: documentation of the value and acceptance of clinical pharmacy. Drug Intell Clin Pharm 1986; **20**: 33–48.
353. Wandless I, Davie JW. Can drug compliance in the elderly be improved? Brit Med J 1977; **1**: 359–61.

354. Gatley MS. To be taken as directed. J Roy Coll Gen Practit 1968; **6**: 39–44.
355. Sherman F, Warrach JD, Libow LS. Child resistant containers for the elderly. J Amer Med Assoc 1979; **241**: 1001–2.
356. Morrow D, Leirer V, Sheikh J. Adherence and medication instructions: review and recommendations. J Amer Geriatr Soc 1988; **36**: 1147–60.
357. Crome P, Akehurst M, Keet J. Drug compliance in elderly hospital inpatients. Trial of the Dosset box. Practitioner 1980; **224**: 782–5.
358. Branch LG, Jette AM. Personal health practices and mortality among the elderly. Amer J Pub Health 1984; **74**: 1126–9.
359. Branch LG, Jette AM. Health practices and incident disability among the elderly. Amer J Pub Health; **75**: 1436–9.
360. Fries JR. Aging, natural death and the compression of morbidity. N Engl J Med 1980; **303**: 130–5.
361. Schneider EL, Reed JD. Life extension. N Engl J Med 1985; **312**: 1159–68.
362. Rudman D, Feller AG, Nagraj HS et al. Effects of human growth hormone in men over 60 years of age. N Engl J Med 1990; **323**: 1–6.
363. Jubb RW. Topical Reviews: Anti Rheumatic Druge and Articular Cartilage. Reports on Rheumatic Diseases (Series 2) No. 20. London: Arthritis and Rheumatism Council For Research, UK, 1992.
364. Editorial. Does topical tretinoin prevant cutaneous ageing? Lancet 1988; **1**: 977–8.

8

Enhancing functional status

General deconditioning with age

Importance

In the adult years, activity is at its highest in the twenties and thirties. There-after, activity levels decline as energetic leisure time pursuits are abandoned. These levels then remain stable until retirement, when a second major decline in activity occurs [1]. There is evidence that a significant proportion of the changes commonly ascribed to the ageing process are, in fact, the biological consequences of this inactivity and disuse [2]. Foremost amongst these changes is cardiovascular deconditioning as manifest by the maximum oxygen consumption, which declines at about 1 per cent per annum with age, but a range of other changes such as reduced red cell mass, loss of lean body mass and osteoporosis have, at least in part, been implicated as being due to disuse that occurs during ageing [2].

There is also increasing evidence that inactivity in later years is associated with an increased susceptibility to certain disabling disorders, such as cardio-vascular disease, stroke and hip fracture, that play a major role in functional decrement. Furthermore, further deconditioning rapidly accompanies the recumbent bed rest [3] and even non-recumbent rest that results from the frequent bouts of intercurrent illness commonly occurring in the elderly population.

Targeting/detection

It is extremely difficult to distinguish between the normal ageing process and the changes due to inactivity and disease. No reliable technique is available to

171

identify those at particular risk of inactivity. Health promotional measures must therefore be applied to the whole of the elderly population.

The inactivity from intercurrent illness that accompanies ageing is more easily targeted by the presence of active rehabilitation programmes in hospital and by the avoidance of overprotection by family carers.

Effectiveness

Physical effects of exercise activity

Physical training programmes have been shown to reduce the decline in maximum oxygen consumption that accompanies ageing [4], to increase muscle strength [5], to improve joint mobility [6] and to improve the sense of balance [7].

Several reviews discuss, in more detail, physical activity programming in older adults [8, 9] and imaginative yet acceptable exercise programmes have been developed for integration into the social life of elderly people [10]. Nevertheless, there is very limited information on the long term compliance with exercise in previously sedentary elderly populations. Group, versus individual, activity and the personality of the activity leader play a significant role in the degree of adherence with such activity programmes [11].

Only isotonic exercises are recommended because isometric exercise is not advantageous and can lead to a dangerous increase in systolic blood pressure. Traditionally it was thought that an improvement in cardiovascular fitness requires a threshold level of aerobic intensity during an exercise session and a minimum frequency of sessions. This led to various exercise prescriptions, one being the dynamic movement of large muscle groups for at least 20 minutes, three or more days per week performed at an intensity of at least 60 per cent of cardiovascular capacity. A further refinement for elderly people was to reach and maintain a pulse rate equal to the formula $(220 - \text{age}) \times 70$ per cent. More recently, however, several studies have shown that low to moderate intensity exercise programmes will result in significant, if less substantial, improvements [12–17].

The health risks associated with exercising are largely unevaluated for the very old population, though the relative risk of sudden death related to the exercise is reduced in those 50 to 69 years compared with younger age groups [18], and Shephard [1] comments that because elderly people are less ambitious exercisers, they tend to sustain less traumatic and less severe overuse injuries.

Neuropsychological effects of exercise activity

Exercise may slow the deterioration in central processing reaction time that occurs with age [20]. An improvement has also been shown in memory and cognition immediately following exercise. The clinical significance of this remains doubtful, however, and a three-month programme of gentle exercise failed to show any lasting effect on neuropsychological function in elderly institutionalised women [21]. However, sustained physical activity on reaching retiral has been shown to be associated with sustained cerebral perfusion and cognition [22] and, recently, a planned programme of walking was also found to improve the communication performance of nursing home patients with established Alzheimer's dementia [23].

The intensity of exercise required to influence higher cortical function is largely unknown and may account for some of the variation in the above findings.

Exercise activity and cardiovascular disease

As a primary preventive measure, exercise in observational studies in subjects up to 84 years of age is associated with a significant reduction in cardiovascular mortality [24]. These studies suggest that the reduction in coronary disease risk associated with exercising may actually be greater for older than for younger subjects. Even in previously sedentary elderly people, the introduction of an exercise programme has been shown to both delay and reduce the likelihood of cardiovascular morbid events [25].

The benefits of exercise in secondary prevention programmes for cardio-vascular mortality are uncertain and the evidence is mostly confined to younger age groups [26–28].

Exercise activity and stroke disease

One study of exercise in middle aged men found a significant correlation between moderate physical activity and reduced risk of stroke disease [29] and a more recent study of subjects over 55 years of age found that both recent and past exercise appeared to contribute independently to prevent further stroke [30]. However, the value of exercise in preventing stroke disease is still to be proven by an interventional trial.

Exercise activity and hip fracture

The impact of exercise activity on hip fracture is summarised on p. 141.

Other effects of exercise activity

Exercise has also been shown to slow age-related changes in serum lipids and insulin levels. Its effect on other parameters is discussed as follows: osteoporosis (see p. 137); falls (see p. 185); and longevity (see p. 150).

The effectiveness of counselling

Information on the long term effectiveness of counselling elderly people to influence their exercise activity patterns is extremely limited.

Cost

Little information is available on the costs of exercise and activity programmes particularly for an older population. The principles behind calculating the cost effectiveness of an exercise programme is, however, discussed in detail by Russell [31].

Memory impairment

Importance

Chronic memory and cognitive impairment, as manifested by senile dementia, is *the* major health problem for the elderly population. Although the precise prevalence in the community varies depending on the populations being screened, a recent careful study reported 3 per cent of the community population aged 65 to 74 years had probable Alzheimer's disease and this proportion rose to 18.7 per cent for those 75 to 84 years and to 47.2 per cent for those over 85 years old [32]. Dementia is a major cause of death in western societies [33]. It is responsible for much morbidity in the form of falls [34], fractures, chronic incontinence of bladder and bowel and psychological distress to the sufferers. Dementia is also a major stressor for family carers [35]. The cost of resourcing the community and institutional care for dementia sufferers is enormous, and in the USA is estimated to cost $30 billion annually [36].

Detection

Detection should be considered in two stages. The first is to determine the existence of significant cognitive impairment. This has been shown to be possible using short, simple screening instruments that can be used by relatively untrained non-medical staff [37]. Two of the most commonly used and best validated are the Mini-mental State Examination [38] and Pfeiffer's Short Portable Mental Status Questionnaire [39]. The appropriate performance of these tests alone is of significant value in inferring the existence of dementia if coupled with corroborative evidence on the timescale for which the disorder has been present.

Nevertheless, depending on the perceived value of trying to establish a more precise diagnosis of the underlying disease state and pathology, an increasingly sophisticated battery of interventions may need to be conducted. Belief in the required extent of this additional workup varies considerably between different health care systems and is not here considered further as an issue of screening.

There appears to be relatively little value in subjecting elderly individuals to a highly sensitive psychological screening battery for mild cognitive impairment. Indeed, there seems little justification to screening investigations that look for various biochemical or neurophysiological markers of early Alzheimer disease [40], because the specificity of these measures is not as yet fully elucidated, and there appears to be significant overlap between the 'normal' and the 'impaired' elderly population. Likewise, screening for age-associated memory impairment (benign senescent forgetfulness) is fraught with methodological problems, some researchers believing most people over 50 years to be affected [41].

Effectiveness

A comprehensive review of the potential for preventing mental disorders in elderly people has recently been provided by Rabins [41a]. When considering memory impairment, the effectiveness of screening (and the knowledge that significant cognitive impairment exists) needs to be evaluated carefully against a number of possible outcomes.

Therapeutic optimism

Earlier hopes that a high proportion of dementia was of a reversible nature have not been sustained. In a careful review of 32 studies on the potential and actual reversibility of dementia, Clarfield [42] concluded that 11 per cent of dementias resolved, either partially (8 per cent) or fully (3 per cent). However, most of these studies came from secondary or tertiary care centres and the true incidence of reversible démentia in the community was probably lower than that reported. It is also significant to note that the commonest reversible causes would not be considered by many as 'dementia' at all. These causes included drugs (28.2 per cent), depression (26.2 per cent) and metabolic factors (15.5 per cent).

With recent advances in medical science it is not unreasonable to assume that the conventional irreversible causes of senile dementia, such as the Alzheimer's and multi-infarct types, might now or in future be amenable to newer therapeutic modalities. However, although some such studies hold a degree of promise for future research [43–45], none is currently at a stage where it holds sufficient utility to merit its widespread application.

Preventing cognitive decline

Although there is currently little that can be done to slow the decline of well established Alzheimer's dementia, the possibility exists that, if identified in its earlier stages, this disorder may prove more responsive to medical intervention. This hypothesis still remains to be proven. In particular, recent attention has focussed on treating the ill-defined concept of age-associated memory impairment. The effects of administering phosphatidylserine to such a group of 'impaired' elderly people has been described [46], but implications of the results await further clarification of the disease entity itself. The area of most optimism may lie in the promise of some reduction in the rate of decline of the multi-infarct variety of dementia by careful lowering of hypertension and the cessation of smoking [46a]. Secondary prevention of multi-infarct dementia has also been successfully demonstrated by Meyer et al. [46b]. They demonstrated better cognitive performance in a group of stroke patients randomised to aspirin prophylaxis than patients receiving placebo up to three years after the event.

Preventing institutionalisation

There is evidence from a number of studies [47–49] that the early detection of dementia, coupled with the prescription of appropriate supportive community services and counselling, does not reduce or delay the number of dementia sufferers being admitted for long term care. Indeed, in two of the studies, greater numbers in the screening and intervention group were admitted than in the control group. It may be that, once problems are detected, individual and societal anxiety about the situation makes it extremely difficult to ignore and take no further perceived protective action.

Although this may be considered an adverse outcome in terms of resource use, it may nevertheless, in many situations, be action that was required and was long overdue because of severe carer burden or recurrent crises.

Reducing carer burden

Regrettably there is little information on the impact of dementia screening and case-finding programmes on carer burden and psychological wellbeing, even though this may be *the* principal reason for their being mounted.

The avoidance of crises

There are also many crises that may arise in undetected dementia sufferers. These include: wandering and getting lost; wandering without clothing; hypothermia; soiling with excrement; malnutrition; fire-induced injury to self or others; and falls and fractures. Future studies gauging the efficacy of screening and case finding would do well to include a comparison of the occurrence of these events between intervention and control groups.

Influence on other management decisions

A final reason for the early detection of dementia is the assistance it gives in influencing other treatment and management decisions. Such decisions include avoiding relocation, taking particular care to avoid iatrogenic insult from drugs, anaesthesia or surgery, the degree of supervision required to ensure compliance with medication, and necessary arrangements to safeguard the various forms of abuse to which the demented population is subject. These issues should also be taken into account when assessing the value of screening and case-finding programmes for dementia.

Cost

No detailed information on costings is available, though Eastwood and Corbin [50], assuming a comprehensive approach, suggested that providing diagnostic services in neuropsychiatric units for all suspected dementia cases would be prohibitive. Assuming an annual incidence of 1 per cent among persons aged over 65 years, and a conservative estimate of $5000 for investigating each patient, they estimated the annual number of new cases in Canada at 22000 and the total cost of specialist diagnosis at not less than $100 million (Canadian 1981 prices). In the light of the previous comments, such a specialist and technological approach seems unjustified at the present time, but no estimates have been made of the more simplistic approaches outlined above.

Table 8.1. *Percentage of patients reporting functional disability and percentage of disabilities underestimated or unrecognised by physicians by practice site*

Functional disability	Patients reporting disabilities(%)			Disabilities underestimated or unrecognised by physicians (%)		
	Hospital-based	Office-based	Total	Hospital-based	Office-based	Total
Basic activities of daily living						
Taking care of self	6	10	8	89	78	81
Moving in and out of a bed or chair	9	8	8	79	74	76
Walking indoors	9	7	8	79	56	67
Instrumental activities of daily living						
Walking one block or climbing one flight of stairs	23	22	22	74	60	66
Walking several blocks	30	33	31	67	60	63
Doing work around the house	21	23	22	83	62	70
Doing errands	22	24	23	81	63	70
Driving a car or using public transportation	18	15	16	79	63	70
Doing vigorous activities	53	65	60	62	39	47
Social activities						
Visiting with relatives or friends	18	12	15	93	86	89
Participating in community activities	22	22	22	89	82	85
Taking care of other people	14	19	17	64	62	63
Total				75[a]	60[a]	66

[a] $P < 0.05$ for difference between rates in two practice types.
Adapted from ref. [54].

Poor mobility

Importance

Numerous surveys have studied the prevalence of disability in the elderly population. However, the different descriptors and criteria used make comparisons difficult. Nevertheless, there is undoubted increase with increasing age and variability depending on the environmental setting studied. In one report, 11 per cent of those 65 to 74 years, and 25 per cent of those over 75 years, had trouble moving around their house [51]. In another, 14 per cent of those 65 to 74 years, 23 per cent of those 75 to 84 years and 40 per cent of those 85 years and over reported difficulty in walking [52]. Similarly, in the acute hospital, impaired mobility was reported in one study in 17 per cent of those 70 to 74 years of age and almost 60 per cent of those over 85 years [53]. The prevalence of immobility is even higher in chronically institutionalised populations, rising to around 80 or 90 per cent in nursing homes and geriatric long stay wards.

Mobility is the physical cornerstone for being able to carry out most other activities of daily living. Immobility is therefore a major cause of dependence, of consumption of community support services and of institutionalisation. Additionally, immobility leads to a wide range of physical complications associated with rest.

Detection

Results from a number of studies indicate that physicians often underestimate or fail to recognise functional disabilities that are reported by their patients. This may lead to deficiencies in care and to patient dissatisfaction with the care offered. Calkins et al. [54], in assessing the ability of doctors to identify mobility problems reported by various groups of patients (60 per cent of whom were over 60 years of age), found the significant discrepancies shown in Table 8.1. Hospital based physicians underestimated these problems more often than did physicians in office based practices within the community.

Neuromuscular impairments elicited in the conventional clinical examination cannot be relied upon to predict mobility problems because the relationship between neuromuscular findings and functional status is not sufficiently predictable to do so. For example, Tinetti [55] found that, although hip and knee flexion are needed to sit down safely, abnormal hip flexion was present in only 15 per cent and abnormal knee flexion in only 30 per cent of elderly subjects who had difficulty sitting down. Therefore additional

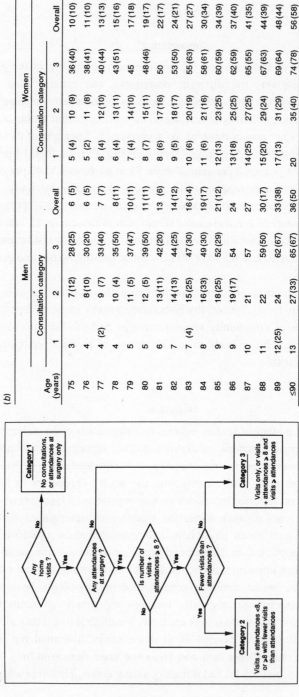

Fig. 8.1. (a) Flowchart for assigning patients to consultation categories, based on consultations, visits and attendances in the previous two years. (b) Forecast percentages and, in parentheses, actual percentages of patients with severe disability ranked according to age, sex, and consultation category. Adapted from ref. [61].

(a)

Any home visits?
No → Category 1
No consultations, or attendances at surgery only
Yes ↓

Any attendances at surgery?
No → Category 3
Visits only, or visits + attendances ≥ 8 and visits > attendances
Yes ↓

Is number of visits + attendances ≥ 8?
No → Category 2
Visits + attendances <8, or ≥8 with fewer visits than attendances
Yes ↓

Fewer visits than attendances?
Yes → Category 2
Visits + attendances <8, or ≥8 with fewer visits than attendances
No → Category 3
Visits only, or visits + attendances ≥ 8 and visits > attendances

(b)

Age (years)	Men				Women			
	Consultation category			Overall	Consultation category			Overall
	1	2	3		1	2	3	
75	3	7 (12)	28 (25)	6 (5)	5 (4)	10 (9)	36 (40)	10 (10)
76	4	8 (10)	30 (20)	6 (5)	5 (2)	11 (8)	38 (41)	11 (10)
77	4 (2)	9 (7)	33 (40)	7 (7)	6 (4)	12 (10)	40 (44)	13 (13)
78	4	10 (4)	35 (50)	8 (11)	6 (4)	13 (11)	43 (51)	15 (16)
79	5	11 (5)	37 (47)	10 (11)	7 (4)	14 (10)	45	17 (18)
80	5	12 (5)	39 (50)	11 (11)	8 (7)	15 (11)	48 (46)	19 (17)
81	6	13 (11)	42 (20)	13 (6)	8 (6)	17 (16)	50	22 (17)
82	7	14 (13)	44 (25)	14 (12)	9 (5)	18 (17)	53 (50)	24 (21)
83	7 (4)	15 (25)	47 (30)	16 (14)	10 (6)	20 (19)	55 (63)	27 (27)
84	8	16 (33)	49 (30)	19 (17)	11 (6)	21 (16)	58 (61)	30 (34)
85	9	18 (25)	52 (29)	21 (12)	12 (13)	23 (25)	60 (59)	34 (39)
86	9	19 (17)	54	24	13 (18)	25 (25)	62 (59)	37 (40)
87	10	21	57	27	14 (25)	27 (25)	65 (55)	41 (35)
88	11	22	59 (50)	30 (17)	15 (20)	29 (24)	67 (63)	44 (39)
89	12 (25)	24	62 (67)	33 (38)	17 (13)	31 (29)	69 (64)	48 (44)
≤90	13	27 (33)	65 (67)	36 (50)	20	35 (40)	74 (78)	56 (58)

simple assessments need to be employed that reproduce daily mobility manoeuvres.

The inclusion of such simple, systematic measurements of functional status into routine clinical practice has been well recommended [56] and several such assessments are available for mobility. The 'Get Up and Go Test' [57], the 'Performance Oriented Assessment of Mobility' [58] and the 'Physical Performance Test' [59] require little time, expertise of equipment to perform and increase provider cognisance of the problem of immobility and of its severity.

However, not all consultations with elderly individuals need or benefit from the inclusion of screening measures for functional disability. To attempt to do so for the whole of the elderly population would merely be inappropriate, time consuming and expensive. Therefore, there is currently considerable interest in the best means of targeting the minority of elderly people who would most benefit from such measures. Clinical experience suggests functional screening may be of value in those referred for long term institutional care or because families are under stress in their caring role. Various targeting strategies for elderly hospitalised patients are also being developed [60]. Refined methods of targeting also need to be developed for the larger number of individuals presenting for consultation at community based, primary care practices. Recently, Hall and Channing [61], in a British general practice, attempted to do this by reviewing their patients living in the community aged 75 years and over and devising a statistical model for predicting disability based on information wholly contained within their medical records. This model, based on age, sex and pattern of consultation (see Fig. 8.1) provided a quick indication of elderly patients' tendency to severe disability that was helpful in screening in day to day conditions.

Effectiveness

A number of strategies are available to promote mobility.

Screening for disability

A recent randomised trial of functional disability screening attempted to evaluate whether feedback to physicians by means of a questionnaire completed each quarter would be used by them to improve patient outcomes. Although 43 per cent of the experimental group physicians reported that they had used the questionnaire to change therapy, patient diaries failed to show any real differences between this group and the control group in terms of management or exercise programmes ordered. There were no significant differences between the groups at exit from the study on any measure of functional status or health outcome [62].

The results of this study enforce the need for caution before widespread screening for functional disability is carried out, but it by no means indicates that *all* functional screening is valueless. Indeed, the subjects studied, although being identified as having at least one disability identified on a 13-item questionnaire, were nevertheless fit enough to attend the physicians' primary care practice. Moreover, only 36 per cent of the experimental group patients were over 70 years of age. This information alone raises the possibility of inadequate targeting of the severely disabled sufficient to show impact of the screening intervention. Furthermore, the data supplied by the 34-item screening questionnaire were presumably unfocussed and in excess of that required to make more limited clinical decisions. The information was also not obtained directly by the physicians but was provided passively to them, a process which may fail to alter clinical behaviour.

Rehabilitation

Several randomised trials have shown the efficacy of rehabilitation in restoring mobility in elderly patients after disabling illness. This is particularly the case with stroke [63] and with hip fracture patients [64]. Rehabilitation, started as late as a year after stroke, has also been shown to improve gait speed [65]. Supervised fitness walking has been shown to increase walking distance and functional status in patients with osteoarthritis of the knee [66].

Functionally orientated care

Traditionally, rehabilitation is associated with the specialised input from a variety of therapy staff. Yet, relatively simple care, orientated towards the restoration of function, has been shown in several trials to be as effective in achieving outcomes for the majority of individuals [67, 68]. The nurses' role in this process is of particular importance and certain models of care, such as Dorothea Orem's self-care deficit theory of nursing practice, seem particularly pertinent to the rehabilitative environment [69].

Maintenance theory

The natural history of functional status associated with many chronic disorders in older people is one of progressive decline. For example, Garroway et al. [70] showed that 12 months after successfully rehabilitating stroke patients from stroke disease, almost a fifth of them had deteriorated to their previous dependent state. Controlled trials have shown that ongoing rehabilitative care can assist in preventing such functional decline after hospital discharge [71].

Reduction of handicap

Reducing handicap from disability may be considered as tertiary prevention. Recently, Hart et al. [72] showed the benefit of a screening programme for locomotor disability and the provision of aids for daily living. This was performed as a randomised controlled trial in a London population of subjects over 85 years living in the community. The percentage improvement for transfers on and off a toilet between initial and follow up assessments was 13 for the control group versus 71 for the intervention group provided with a raised toilet seat.

Cost

Few detailed costings are available. One estimate of the cost for screening the London population of 85 year olds referred to above [72], and for providing aids for daily living, concluded that the cost–benefit (product of the prevalence of disability, the percentage benefit conferred and the costs incurred) for the transferring disability screened was £73.60 (1990 prices). Screening for more than one disability concurrently was more cost effective.

Falls

Importance

Estimates of the likelihood of falling amongst community-living elderly people range from 24 to 62 falls per 100 [73]. The incidence of falls in institutionalised elderly people depends on the frailty of the population studied and their level of permitted activity. The incidence of falls in a geriatric hospital population has been calculated as 422 per 1000 patient bed days [74]. The incidence in more active elderly people in nursing homes and in residential homes is twice that level [75].

Falls lead to hypothermia, pneumonia, subdural haematoma, loss of confidence, the imposition of rest, worsened mobility and institutionalisation. The most common severe outcome from falls is hip fracture, the incidence of the latter doubling every five years after age 60 [76]. Falls are the leading source of injury-related deaths, which, in turn, is the sixth most common cause of death in those 75 years and older [77].

Targeting/Detection

The natural history of falls in old age remains unclear. Evidence suggests that there may be two categories of fallers. The first and, probably, larger group are those presenting after a single fall. This group may be more prone to serious injury such as hip fracture. The one-off nature of the event and the absence of lag time before injury may limit the impact of preventive measures. The second, and probably smaller group, are those presenting with recurrent falls, who may suffer less severe injury but rather experience anxiety, worsened mobility and eventually demand for long term institutionalisation.

Detection measures for those at risk of falling either singly or multiply consist of direct observation of the performance of the position changes and gait manoeuvres used during daily activities. Again, simple tests of balance and gait, such as the 'Get Up and Go Test' [57] or the 'Performance Oriented Assessment of Mobility' [58] can be useful.

Various risk profiles have also been drawn up to identify the risk of more falls in elderly people with recurrent (non-syncopal) falls. These have been based on retrospective clinical data, clinical features and gait pattern analysis. Using some of these data, the proportion of subjects in one study with two or more falls per year increased from 0.10 for those with none or one of the risk factors to 0.69 for those with four or more risk factors [78].

Effectiveness

A number of strategies are available to reduce the risk of falling in elderly people. The efficacy of these programmes has been well reviewed by Campbell [79] who concluded that, although the factors that increase the risk of falling have been identified, programmes of primary prevention or post-fall rehabilitation have not been tried and proved.

Professional assessment and treatment

The benefit of professional assessment and treatment of underlying causes in elderly people who fall (particularly with syncope) is well documented [80] and should always be the first health maintenance measure employed.

Reducing adverse medication

Reduction in the frequency of subsequent falls can be expected by reducing or discontinuing medications that cause parkinsonism, postural hypotension, drowsiness and impaired psychomotor responsiveness. A recent extensive study from the USA implicated long-acting hypnotics, antidepressants and certain antipsychotic medications as being significantly associated with fracture inducing falls. Short-acting hypnotics were not so implicated [81].

Fall rehabilitation programmes

There is little evidence to support the use of formal fall rehabilitation programmes. One well-designed controlled trial of fall evaluation and rehabilitation in an institutional setting failed to show any difference in subsequent fall rate in the actively treated group compared with controls [82]. Similarly, in another study there was no difference in subsequent fall rates between those given short term or long term physiotherapy [83]. In a recent primary preventive study the effectiveness of exercise and cognitive-behavioural programmes held in 'senior centres' in a community in the USA were compared with discussion control programmes [83a]. No significant difference was observed in time to first fall and secondary outcome measures such as strength, balance, fear of falling and perceived health did not significantly change. A further community study in which a community nurse was used to correct nutritional deficiencies, counsel on smoking and alcohol reduction, refer for appropriate medical conditions, assess and correct environmental hazards and refer for exercise therapy, found no significant differences in the fall or fracture rates between the intervention and control groups [84]. It is suggested that these disappointing results may be due to increased activity rates in the intervention groups with consequent increased predisposition to fall. 'Thus in our present state of knowledge, a falls rehabilitation programme for older people is either a research undertaking or an act of good faith' [79].

Other types of exercise

Exercise is considered to be of importance and can be thought of in four categories. Firstly, general exercise throughout old age, which has been shown to improve balance, sensory feedback, posture and mobility. Secondly, a course of rehabilitation, which often follows a period of enforced rest because of illness. This exercise avoids the 'hypokinetic state' of unsteady gait and recurrent falls that so often accompany reduced activity. Thirdly, exercise (emphasising balance, sensory feedback and gait training techniques) can be of benefit to recurrent fallers. Lastly, various specific exercise techniques are proposed for the minority of elderly people who fall because of true ataxia or peripheral neuropathy [85].

Elimination of home hazards

Home hazards are implicated in about 17 per cent of non-syncopal falls in elderly people [78]. Several checklists are available for their identification [80]

Table 8.2. *Fall proofing checklist*

Lighting
Adequate illumination, particularly of stairs and landings
Avoidance of shadows
Easily-accessible switches at doors of rooms
Light switches at top and foot of stairs
Use of nightlights in bedrooms and access corridors to toilets

Footwear
Use of proper shoes rather than slippers
Low heels
Non-skid soles

Carpets
Preferably wall-to-wall or edges tacked down completely
Thick, shock-absorbent underlay
Non-skid backing to carpets and rugs
Minimise use of scatter rugs

Floors
No highly-polished surfaces
Use of non-slip polish
Remove wooden thresholds from doorways

Bathroom
Non-skid rubber mats in shower or bath
Use of handrails by bath and toilet
Use of raised toilet seat
Use of bath seat/shower chair
Wipe water/spills from floor promptly

Kitchen
Easy access to storage areas to avoid stretching/bending
Wipe water/spills from floor promptly

Stairs
Windows in doors leading to stairwells to allow visualisation of stairs
Clear delineation of top and bottom steps
Non-skid treads
Steps in good repair
Handrails bilateral, graspable, end projecting beyond last step and shaped to signify
    bottom of stairway

Miscellaneous
Control pets and children to avoid collisions and avoidance reactions
Avoid chairs on castors
Ensure wheelchair brakes on before transferring
Avoid flex or cable extensions at floor height that can be tripped over

---

Kennie DC, Reid JR. Brit J Hosp Med 1990; **44**: 112.

(see Table 8.2). Elimination of hazards that make activities of daily living more difficult (e.g. poor lighting, inaccessible storage space, low seats and chairs) may be particularly beneficial in reducing the risk of falls [78]. The type of surface on which the old person falls has not been shown to be of importance [86].

The potential benefit of this preventive strategy may be restricted by the extent to which elderly people are reluctant to make lifestyle changes to reduce their chances of falling. One study found that the interventions of a community nurse (health visitor) were welcomed when such visits were confined to medical matters or the correct taking of drugs but were rejected in the majority of cases when they included environmental manipulation and devising systems for alerting others to the consequences of falls [87].

Adequate supervision in institutions

An important strategy to minimise falls in the institutionalised elderly population is to ensure adequate staffing ratios at times of maximal activity in the mornings and evenings [88]. This usually corresponds to changes in shifts. Management should therefore ensure adequate overlap of personnel at these times.

It is important to appreciate that there are limits to the extent to which falls can and should be prevented in the institutionalised elderly population. Falls can be completely eliminated by sufficient chemical or physical restraint. However, this is an unacceptable form of care and leads to physical complications and minimal discharge rates. The prevention of falls and the maintenance of mobility are therefore competing health promotional strategies and an appropriate balance must be achieved between them.

Use of dispersed alarms

The installation of an alarm system within the faller's house (particularly a body-worn device) can do much to alleviate anxiety and can prevent the complications of a 'long lie' after further falls [89]. However, the benefit of such a strategy is still to be proven in a randomised controlled trial. When selecting an alarm device it is essential to concentrate not just on the 'hardware' but on the nature, reliability and speed of the response to the emergency call.

Cost

No information is available on the costs of fall prevention.

Table 8.3. *Self-care and house-care abilities by living arrangements*

			Private households					Private households		
	Self-care scale					House-care scale				
Incapacity categories	Scale score	Activities	Lives alone (%)	Lives with spouse only (%)	Lives with others (%)	Scale[a] score	Activities	Lives alone (%)	Lives with spouse only (%)	Lives with others (%)
No incapacity	0	No difficulty with any listed activity	89.1	93.6	85.9	0	No difficulty with any listed activity	64.7	74.8	63.3
Long interval	1–5	Difficulty with: washing hair, dressing, washing hands or face / Unable to: wash hair, wash or bath all over	10.5	4.6	10.7	1–7	Difficulty with: ironing clothes, light housework, preparing/cooking meal / Unable to: do heavy shopping, wash clothes, iron clothes	31.0	20.6	29.1
Short interval	6–8	Unable to: dress, put on shoes and socks, wash hands or face	0.3	1.3	1.6	8–10	Unable to: make bed, prepare/cook meal, do light housework	4.1	4.1	5.5
Critical interval		Chairfast or bedfast	0.1	0.5	1.9		Chairfast or bedfast	0.1	0.6	2.1

Source: ref. [90].

Inability to perform the activities of daily living

Importance

The inability to perform the personal or domestic activities of daily living (ADL) is a cause of much distress to elderly people and results in much carer fatigue and breakdown. The inabilities result in the use of many community support services and eventually may be a major factor dictating institutionalisation.

Using the terms 'self care' and 'house care' as substitutes for the personal and domestic activities of daily living respectively, the prevalence of these disabilities was carefully analysed in one Scottish survey [90] and the results are shown in Table 8.3.

In another study, Hart et al [72] found that 10.6 per cent of elderly people over 85 years living in the community had difficulty putting on their shoes. Hunt [91] found that between 13 and 25 per cent of people aged over 85 years were unable to carry out mealmaking domestic activities of daily living such as opening jars, carrying a saucepan or making a cup of tea. In Hart's study [72] between 5 and 6 per cent had problems with mealmaking such as pouring a teapot, turning on a tap or carrying a saucepan.

Detection

Most nursing and social work assessments of elderly people already include data on the activities of daily living. Regrettably this is not the case with medical assessments. Many standardised functional assessment instruments are available but are considered too lengthy and overinclusive for routine use in the clinical setting. Recently, the American College of Physicians Subcommittee on Aging commissioned Feinstein and colleagues at Yale University School of Medicine to develop a simple, practical and sensible approach to screening assessment for these issues. This work has now been published [92] and recommends that the elderly person be asked about their ability to do four tasks: 'Can you transfer out of bed?'; 'Can you dress yourself?'; 'Can you prepare meals?'; 'Can you shop?'. Successful performance of these tasks usually reflects independence in other personal and domestic activities of daily living. For frail or cognitively impaired individuals the responses should, wherever possible, be corroborated by a member of the family or other carer.

Table 8.4. *Cumulative total and monthly costs to society as a whole: 1977 prices over four years with and without annual discounting of future costs*

	Excluding annual discounting		Including annual discounting	
Year/s	Matched experimental group	Matched control group	Matched experimental group	Matched control group
Total cost (£)				
1	2669	2498	2669	2498
1, 2	5101	4513	4985	4417
1, 2, 3	7349	6273	7024	6013
1, 2, 3, 4	9139	7605	8570	7164
Costs per month (£)				
1	223	247	223	247
1, 2	234	262	229	258
1, 2, 3	242	267	233	260
1, 2, 3, 4	245	268	233	259

Adapted from ref. [94].

Effectiveness

Screening for the provision of aids

Hart et al. [72] have shown the benefit of a screening programme for the provision of aids for daily living. This was performed as a randomised controlled trial in a London population of subjects over 85 years living in the community. The impact of four types of aid was studied: (a) pouring from a teapot using a tea tipper; (b) turning on a tap using a tap turner; (c) carrying a saucepan using a double-handled saucepan; and (d) putting on shoes using a shoe horn and elastic laces. The percentage improvements between initial and follow up assessments were: (a) 100 versus 33; (b) 100 versus 0; (c) 88 versus 0; and (d) 50 versus 13 for the intervention and control groups, respectively.

Care managed community services

Appropriately targeted services to those unable to carry out their activities of daily living have been shown in a number of controlled studies to prevent or delay institutionalisation. When the mechanism of delivery of these services has been flexible and coordinated through a case-managed approach they have also resulted in improved wellbeing and reduced carer stress [93].

Cost

Hart et al. [72], after screening the London population of over 85-year-olds referred to above and providing aids for daily living, concluded that the cost benefit (product of the prevalence of disability, the percentage benefit conferred and the costs incurred) for the teapot pourer, tap turner, double handled saucepan and shoe horn plus elastic laces were £78.30, £47.80, £52.50 and £88, respectively (1990 prices). Screening for more than one disability concurrently was most cost effective.

In one English study, the introduction of care-managed community services to offset the handicap of being unable to carry out the activities of daily living has been shown to result in a reduction in costs per person per month (see Table 8.4), though the longer lifespans of the recipients result in an increase in costs overall [94]. Poor targeting of support services may also allow inclusion of those with minimal handicap [95] and a consequent escalation of costs for minimal return.

Feeding/eating dependency

Importance

Feeding or eating dependency is virtually unknown in elderly people under 80 years of age living in the community, but rises to 6.5 per cent of those over 85 years of age [96]. However, loss of independent feeding or eating capacity is a much more significant problem for frail elderly people in institutions, some surveys reporting prevalence rates of 32 to 50 per cent [97, 98]. Deficient nutrient intake in institutionalised elderly populations is largely confined to this subgroup [99].

Detection

Although feeding or eating dependency correlates highly with impaired mobility and cognition, upper extremity dysfunction and abnormalities of the oral and pharyngeal stages of swallowing [97], the only reliable detection manoeuvre for feeding/eating dependency appears to be close observation by nursing staff (or other care staff) who make the time to monitor feeding habits. Yet, in busy, poorly run or inadequately staffed institutions, feeding/eating dependency may be missed or underreported and regular weighing, with more careful scrutiny of those with weight loss, may form an alternative approach. Scientific validation of both these detection strategies is lacking.

Table 8.5. *The promotion of social activities*

Transport and access
Site public facilities appropriately
Improve access to public buildings
Ramp kerbs
Space out regular sitting areas
Improve bus services
Provide dial-a-lift services for the more disabled

A supportive environment
Locate public toilets conveniently
Plan for the elderly in traffic management (e.g. prolonged phasing of pedestrian
  lights)
Ensure effective community policing
Improve home security and alarm provision
Provide personal attack alarms
Develop victim support schemes

Leisure
Provide mobile library services for the housebound
Provide library services to the institutionalised
Provide large print books
Provide spoken cassettes
Provide library information services for the needs of the elderly

Continuing education
Provide pre-retirement education courses
Provide self education groups
Ensure curriculum development groups for services to retired people
Establish models such as the University of the Third Age.

Sport
Encourage sport before retirement
Provide a range of activities to cater for older women
Ensure special sessions for elderly people (e.g. at swimming pools)
Increase the attention paid to privacy in changing areas

Effectiveness

Little information is available on the extent to which the weight loss and nutritional deficiencies associated with feeding/eating dependency can be prevented. It is likely that success will be limited because of the practical and ethical issues surrounding the enhanced nutritional support of those with feeding/eating dependency and food refusal [100].

Cost

Little information on costs is available though it has been estimated that the cost of managing feeding or eating dependency is 25 per cent of the cost of caring for a *totally* dependent individual [101].

Impaired social functioning

Importance

There is evidence that a sizeable proportion of the older population experiences lessened social functioning with age. This is manifest in a wide range of interpersonal relationships, interests, leisure pursuits, hobbies and sport [1, 102]. Detailed estimations of the extent of these disabilities is, however, lacking.

Detection

Because many of the elderly population have low expectation of social activity, they rarely make spontaneous comment on limitations in this area. This may alter with the changing expectations of successive generations. Social values and desires can be elicited only if the elderly person is given time to discuss the issues and once rapport has been established.

Effectiveness

A wide range of measures are available to promote social activity and inter-action. Some are itemised in Table 8.5. There is little information on the extent to which these measures influence social functioning and/or the quality of life. Public advocacy is nevertheless a reflection of their perceived value.

Cost

Costs must be significant, but have not been detailed.

Incontinence

Importance

The prevalence of urinary incontinence in elderly men and women living in the community is 7 and 12 per cent respectively [103]. Its prevalence in British residential homes averages 16.6 per cent [104] and among elderly patients in nursing homes in the USA it reached 50 per cent [105]. During acute medical or surgical hospitalisations, 35 per cent of patients over 65 years of age are likely to be incontinent at some time during their stay.

Incontinence is a major problem for elderly people and their carers.

Incontinence increases, by a factor of almost six, their predisposition to pressure sores and skin disorders [106]. It acts as a major barrier to the discharge of hospitalised patients [107] and is a major factor in dictating the level of care at which elderly persons are able to be cared for. It results in much embarrassment and social distress to the sufferers [108], and is a major stress factor on family attendants [109]. Estimates of the economic impact of incontinence in elderly people have varied considerably depending on the different methodologies and data sources used. In reviewing the economic evidence, Hu [110] concluded that the total economic costs for the USA in 1984 were $8.1 billion. Costs incurred by nursing homes were $1.8 billion and community costs were $6.3 billion.

Detection

There are difficulties in detecting incontinence. Elderly people are reluctant to admit to it. This results in self reported rates of incontinence being almost half the real prevalence [103]. Prevention therefore depends on better public awareness that incontinence is a common, treatable problem. A further difficulty arises from the significant under-recording of this problem by physicians even when it is known to be present [111, 112].

Effectiveness

A number of preventive strategies have been attempted for incontinence.

Medical treatment

A wide range of drug treatments have been used for the maintenance of continence. These have been comprehensively reviewed by Ouslander and Sier [113]. Unfortunately, there are numerous methodological deficiencies in many of the trial reports of their efficacy but, nevertheless, several treatments show significant benefit for selected groups of elderly people. Surgical treatment for stress incontinence in elderly women can also be successful in selected cases [114].

Toileting schedules

Hadley [115] has reviewed evidence of the efficacy of bladder training and related therapies in older people and concluded there was evidence to support the use of some, but not all, regimens. More recently, Hu et al. [116] conducted a randomised controlled trial of behavioural therapy in an elderly nursing home population using an hourly check and prompt to toilet, coupled with positive social reinforcement. At the end of a three-month training period the treatment patients' wet episodes had been reduced by 0.6 episodes per day, a 26 per cent reduction over baseline. More cognitively intact residents, those with normal bladder capacity, and those with a high frequency of response during baseline responded best to this programme.

Improved nursing intervention

There are various descriptive reports in the literature of the benefit of nursing input to the promotion of continence. Much of this has centred around the employment of a specialist continence advisor who teaches 'best practice' to the community nursing staff and members of the primary health care team [117]. The continence nurse advisor may also be responsible for the purchasing of catheters and continence aids in the locality. Recently, O'Brien et al. [118] showed the benefit of a non-specialist nurse supervising pelvic floor exercises and bladder retraining. In a randomised controlled trial of subjects (including a younger population) in the community, 97 per cent of the women in the intervention group reported improvement, compared with 5 per cent in the control group.

Reduction of handicap

A range of undergarments, external collection devices and environmental aids are employed to reduce handicap from incontinence. The effectiveness of most of these has not been subjected to scientific scrutiny, though some evidence substantiates the use of certain absorbent undergarments and pads [119, 120].

Improving other aspects of function

Other techniques, such as improving the person's mobility and improving access to, and stability at, the toilet, may also be effective but have not so far been the subject of scientific scrutiny.

Cost

Only a limited amount of information is available on the costs of continence promotion programmes. It is likely that the labour costs of behaviour therapy will be higher than the savings in laundry costs to a nursing home. Schnelle et al. [121] point out that a successful rehabilitation continence programme will produce direct savings only if compared with the cost that occurs if patients are changed on a basis that matches actual continence frequency. In reality, nursing home staff often minimise the direct cost of incontinence by not changing patients at anything like that frequency. This can be seen from their

Table 8.6. Cost breakdown – all patients

Condition	N	Frequency of change per diem	Frequency of toileting per diem	Labour cost per diem ($)	Laundry cost per diem ($)	Total cost per diem ($)
Non-experimental condition						
Nursing home changes	92	1.34	0.49	0.76	0.76	1.52
(Range)		(0–4)	(0–1)	(0.00–1.49)	(0.00–2.28)	(0.00–3.77)
Experimental conditions						
Baseline	92	3.26	0.49	1.47	1.86	3.33
(Range)		(1–5)	(0–2)	(0.42–2.93)	(0.57–2.85)	(0.99–5.78)
One-hour treatment	92	2.02	2.59	2.15	1.15	3.30
(Range)		(0–4)	(1–5)	(0.54–3.42)	(0.00–2.28)	(0.54–5.70)

All prices are in US dollars.
Adapted from ref. [121].

costing data shown in Table 8.6, where usual frequency of change is shown in the non-experimental condition section and the change frequency that matches continence frequency is shown in the baseline section under experimental conditions. Because nursing homes may not realise savings for keeping patients continent, reimbursement incentives may need to be utilised to implement continence programmes in order to achieve their effect on quality of life.

A number of evaluations with small numbers of patients have suggested that the use of launderable, absorbent sheets may achieve significant savings in management costs [122].

Some descriptive data are available to suggest that the employment of a continence nurse advisor may permit savings by the development of a rational purchasing policy for catheters, continence aids and other sundries.

Nocturia

Importance

Noctural frequency is one of the most prevalent symptoms in the elderly population being reported in around 80 per cent of people over 65 years [123]. It increases in severity with increasing age. Nocturia presents many problems, resulting in insomnia, subsequent day-time somnolence and caregiver stress [123a]. Those reporting nocturia at least twice per night have also been shown to be at greater risk of reporting falls [123b].

Detection

Nocturia is easily identified by questioning but is commonly omitted from assessment enquiry. Health professionals' awareness of this problem needs improvement.

Effectiveness

Despite the stress caused by this symptom, there is very little published information on treatment or preventive strategies. Commonly employed techniques tend to address the often multifaceted underlying aetiology. Predominant amongst these are measures to minimise the disproportionate nocturnal urine production that occurs in elderly people (particularly attempts to minimise peripheral oedema that may return to the circulation on recumbency and cause diuresis) and measures to prevent uninhibited bladder contractions [124].

Cost

No information is available on costs.

Constipation

Importance

Constipation is no more prevalent in elderly people living in the community than in the young [125]. However, it is present in the majority of elderly people who are institutionalised or immobile [126, 127]. It can result in impaction with overflow soiling and may aggravate haemorrhoids and diverticular disease [128]. Additionally, the absence of a regular bowel motion can cause considerable psychological distress to old people because of a lifelong misperception that this has adverse effects on health.

Detection

Detection depends on an accurate history of bowel function either from the elderly person or from their care attendant. If faecal impaction is not to be missed, it should be supplemented by a rectal examination though, even then, higher colonic impaction may not be identified.

Effectiveness

Although very little scientific evidence is available, a number of strategies are regularly employed in clinical practice to prevent constipation. Dietary fibre supplements may benefit, for they bulk the stools. Eating an extra gram of fibre daily adds about 5 grams to the 24-hour stool weight. Because of this effect, fibre supplements have been shown to improve bowel transit times [129]. Nevertheless, the effect of fibre supplements in elderly individuals may be limited because this population has difficulty in complying with fibre-rich diets and additives. Also, the bulking effect of fibre diminishes as intestinal transit slows down, being least effective in the people who need it most. Other strategies, used particularly for those in institutions, are a diet containing adequate fruit and vegetables, the maintenance of physical activity, an adequate fluid intake, and the avoidance of constipating drugs.

Table 8.7. *Eye changes and disorders with age*

	Visual acuity[a] (total both sexes)		Senile macular[b] degeneration (%)		Cataract[c] (%)		Ocular hypertension[d] (%)	
Age group	20/25 (6/9)	20/40 (6/12)	Male	Female	Male	Female	Male	Female
60–64							8.8	15.6
65–69							10.4	12.0
65–74	91.9	97.5	46	48	16	19		
70–74							11.8	18.6
75–85	69.1	87.0	49	50	42	49		

[a] Corrected visual acuity in better eye.
[b] Total of all severity grades.
[c] Posterior or cortical lens changes or nuclear sclerosis and visual acuity 6/9 or less or aphakia.
[d] Intra-ocular pressure 21 mmHg or more on one occasion.
Data extracted from:
Kim MM, Liebowitz HM, Colton T et al. Amer J Opthalmol 1978; **85**: 28
Sperduto RD, Spiegel D. Amer J Ophthalmol 1980; **80**: 86
Hollows FC, Graham PA. Brit J Ophthalmol 1966; **50**: 570.

Cost

No information on costs is available.

Poor vision

Importance

Impaired vision in elderly people can manifest itself in many ways [130]. One of the most important and studied parameters is visual acuity. Although most individuals even in old age will have well-preserved visual acuity (see Table 8.7) recent American surveys suggest nearly 13 per cent of those over 65 years will have some visual impairment and almost 8 per cent will suffer from severe impairment, such as blindness in both eyes or inability to read newsprint even with glasses [131]. These figures are not surprising in view of the high prevalence of senile macular degeneration, cataract and open angle glaucoma in this population [132, 133] (see Table 8.7).

Impaired vision is a known risk factor for falls and fracture of the femur [134]. Poor vision may also restrict activity, result in social isolation and lower morale and self esteem. It contributes to road traffic accidents and aggravates paranoid and delusional states. It may also accelerate cognitive decline. However, the impact of poor vision must be seen in a context where many elderly people consider poor vision an inevitable and irremediable accompaniment of ageing. Usually other chronic illness or disability takes priority in discussions with health care professionals [135, 136]. Only when poor sight is the sole handicap does it play a major role in perceived difficulties [137]. These attitudes must explain in part the significant lack of self reporting of visual problems in this older age group.

Detection

Little attention has been paid to appropriate targeting of the elderly population for primary preventive measures as these are still in their infancy (see below).

The detection of visual impairment necessary before implementing secondary preventive measures can be achieved by simple manoeuvres using relatively untrained personnel. Cullinan [138] suggests the first stage is to take an adequate history relevant to elderly people including specific questions about *near* vision (reading, sewing, etc.) and *distance* vision (mobility inside and outside the house, watching television, etc.). These enquiries can be formalised by using the Activities of Daily Vision Schedule [139]. This should be followed by near-vision testing under good illumination using near-vision sight testing cards. It is suggested that if an elderly person can do no better than read print size N12 in good light and has not been to an optician within the last two years, then such a referral should be made. Likewise, distance vision may be assessed, again in good light, using the distance-vision (Snellen) card. Referral for specialist opinion is suggested for anyone with vision of less than 6/18 equivalent and, in general, anyone with a visual acuity of 6/9 to 6/18 in the better eye and who has not been to an optician within the last two years should be so referred.

More detailed ophthalmoscopic examination of the eye and visual field testing may be useful but require additional expertise and equipment. The value of tonometry for glaucoma is discussed elsewhere.

Effectiveness

Health promotional strategies to prevent poor vision are as follows.

Primary prevention

Primary preventive measures are in their infancy. Perhaps most work has focussed on cataract prevention and this has been ably reviewed by Harding [140]. In humans, aspirin-like analgesics have been identified as protective factors against cataract in a number of case-control studies, but several other anti-cataract agents are currently being scrutinised. Recent research that implicates smoking increasingly as a risk factor for nuclear cataract and possibly for posterior capsular cataract raises the opportunity for prevention through quit smoking programmes [140a].

Population screening

There is no evidence available to assess the efficacy of widespread screening for visual impairment in the elderly population. It is known, however, that mounting a mass-screening programme in general practice for impaired visual acuity in middle aged persons failed to show any difference between the control and screened group in follow up five years later [141]. This outcome may be different in elderly people in whom there is a high prevalence of unrecognised visual loss. For example, in a random sample of people over 65 years in London, the prevalence of blindness was found to be 1 per cent using WHO criteria and 3.9 per cent using American criteria. The prevalence of low vision or visual impairment was similarly found to be 7.7 per cent using WHO criteria and 10.6 per cent using American criteria. Only 50 per cent of those with low vision were known by their general practitioner to have an eye problem [142]. In another British study of patients aged 60 to 75 years registered with their general practice, 26 per cent had not received an eye check by an optometrist within the previous three years (those with mobility problems being less likely to have had their eyes checked), and of these an appointment for a screening appointment was accepted by 44 per cent [142a].

Further evidence for the potential value of screening the vision of elderly people comes from a geriatric day centre where screening revealed that one-third of attendees had unrecognised visual loss [143]; an outpatient clinic screening programme, which showed 12 per cent of elderly patients had previously undiagnosed conditions, most of which were treatable [144]; and a continuing care ward study where screening led to improvement in vision in 21 per cent of patients [145].

Specific treatment measures

After generalised or opportunistic screening, specialist referral to prevent progress of disease is increasingly worthwhile as the major eye disorders (cataract, macular degeneration, glaucoma and diabetic retinopathy) that lead to loss of vision in elderly people become amenable to treatment. For example, one prospective study from the USA of elderly patients undergoing cataract surgery with intraocular lens implantation found that visual acuity in the surgical eye improved from a mean of 20/100 before surgery to 20/40 four months after surgery. This improvement was maintained at one year. Positive changes were reported in some subjective measures of patient function but these were modest. However, marked changes occurred in objective measures of function and these were maintained at one year [146, 147]. Likewise, laser photocoagulation therapy has been shown in various controlled trials [148, 149] to benefit certain types of disciform macular degeneration, though there is a 10 to 12 per cent per year risk of recurrence in the same eye and also of involvement in the opposite eye, so that ongoing supervision is required. Laser photocoagulation also fails to be of benefit when degeneration occurs close to the fovea [150].

Improvement of lighting

General levels of lighting are often poor in elderly people's homes yet three times the amount of light is needed for the older retina to achieve the same resolution as in the younger eye. This provides an opportunity for prevention. One study of people of average age 76 years with visual acuity 6/18 (Snellen) or less has shown that an improvement in the ambient level of lighting at home improved visual acuity in 82 per cent of subjects [151]. This augmentation could be achieved by simple measures such as the provision of a 60 watt bulb in a small adjustable lamp close to the area where reading or other similar activities took place.

Provision of low-vision aids

A considerable number of 'low-vision aids' are available to assist in reducing the handicap from visual disability. Clinical experience strongly supports their value. However, there have been few scientific studies reporting their efficacy in elderly populations and it is known that many old people often quickly discard the aids that someone else has felt appropriate for them.

Cost

Although not specifically targeted on elderly populations, several cost effectiveness analyses have been performed on screening *diabetics* for the presence of diabetic retinopathy [152]. When considering three different populations of diabetic patient, screening strategies seemed to be cost saving for type I and type II diabetics taking insulin but, for type II diabetics who did not take insulin (the majority situation in the elderly population), annual screening ophthalmoscopic examinations yielded additional years of sight at a cost of about $1500 per year of sight saved [153].

Deafness

Importance

Hearing loss prevalence estimates indicate that 25 to 40 per cent of individuals over 65 years of age are hearing impaired, with more than 90 per cent of persons in their ninth decade of life exhibiting a hearing handicap [154]. There is a significant association between impaired hearing and reduction of outdoor activities, loss of friends, anxiety, depression, cognitive impairment and the precipitation and aggravation of paranoid traits [155, 156].

Detection

Deafness is much under-reported by elderly people. Over a third of a sample of hearing-impaired elderly people had not told their GP about their hearing loss even though they saw him or her regularly. More active screening for hearing impairment therefore seems advisable. Fortunately, there are several well-validated methods for such screening in this older population [157].

One such method is to use the Hearing Handicap Inventory for the Elderly (HHIE) – Screening Version. A score of over 8 on this questionnaire has a sensitivity of 72 per cent and specificity of 77 per cent [157]. A recent study of a slightly younger, community-living population using a different screening questionnaire nevertheless suggests that distributing such questionnaires by post and then inviting those with problems for audiometric testing may be quite an effective strategy. Only two postings were required to detect 96 per cent of those who accepted hearing aids [158].

Another method of screening is to use the Welch–Allyn audioscope (a hand-held otoscope with a build-in audiometer) which has a sensitivity of 94 per cent and a specificity of 72 per cent [157]. Any significant hearing impairment should be followed up by otoscopic and, if necessary, more complete audio-logical assessment. Even simpler assessments of hearing impairment can be effective. For example, free-field voice testing (the whispered voice test) can reliably exclude significant hearing impairment (mean pure tone threshold at 0.5, 1, and 2 kHz worse than 30 dB) with a sensitivity of 100 per cent and a specificity of 84 per cent [159]. It has also been shown that in a long stay institutional setting there is good correlation between nurses' subjective impression of a patient's hearing loss and impairment as measured by more objective means [160].

Effectiveness

A number of strategies are available to prevent hearing impairment in elderly individuals.

Provision of a hearing aid

Amplification of sound by the provision of a hearing aid not only improves hearing in the majority of elderly deaf people but, in a randomised controlled trial, has been shown to bring about significant improvements in social and emotional function, in communication function, in cognitive function and in depression (see Table 8.8). The benefits of hearing aids were experienced as early as six weeks after their provision [161].

Because many institutionalised and cognitively impaired elderly people are unable or unwilling to comply with aural rehabilitation, a prognostic rating [162] should be made on the likelihood of a hearing aid being used before proceeding to the provision of an aid.

Improved access for hearing aid provision

Although specialist assessment by an otolaryngologist does not necessarily create delays in being provided with a hearing aid [163], in many parts of the British NHS significant waiting times do exist for this service [164]. It may therefore be that accelerated referral through less professional channels to a hearing-aid dispenser would have significant advantages for many. An outstanding concern, however, is that lack of professional assessment may result in missed pathology that would require other treatment. There is debate as to the extent of this issue [163], but simple exclusion criteria for such accelerated referrals are available and probably reduce much of the risk. In fact, the pick up rate of potentially serious, coexistent ear pathology in some studies specifically in older populations has been surprisingly low [165].

Removal of ear wax

Removal of impacted cerumen from the auditory canals meets with variable results, but often can have significant impact in reducing the resultant handicap in communication. Wax is most commonly removed by ear syringing, a procedure that is not without iatrogenic consequences, complications arising in about 1 per 1000 ears syringed [166].

Table 8.8. *Average differences between groups in quality-of-life change scores*

Scale	Change[a]	95% confidence interval	p-value
HHIE	34.0	(27.3, 40.8)	<0.0001
QDS	24.2	(17.2, 31.2)	<0.0001
SPMSQ	0.28	(0.08, 0.48)	0.008
GDS	0.80	(0.09, 1.51)	0.03
SELF	1.9	(−1.6, 5.4)	0.27

HHIE, Hearing Handicap Inventory in the Elderly; QDS, Quantified Denver Scale; SPMSQ, Short Portable Mental Status Questionnaire; GDS, Geriatric Depression Scale; and SELF, Self Evaluation of Life Function scale.
[a] A positive change indicates an advantage for the hearing aid group.
Adapted from ref. [161].

Health education of the elderly public

Publicity campaigns designed, through the use of posters and leaflets displayed in waiting areas, to encourage earlier presentation by elderly people with complaints of hearing loss have been shown, at least in younger populations, to double the incidence of presentation of loss of hearing. However, half of those complaining claimed they had failed to notice these messages and the beneficial effect was lost as soon as the posters were removed [167].

Education of health care providers

A barrier to treatment is the negative attitude of many doctors to the problem of hearing loss. Over half of the persons who have discussed their hearing problem with health care providers are told that their hearing loss is minor or that it cannot be improved with a hearing aid [168]. As a consequence, only about 50 per cent of hearing-impaired elderly people who go to their family doctor are referred for specialist help. It may be that this problem could be minimised by education to increase physician awareness coupled with explicit screening and referral protocols.

Special measures for institutionalised populations

A report by the UK Advisory Committee on Services for Hearing Impaired People [169] highlighted that very rarely were the difficulties that stemmed from hearing loss in institutionalised populations understood by all staff. It is, therefore, suggested that a 'key worker' be made available with a special commitment to the hearing impaired in the residential setting.

The use of communication and environmental aids

A large number of relatively simple assistive listening devices are available to reduce the handicap from hearing disability [170]. Although clinical experience suggests their considerable value, there is a dearth of hard scientific evidence on their proven efficacy in the elderly population.

Cost

In the recent randomised trial in the USA on the use of hearing aids, the cost of identifying hearing impaired persons, providing formal audiological testing with subsequent hearing-aid fitting and orientation sessions, and one follow up examination was calculated at approximately $1000 per hearing aid dispensed. When the Hearing Quality Adjusted Life Years (HQALYs) for persons receiving hearing aids were projected, based on percentage improvements as assessed by the HHIE, cost effectiveness was estimated at $200 per HQALY gained [161].

Insomnia

Importance

Many changes to the extent and nature of the sleep cycle may be considered a normal part of the ageing process. Yet around 40 per cent of elderly women in the UK complain of insomnia. On average, 10 to 15 per cent of the elderly population living at home consume prescribed hypnotic drugs, and the equivalent figure averages about 35 per cent for those in various types of institution [171]. For a significant proportion of these, the insomnia leads to psychological distress, subsequent day-time somnolence and carer stress.

Detection

Questioning will elicit the complaint of insomnia which is probably the issue of most concern to the health care provider. There is, however, a poor correlation between this complaint and the true sleep pattern [172]. Corroboration from an independent source or more extensive investigation may at times be required.

Effectiveness

Hypnotic agents

Hypnotics rarely benefit chronic insomnia, as tolerance to their effects usually develops within a few weeks. Problems associated with somnolence and from the side effects of the drugs are also greater in elderly people than in the young [173, 174]. For these reasons hypnotic therapy is usually recommended only for short courses of a few weeks duration to cover times of emotional upset or concurrent medical illness.

Other measures

Of more practical benefit for the majority of chronic elderly insomniacs are counselling, the prescription of comfort measures and the treatment of aggravating physical and psychiatric problems [171, 175]. It is also known that subjects who are awake for only four hours before their usual bedtime take three times longer to go to sleep and that exercise earlier in the day may enhance subsequent sleepiness. An increase in day-time activity and the avoidance of napping in the late afternoon and evening may therefore be useful strategies in avoiding insomnia. Most of these techniques, however, have not been subjected to rigorous scientific scrutiny.

Cost

No detailed information on costs is available, though there is a considerable (and inappropriate) expenditure on hypnotic drugs for the elderly population.

References

1. Shephard RJ. Activity Patterns of the Elderly: Physical Activity and Aging. Chicago: Croom Helm, 1978.
2. Bortz WM. Disuse and Aging. J Amer Med Assoc 1982; **248**: 1203–8.
3. Basey EJ, Fentem PH. Extent of deterioration in physical condition during post-operative bed rest and its reversal by rehabilitation. Brit Med J 1974; **4**: 194–6.
4. De Vries, H. Physiological effects of an exercise training regimen upon men aged 52–88. J. Gerontol 1970; **25**: 325.
5. Aniansson A. Muscle Function in Old Age with Special Reference to Muscle Morphology Effect of Training Capacity on Activities of Daily Living. Department of Rehabilitation Medicine in Geriatric and Long Term Medicine. Sweden: University of Goteberg, 1980.

6. Frekany GA, Leslie DK. Effects of an exercise programme on selected flexibility measurements of senior citizens. Gerontology 1975; **21**: 182.
7. Vanfraechem J, Vanfraechem R. Studies of the effect of a short training period on aged subjects. J Sports Med Phys Fitness 1975; **21**: 182.
8. Mahler DA, Cunningham LN, Curfman GD. Aging and exercise performance. In: Mahler DA (ed) Clinics in Geriatric Medicine: Respiratory Diseases, vol. 2, pp. 433–52. Philadelphia, PA: WB Saunders, 1986.
9. Shephard RJ. The scientific basis of exercise prescribing for the very old. J Amer Geriatr Soc 1990; **38**: 62–70.
10. Harris R, Frankel L, Harris S. Guide to Fitness After Fifty. London: Plenum Press, 1977.
11. Franklin B. Exercise program compliance: important strategies. In: Storlie J, Jordin H (eds) Behaviour Management of Obesity, pp. 103–35. New York: Spectrum, 1984.
12. DeVries HA. Exercise intensity threshold for improvement of cardiovascular-respiratory function in older men. Geriatrics 1971; **25**: 94.
13. Seals DR, Hagberg JM, Hurley BF et al. Endurance training in older men and women. i. Cardiovascular responses to exercise. J Appl Physiol; Respir Environ Exercise Physiol 1984; **57**: 1024.
14. Sidney KH, Shephard RJ. Frequency and intensity of exercise training for elderly subjects. Med Sci Sports Exerc 1978; **10**: 125.
15. Emes CG. The effects of a regular program of light exercise on seniors. J Sports Med Phys Fitness 1979; **19**: 185–9.
16. Badenhope DT, Cleary P, Schaal SF et al. Physiologic adjustments to higher or lower intensity exercise in elders. Med Sci Sports Exerc 1983; **15**: 496–502.
17. Haskell WL, Montoye HJ, Orenstein D. Physical activity and exercise to achieve health-related physical fitness components. Pub Health Rep 1985; **100**: 202–12.
18. Vuori I, Suurnakki L, Suurnakki T. Risk of sudden cardiovascular death (SCVD) in exercise. Med Sci Sports Exerc 1982; **14**: 114–15.
19. Shephard RJ. The scientific basis of exercise prescribing for the very old. J Amer Geriatr Soc 1990; **38**: 62–70.
20. Gorman KM, Posner JL. Benefits of exercise in old age. In: Kaye D, Posner JD (eds) Clinics in Geriatric Medicine: Common Clinical Challenges in Geriatrics, vol. 4. Philadelphia, PA: WB Saunders, 1988.
21. Molloy DW, Beerschoten DA, Borrie MJ et al. Acute effects of exercise on neuropsychological function in elderly subjects. J Amer Geriatr Soc 1988; **36**: 29.
22. Rogers RL, Meyer JS, Mortel KF. After reaching retirement age physical activity sustains cerebral perfusion and cognition. J Amer Geriatr Soc 1990; **38**: 123–8.
23. Friedman R, Tappen RM. The effect of planned walking on communication in Alzheimer's disease. J Amer Geriatr Soc 1991; **39**: 652–4.
24. Paffenbarger RS, Hyde RT, Wing AL et al. Physical activity, all-cause mortality and longevity of college alumni. N Engl J Med 1986; **314**: 604.
25. Posner JD, Gorman KM, Gitlin LN et al. Effects of exercise training in the elderly on the occurrence and time to onset of cardiovascular diagnosis. J Amer Geriatr Soc 1990; **38**: 205–10.
26. Kallio V, Hamalainen H, Hakkila J et al. Reduction in sudden deaths in multi-factoral intervention programme after acute myocardial infarction. Lancet ii; 1979: 1091.

27. Rechnitzer PA, Cunningham DA, Andrew GM et al. Relation of exercise to the recurrence rate of myocardial infarction in men: The Ontario Exercise-Heart-Collaborative-Study. Amer J Cardiol 1983; **51**: 65.

28. Wilhelmsen L, Sanne H, Elmfeldt D et al. A controlled trial of physical training after myocardial infarction: effects on risk factors, non-fatal infarction and death. Prev Med 1975; **4**: 491.

29. Wannamethee G, Shaper AG. Physical activity and stroke in British middle aged men. Brit Med J 1992; **304**: 597–601.

30. Shinton RA, Sagar G. Lifelong activity and stroke. Paper presented at British Geriatrics Society Meeting, London, 1992.

31. Russell LB. Is Prevention Better Than Cure? Washington, DC: The Brookings Institution, 1986.

32. Evans DA, Funkenstein H, Albert MS et al. Prevalence of Alzheimer's disease in a community population of older persons. J Amer Med Assoc 1989; **262**: 2551–6.

33. Weiler PG. The public health impact of Alzheimer's disease. Amer J Pub Health 1987; **77**: 1157–8.

34. Buchner DM, Larson EB. Falls and fractures in patients with Alzheimer-type dementia. J Amer Med Assoc 1987; **257**: 1492–5.

35. Rabins PV. Psychosocial aspects of dementia. J Clin Psychiatry (suppl) 1988; **49**: 29–31.

36. Hay JW, Ernst RL. The economic costs of Alzheimer's disease. Amer J Pub Health 1987; **77**: 1169–75.

37. Fillenbaum GG. Comparison of two brief tests of organic brain impairment: the MSQ and the Short Portable MSQ. J Amer Geriatr Soc 1980; **28**: 381–4.

38. Folstein MF, Folstein SE, McHugh PR. 'Mini-mental state'. A practical method for grading the cognitive state of patients for the clinician. J Psych Res 1975; **12**: 189–98.

39. Pfeiffer E. A short portable mental status questionnaire for the assessment of organic brain deficit in elderly patients. J Amer Geriatr Soc 1975; **23**: 433–41.

40. Thienaus OJ, Hartford JT, Skelly MF, Bosmann HB. Biologic markers in Alzheimer's disease. J Amer Geriatr Soc 1985; **33**: 715–26.

41. McEntee WJ, Crook TH. Age-associated memory impairment: a role for catecholamines. Neurology 1990; **40**: 526–30.

41a. Rabins PV. Prevention of mental disorder in the elderly: current perspectives and future prospects. J Amer Geriatr Soc 1992; **40**: 727–33.

42. Clarfield AM. The reversible dementias: do they reverse? Annals Intern Med 1988; **109**: 476–86.

43. Reisberg B (ed). Pharmacologic investigations into the treatment of Alzheimer's disease. In: Alzheimer Disease, pp. 327–95. New York: The Free Press, 1983.

44. Crapper McLachlan DR, Dalton AJ, Kruck TPA et al. Intramuscular desferrioxamine in patients with Alzheimer's disease. Lancet 1991; **337**: 1304–8.

45. Battaglia A, Bruni G, Ardia A, Sacchetti G. Nicergoline in mild to moderate dementia: a multicenter, double-blind, placebo-controlled study. J Amer Geriatr Soc 1989; **37**: 295–302.

46. Crook TH, Tinkleberg J, Yesavage J et al. Effects of phosphatidylserine in age-associated memory impairment. Neurology 1991; **41**: 644–9.

46a. Meyer JS, Judd BJ, Tawaklna T. Improved cognition after control of risk factors for multi-infarct dementia. J Amer Med Assoc 1986; **256**: 2203–9.

46b. Meyer JS, Rogers RL, McClintic K et al. Randomized clinical trial of daily aspirin therapy in multi-infarct dementia. J Amer Geriatr Soc 1989; **37**: 549–55.
47. O'Connor DW, Pollitt PA, Brook CPB et al. Does early intervention reduce the number of elderly people with dementia admitted to institutions for long term care? Brit Med J 1991; **302**: 871–5.
48. Blenkner M, Bloom M, Nielsen M. A research and demonstration project of protective services. Social Casework 1971; **52**: 483–99.
49. Askham J, Thompson C. Dementia and Home Care. London: Age Concern, 1990.
50. Eastwood MR, Corbin S. Investigation of suspect dementia. Lancet 1981; **i**: 1261.
51. Abrams M. Beyond Three Score and Ten: A First Report on a Survey of the Elderly. Age Concern Research Unit. London: Age Concern Publications, 1978.
52. Dawson D, Hendershot G, Fulton J. Aging in the 80s: functional limitations of individuals aged 65 years and over. Advance data from vital and health statistics of the National Center for Health Statistics 1987; **133**: 1–11.
53. Warshaw GA, Moore JT, Friedman SW et al. Functional disability in the hospitalised elderly. J Amer Med Assoc 1982; **248**: 847–50.
54. Calkins DR, Rubenstein LV, Cleary PD. Failure of physicians to recognise functional disability in ambulatory patients. Annals Int Med 1991; **114**: 451–4.
55. Tinetti ME, Ginter SF. Identifying mobility dysfunctions in elderly patients. J Amer Med Assoc 1988; **259**: 1190–3.
56. American College of Physicians: Health and Public Policy Committee. Comprehensive functional assessment for elderly patients. Annals Intern Med 1988; **109**: 70–2.
57. Mathias S. Balance in elderly patients: the 'get up and go test'. Arch Phys Med Rehabil 1986; **67**: 387–9.
58. Tinetti ME. Performance-oriented assessment of mobility problems in elderly patients. J Amer Geriatr Soc 1986; **34**: 119–26.
59. Reuben DB, Siu AL. An objective measure of physical function of elderly out-patients. The physical performance test. J Amer Geriatr Soc 1990; **38**: 1105–12.
60. Winograd CH. Targeting strategies; an overview of criteria and outcomes. J Amer Geriatr Soc 1991; **39**: 25S–35S.
61. Hall RGP, Channing DM. Age, pattern of consultation and functional disability in elderly patients in one general practice. Brit Med J 1990; **301**: 424–8.
62. Rubenstein LV, Calkins DR, Young RT et al. Improving patient function: a randomised trial of functional disability screening. Annals Intern Med 1989; **111**: 836–42.
63. Garroway AM, Akhtar AJ, Prescott RJ et al. Management of acute stroke in the elderly: preliminary results of a controlled trial. Brit Med J 1980; **280**: 1040–3.
64. Kennie DC, Reid J, Richardson I et al. Effectiveness of geriatric rehabilitative care after fractures of the proximal femur in elderly women: a randomised clinical trial. Brit Med J 1988; **297**: 1083–6.
65. Wade DT, Collen FM, Robb GF, Warlow CP. Physiotherapy intervention late after stroke and mobility. Brit Med J 1992; **304**: 609–13.
66. Kovar PA, Allegrante JP, MacKenzie R et al. Supervised fitness walking in patients with osteoarthritis of the knee. Annals Intern Med 1992; **116**: 529–34.
67. Stern PH, McDowell F, Miller JM, Robinson M. Factors influencing stroke rehabilitation. Stroke 1971; **2**: 213–18.

68. Feldman DJ, Lee PR, Unterecker J et al. A comparison of functionally oriented medical care and formal rehabilitation in the management of patients with hemiplegia due to cerebral vascular disease. J Chron Dis 1962; **15**: 297–310.

69. Orem D. Nursing: Concepts of Practice. New York: McGraw-Hill, 1980.

70. Garraway WM, Akhtar AJ, Hockey L, Prescott RJ. Management of acute stroke in the elderly: follow-up of a controlled trial. Brit Med J 1980; **281**: 827–9.

71. Smith DS, Goldenberg E, Ashburn A et al. Remedial therapy after stroke: a randomised controlled trial. Brit Med J 1981; **282**: 517–20.

72. Hart D, Bowling A, Ellis M, Silman A. Locomotor disability in very elderly people: value of a programme for screening and provision of aids for daily living. Brit Med J 1990; **301**: 216–20.

73. Cambell AJ, Reinken J, Allan BC, Martinez GS. Falls in old age: a study of frequency and related clinical factors. Age Ageing 1981; **10**: 264–70.

74. Morris EV, Isaacs B. The prevention of falls in a geriatric hospital. Age Ageing 1980; **9**: 181–5.

75. Wild D. A prospective study of falls in residential homes. Report to the Department of Health and Social Services. Birmingham: University of Birmingham, 1981.

76. Alffram PA. An epidemiological study of cervical and trochanteric fractures of the femur in an urban population. Acta Orthopaed Scand 1964: Suppl 65.

77. National Safety Council. Accident Facts Chicago, Illinois, 1983.

78. Tinetti ME, Speechley M, Ginter SF. Risk factors for falls among elderly persons living in the community. N Engl J Med 1988; **319**: 1701–7.

79. Campbell AJ. Role of rehabilitation in fall recovery and prevention. Rev Clin Gerontol 1992; **2**: 53–65.

80. Tinetti ME, Speechley M. Prevention of falls among the elderly. N Engl J Med 1989; **320**: 1055–9.

81. Ray WA, Griffin MR, Schaffner W et al. Psychotropic drug use and the risk of hip fracture. N Engl J Med 1987; **316**: 363–9.

82. Rubenstein LZ, Robbins AS, Josephson KR et al. The value of assessing falls in an elderly population. A randomized clinical trial. Annals Intern Med 1990; **113**: 308–16.

83. Obony OT, Drummond M, Isaacs B. Domiciliary physiotherapy for old people who have fallen. Int Rehabil Med 1984; **5**: 157–60.

83a. Reinsch S, MacRae P, Lachenbruch PA, Tobis JS. Attempts to prevent falls and injury: a prospective community study. Gerontologist 1992; **32**: 450–6.

84. Vetter NJ, Lewis PA, Ford D. Can health visitors prevent fractures in elderly people? Brit Med J 1992; **304**: 888–90.

85. Overstall P. Falls. In: Pathy MSJ (ed) Principles and Practice of Geriatric Medicine, pp. 701–9. Chichester: John Wiley and Sons, 1985.

86. Grisso, JA, Kelsey JL, Strom BL et al. Risk factors for falls as a cause of hip fracture in women. N Engl J Med 1991; **324**: 1326–31.

87. McCabe J. Mind you don't fall. Nursing Mirror 1985; **26**: 160.

88. Sehested P, Severin-Nielsen T. Falls by hospitalised elderly patients: causes and prevention. Geriatrics April 1977; 101–8.

89. McWhirter M. A dispersed alarm system for the elderly and its relevance to local general practitioners. J Roy Coll Gen Pract 1987; **37**: 244–7.

90. Bond J, Carstairs V. Services for the Elderly. Scottish Health Service Studies No. 42. Edinburgh: Scottish Home and Health Department, 1982.

91. Hunt A. The elderly at home. Survey for the Department of Health and Social Security. London: HMSO, 1978.
92. Lachs MS, Feinstein AR, Cooney LM et al. A simple procedure for general screening for functional disability in elderly patients. Annals Int Med 1990; **112**: 699–706.
93. Challis D, Davies B. Case Management in Community Care. Aldershot: Gower, 1986.
94. Chesterman J, Challis D, Davies B. Long term care at home for the elderly: a four year follow up. Brit J Social Wrk 1987; **18**: 43–53.
95. Kane RL, Kane RA. Alternatives to institutional care of the elderly: beyond the dichotomy. Gerontologist 1980; **20**: 249–59.
96. Branch LG, Fowler FJ. The health care needs of the elderly and chronically disabled in Massachusetts. Submission to Massachusetts Department of Health by Survey Research Program, a joint facility of the University of Massachusetts, Boston, and Joint Center for Urban Studies of MIT and Harvard University, March 1975.
97. Siebens H, Troupe E, Siebens A et al. Correlates and consequences of eating dependency in institutionalised elderly. J Amer Geriatr Soc 1986; **34**: 192–8.
98. Zimmer JG. Characteristics of patients and care provided in health-related and skilled nursing facilities. Med Care 1975; **13**: 992.
99. Maclennan WJ, Martin P, Mason BJ. Causes for reduced dietary intake in a long-stay hospital. Age Ageing 1975; **4**: 175–80.
100. Norberg A, Norberg B, Pexell G. Ethical problems in feeding patients with advanced dementia. Brit Med J 1980; **281**: 847.
101. Kottkee FJ. Historia Obscura Hemiplegiae. Arch Phys Med Rehab 1974; **55**: 4.
102. Gordon C, Gaitz CM, Scott J. Leisure and Lives. In: Binstock RH, Shanas E (eds) Handbook of Aging and the Social Sciences. New York: Van Nostrand Reinhold, 1976.
103. Thomas M. Prevalence of urinary incontinence. Brit Med J 1980; **281**: 1243–6.
104. Milne JS. Prevalence of incontinence in the elderly age groups. In: Willington SL (ed) Incontinence in the Elderly. London: Academic Press, 1976.
105. Ouslander JG, Kane RL, Abrass IB. Urinary incontinence in elderly nursing home patients. J Amer Med Assoc 1982; **248**: 1194–8.
106. Lothian PT. Underpads in the prevention of decubitae. In: Kenedi RM (ed) Tissue Viability and Clinical Applications. London: Macmillan, 1975.
107. Weissert W. Determinants of Institutionalisation of the Aged. Working Paper No. 1466. Washington, DC: The Urban Institute, 1982.
108. Ory M et al. Psychosocial factors in urinary incontinence. In: Ouslander J (ed) Clinics in Geriatric Medicine. Philadelphia, PA: WB Saunders, 1986.
109. Sanford JRA. Tolerance of debility in elderly dependants by supporters at home: its significance for hospital practice. Brit Med J 1975; **3**: 471–3.
110. Th-wei Hu. The economic impact of urinary incontinence. In: Ouslander J (ed) Clinics In Geriatric Medicine, vol. 1, part 4. Philadelphia, PA: WB Saunders, 1986.
111. Ouslander JG, Kane RL, Abrass IB. Urinary incontinence in elderly nursing home patients. J Amer Med Assoc 1982; **248**: 1194–8.
112. Ribeiro BJ, Smith SR. Evaluation of urinary catheterisation in urinary incontinence in a general nursing home population. J Amer Geriatr Soc 1985; **33**: 479–81.

113. Ouslander JG, Sier HC. Drug therapy for geriatric urinary incontinence. In: Ouslander J (ed) Clinics In Geriatric Medicine, vol. 2, part 4. Philadelphia, PA: WB Saunders, 1986.

114. Schmidbauer CP, Chiang H, Raz S. Surgical treatment for female geriatric incontinence. In: Ouslander J (ed) Clinics in Geriatric Medicine, vol. 2, part 4, pp. 759–76. Philadelphia, PA: WB Saunders, 1986.

115. Hadley EC. Bladder training and related therapies for urinary incontinence in older people. J Amer Med Assoc 1986; **256**: 372–9.

116. Hu TW, Igou JF, Kaltreider L et al. A clinical trial of a behavioural therapy to reduce urinary incontinence in nursing homes. J Amer Med Assoc 1989; **261**: 2656–62.

117. Duffin H, Castleden CM. The continence nurse adviser's role in the British health care system. In: Ouslander JG (ed) Clinics in Geriatric Medicine: Urinary Incontinence, vol. 2, part 4. Philadelphia, PA: WB Saunders, 1986.

118. O'Brien J, Austin M, Sethi P, O'Boyle P. Urinary incontinence: prevalence, need for treatment and effectiveness of intervention by nurse. Brit Med J 1991; **303**: 1308–12.

119. Bainton D, Blannin JD, Shepherd AM. Pads and pants for urinary incontinence. Brit Med J 1983; **285**: 419–21.

120. Watson AC. A trial of Molnlycke pants and diapers. Nursing Times 1980; **76**: 1017–19.

121. Schnelle JR, Sowell VA, Hu TW, Traughber B. Reduction of urinary incontinence in nursing homes: does it reduce or increase costs? J Amer Geriatr Soc 1988; **36**: 34–9.

122. Williams TF, Foerster JE, Proctor JK et al. A new double-layered launderable bed sheet for patients with urinary incontinence. J Amer Geriatr Soc 1981; **24**: 520–4.

123. Hale WE, Perkins LL, May FE et al. Symptom prevalence in the elderly. J Amer Geriatr Soc 1986; **34**: 333–40.

123a. Barker JC, Mitteness LS. Nocturia in the elderly. Gerontologist 1988; **28**: 99–104.

123b. Stewart RB, Moore MT, May FE et al. Nocturia: a risk factor for falls in the elderly. J Amer Geriatr Soc 1992; **40**: 1217–20.

124. Ouslander JG, Sier HC. Drug Therapy for Geriatric Urinary Incontinence. In: Ouslander JG (ed) Clinics in Geriatric Medicine: Urinary Incontinence, vol. 2, part 4. Philadelphia, PA: WB Saunders, 1986.

125. Connell AM, Hilton C, Irvin G et al. Variations in bowel habit in two population samples. Brit Med J 1965; **11**: 1095–9.

126. Brocklehurst JC, Khan Y. A study of faecal stasis in old age and use of Dorbanex in its prevention. Gerontologia Clinica 1960; **11**: 293–300.

127. Brocklehurst JC, Kirkland JL, Martin J, Ashford J. Constipation in long stay elderly patients: its treatment and prevention by Lactulose, Poloxalkol, Dihydroxyanthroquinolone and Phosphate enema. Gerontology 1983; **29**: 181–4.

128. Burkitt D, Meisner P. How to manage constipation with high fiber diet. Geriatrics 1979; **33**: 38.

129. Cleave TL. Natural bran in the treatment of constipation. Brit Med J 1941; **i**: 461.

130. Kahn HA, Leibowitz HM, Ganley JP et al. The Framingham Eye Study. I. Outline and major prevalence findings. Epidemiol 1977; **106**: 17–32.

131. Nelson KA. Visual impairment among elderly Americans: statistics in transition. J Vis Impair Blind 1987; **81**: 331–4.

132. Kini MM, Leibowitz HM, Colton T et al. Prevalence of senile cataract, diabetic retinopathy, senile macular degeneration and open angle glaucoma in the Framingham eye study. Amer J Ophthalmol 1978; **85**: 28–34.

133. Sperduto RD, Seigel D. Senile lens and senile macular changes in a population-based sample. Amer J Ophthalmol 1980; **90**: 86–91.

134. Felson DT, Anderson JJ, Hannan MT et al. Impaired vision in hip fracture. J Amer Geriatr Soc 1989; **37**: 495–500.

135. Keegan D, Ash D, Greenough T. Adjustment to Blindness. Canad J Ophth 1975; **11**: 22.

136. Calnan S. Elderly people with poor sight at home. M Phil Thesis. Dept of Preventive Medicine, St Bartholomew's Hospital Medical College, 1981.

137. Cullinan TR. The epidemiology of visual disability. Studies of visually disabled people in the community. University of Kent: HSRU Report No. 28, 1977.

138. Cullinan T. Visual Disability in the Elderly. London: Croom Helm 1986.

139. Mangione CM, Phillips RS, Gilbert MM et al. Change in visual functional status following cataract extraction and intraocular lens implantation in elderly adults. Clin Res 1991; **39**: 604A.

140. Harding J. Cataract: biochemistry, epidemiology and pharmacology. London: Chapman and Hall, 1991.

140a. West S. Does smoke get in your eyes? J Amer Med Assoc 1992; **268**: 1025–6.

141. Stone D, Shannon DJ. Screening for impaired visual acuity in middle age in general practice. Brit Med J 1978; **2**: 859–61.

142. Wormald RPL, Wright LA, Courtney P et al. Visual problems in the elderly population and implications for services. Brit Med J 1992; **304**: 1226–9.

142a. Webster E, Wilson A and Barnes G. Eye tests in the elderly: factors associated with attendance and diagnostic yield in non-attenders. J Roy Soc Med 1992; **85**: 614–15.

143. McMurdo MET, Baines PS. The detection of visual disability in the elderly. Health Bull (Scot) 1988; **46**: 327–9.

144. Long CA, Holden R, Mulkernin E, Sykes D. Opportunistic screening of visual acuity of elderly patients attending outpatient clinics. Age Ageing 1991; **20**: 392–5.

145. Fenton PJ, Larson EB, Rees TS et al. Evaluation of vision in slow stream wards. Age Ageing 1975; **4**: 43–8.

146. Appelgate WB, Miller ST, Elam JT et al. Impact of cataract surgery with lens implantation on vision and physical function in elderly patients. J Amer Med Assoc 1987; **257**: 1064–6.

147. Elam JT, Graney MJ, Appelgate WB et al. Functional outcomes 1 year following cataract surgery in elderly persons. J Gerontol 1988; **43**: M122.

148. Macular Photocoagulation Study Group. Argon laser photocoagulation for senile macular degeneration. Results of a randomised clinical trial. Arch Ophthalmol 1982; **100**: 912–18.

149. Moorfields Macular Study Group. Treatment of senile disciform macular degeneration: a single blind randomised trial by argon laser photocoagulation. Brit J Ophthalmol 1982; **66**: 745–53.

150. Macular Photocoagulation Study Group. Krypton laser photocoagulation for neovascular lesions of age-related macular degeneration: results of a randomized clinical trial. Arch Ophthalmol 1990; **108**: 816.

151. Cullinan T, Silver J, Gould E, Irvine D. Visual disability and home lighting. Lancet 1979; **1**: 642–4.
152. Singer DE, Nathan DM, Fogel HA, Schachat AP. Screening for diabetic retinopathy. Annals Intern Med 1992; **116**: 660–71.
153. Dasbach EJ, Fryback DG, Newcomb PA et al. Cost-effectiveness of strategies for detecting diabetic retinopathy. Med Care 1991; **29**: 20–39.
154. Davis A. The epidemiology of hearing disorders. In: Hinchliffe R (ed) Hearing and Balance in the Elderly, pp. 1–43. Edinburgh: Churchill Livinstone, 1983.
155. Herbst KG. Psychosocial consequences of disorders of hearing in the elderly. In: Hinchliffe R (ed) Hearing and Balance in the Elderly, pp. 174–200. Edinburgh: Churchill Livingstone, 1982.
156. Uhlmann RF, Larson EB, Rees TS et al. Relationship of hearing impairment to dementia and cognitive dysfunction in older adults. J Amer Med Assoc 1989; **261**: 1916–19.
157. Lichtenstein MJ, Bess FH, Logan SA. Validation of screening tools for identifying hearing impaired elderly in primary care. J Amer Med Assoc 1988; **259**: 2875–8.
158. Stephens DG, Callaghan DE, Hogan S et al. Hearing disability in people aged 50 to 65: effectiveness and acceptability of rehabilitative intervention. Brit Med J 1990; **300**: 508–11.
159. MacPhee GJA, Crowther JA, McAlpine CH. A simple screening test for hearing impairment in elderly patients. Age Ageing 1988; **17**: 347–51.
160. Whitham G, Gilchrist W, Williams BO. Prevalence of deafness and the nurse/patient appreciation of hearing problems in long stay elderly patients. Paper presented to Scottish Branch of the British Geriatrics Society, 1980.
161. Mulrow CD, Aguilar C, Endicott JE. Quality of life changes and hearing impairment. Annals Intern Med 1990; **113**: 188–94.
162. Rupp RR. A feasibility scale for predicting hearing aid use (FSPHAU) with older individuals. J Acad Rehabil Audiol 1977; **10**: 81.
163. Watson C, Crowther JA. Provision of hearing aids: does specialist assessment cause delay? Brit Med J 1989; **299**: 437–9.
164. Johnson J, Grover B, Martin MA. A survey of National Health Service hearing aids services. London: Royal National Institute for the Deaf, 1984.
165. Narula A, Setchfield N, Bradley P. Audiological survey in acute geriatric unit. Paper presented to the Scottish Branch of the British Geriatrics Society, 1980.
166. Sharp JF, Wilson JA, Ross L, Barr-Hamilton RM. Ear wax removal: a survey of current practice. Brit Med J 1990; **301**: 1251–3.
167. King RL, Barry B, Brooks DN. Effectiveness of publicity campaign encouraging earlier referral of hearing loss in adults. Brit Med J 1987; **294**: 1342–3.
168. NATTRASS. Sound sense: how local groups can help hard of hearing people. London: Age Concern, 1982.
169. Department of Health and Social Security: Advisory Committee on Services for Hearing Impaired People. Report of a Sub-Committee appointed to consider the role of Social Services in the care of the deaf of all ages. London: ACSHIP, DHSS, 1977.
170. Andrews K. Deafness and hardness of hearing. In: Andrews K (ed) Rehabilitation of the Older Adult, pp. 201–12. London: Edward Arnold, 1987.
171. Kevin and Morgan. Sleep and Ageing. London: Croom Helm, 1987.
172. Gerard P. Subjective characteristics of sleep in the elderly. Age Ageing 1978; **7** (Suppl): 55–9.

173. Greenblatt DJ, Allen MD. Toxicity of nitrazepam in the elderly: a report from the Boston Collaborative Drug Surveillance Program. Brit J Clin Pharmacol 1978; **5**: 407–13.
174. Greenblatt DJ, Allen MD, Shader RI. Toxicity of high dose flurazepam in the elderly. Clin Pharmacol Ther 1977; **21**: 355–61.
175. Kennie DC. Insomnia. In: The Aging Process 2. Home Study Program No. 21, pp. 21–4. Kansas City, KA: American Academy of Family Physicians, 1980.

9

Strengthening support systems

Imposed burden on family carers

Importance

The impact of the caring role on the health and wellbeing of family and other informal carers is considerable. While the caring bond may be of mutual benefit and enhance relationships there is now well-documented evidence that caring for elderly people can have numerous adverse effects (see Fig. 9.1). Many researchers have produced evidence that such caring can produce increased levels of anxiety, embarrassment, guilt, low morale and depression [1–3]. Several studies attest to a significant degree of physical ill-health in carers [3, 4], and diabetes, arthritis, anaemia and the use of psychotropic medication have been shown to be more common than in non-carers [6]. This may be because the caring role is causal or because many carers themselves are elderly. Caregiving undoubtedly involves a degree of financial penalty incurring both direct and indirect (or opportunity) costs [7, 8]. Caring can also jeopardise opportunities for employment, many younger relatives giving up work or restricting their working hours to continue with the role [9, 10]. If they remain at work their performance often suffers significantly [11].

The impact of caring on carers can have a subsequent negative effect on their families, on the elderly people themselves and on society at large. For example, caregiving often involves spending time away from the carer's own family and family disharmony frequently accompanies the caregiving role [12]. The burden of caring often results in demand for community services or institutionalisation and, if these services and facilities are not forthcoming, to various types of elder abuse.

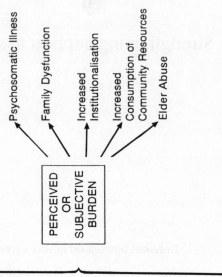

CAREGIVER STRESS : CAUSE AND EFFECT

MEASURABLE OR OBJECTIVE BURDEN

* Relating to Patient Characteristics:
  e.g. immobility, incontinence, insomnia

* Relating to Interference with Social Functioning
  e.g. inability of caregiver to get out of house or go on holiday

* Relating to the Caregiver's Limitations from:
  i) Physical stress e.g. backache, cardiac disease
  ii) Psychodynamic stress e.g. anxiety, guilt, fatigue, role reversal

'MODULATING' VARIABLES

* Previous strength of relationship between patient and caregiver

* Conflicting goals, ambitions and duties

* Social class

* Ethnic grouping

* Caregiver's own support system

* Rapidity of onset of patient's dependency

* Duration of burden of caring

* Caregiver's perception of an end to the caregiving role

PERCEIVED OR SUBJECTIVE BURDEN

OUTCOMES

Psychosomatic Illness

Family Dysfunction

Increased Institutionalisation

Increased Consumption of Community Resources

Elder Abuse

Fig. 9.1. The causes and effects of caregiver stress. The different burdens may be modified by any of several variables that modulate the clinical or social outcome.

Detection

Identifying the impact of the caring role on carers is a skill infrequently taught to health care professionals. It is unusual for elderly persons themselves (particularly if they are demented) to express or identify carers' problems during assessment and a further direct interview with the caregiver is usually required. This interview may be unstructured or semistructured or may contain a rating scale to elicit caregiver stress. Recently, ten such scales for measuring burden and stress amongst the caregivers of dementia sufferers have been reviewed [13]. Some of these scales measure objective burden, others measure subjective feelings. Most measure a combination of such parameters. Little attempt has yet been made to correlate the various outcomes of the caring role with individual aspects of each of these components, and consequently accurate targeting of strategies to those who would benefit is still a matter of clinical judgement rather than of scientific fact.

Effectiveness

Although several strategies are in high demand from the caring public and have been employed for many years in an attempt to reduce carer burden and stress, research on their efficacy is in its infancy. Initially research concentrated on whether or not the strategy would help to prevent or delay institutionalisation and only recently have attempts been made to evaluate whether or not the measures improve wellbeing in the carers themselves. Although carers are a heterogeneous group, most information is available on those looking after dementia sufferers. The strategies may be summarised as follows.

Development of a Carers' Charter

In some areas a Carers' Charter has been developed that sets out their basic rights (see Fig. 9.2). Although no attempt has been made to evaluate the impact of such Charters, their development has helped to focus attention on the plight of carers, to reprioritise the allocation of resources and to serve as a basis for future audit and quality control.

Community services for elderly people

Public demand, as well as the evidence from some research, suggests that formal community services (home helps, home health aids, mobile meal services, community nursing, etc.), at least of some types and under some circumstances and when delivered as a coordinated package, do alleviate stress and do aid in raising the morale of family carers [14].

Night nursing service

There has been little evaluation of the impact of night nursing services on carers. However, one scheme emphasised the importance of a night nursing service to relatives by giving them short breaks that enabled them to cope with the elderly person at home for a longer period than would otherwise have been possible [15]. This report also alluded to a survey of the attitudes of patients' relatives, but did not give details.

Dispersed community alarm services

Little evidence is available on the impact of dispersed alarm systems on carers. Yet, families are the major procurors of this service and the presence of an alarm (and subsequent response backup) may minimise or even eliminate the need for a carer to visit frequently. The presence of an alarm system may also reduce the anxiety of leaving a frail elderly person on his or her own.

In-home respite services

In the UK, these services are exemplified by the Crossroads Care Attendant Schemes which provide sessions of time where someone substitutes for the family carer whilst the latter either recuperates or attends to other tasks. In one evaluative study, the interval from the dementia sufferer's admission to institutional care to death (what was known as the 'death interval') for those receiving such in-home respite service was 12.7 months as distinct from 17.6 months for a control group. This suggests that, by the time of admission, those receiving in-home care were more dependent and had been maintained in the community for a longer period [16].

Day care

Several published studies have described the positive impact of day care programmes on the families of frail elderly people [17–19]. Gilleard's study of stress and outcome at a psychogeriatric day care unit showed significant improvement in the supporters' General Health Questionnaire score at three months follow up compared with on initial attendance, the score reducing from 13.2 to 7.1 [20]. A further published report from California found that day health care programmes had a significant impact on carers. Of those interviewed, almost half indicated that personal respite was a major reason for selecting this type of programme and after six months 92 per cent of carers indicated that the programme had helped them maintain themselves in their caring role [21].

CARER'S CHARTER

*Our philosophy is based on the belief
that you have a right to:*

*A range of information services pertinent to your caring role
and the problems of your dependants.*

*Counselling, training and support services to assist you in
your caring role.*

*Choose the extent of your involvement in the caring
partnership with the Health Board's provider units.*

*Time off (respite) for yourself and the choice to fill this time
with rest, recreation or purposeful self-fulfilling activity.*

*Promptness in receiving services for your dependants and for
yourself.*

*Prompt and sensitive intervention when a crisis has
developed due to the caring burden becoming excessive.*

*Choose a caring partnership with Health Board staff once
your dependants have had to go into care and the right to be
provided with a range of practical options for so doing.*

*Physical and psychological support (if applicable) in the
terminal or bereavement phases of your caring role.*

*Be consulted in policy making and planning for resources for
carers and their dependants.*

*Equal consideration (and at times more consideration) to the
person cared for when their condition impinges on your own
rights.*

Fig. 9.2. A carers' charter

Institutional respite care

Institutional respite care (in hospital, in nursing home or in residential home, depending on the health care system and dependency of the elderly person concerned) was initiated by De Largy [22] in the UK. Since then a number of descriptive schemes suggesting benefit have been outlined. However, more formal evaluation was attempted by Robertson [23], who found that the planned intermittent use of an institutional bed allowed caregivers to place their frail elders when medical procedures, surgery or a vacation was needed. A further retrospective evaluative study by Dunn [24] suggested that such institutional respite delayed the need for long term institutional care. Scharlach [25] has also demonstrated improvement in carers' health and in their sleep pattern due to institutional respite care. Contrarily, a recent controlled trial of various types of respite for the carers of Alzheimer's patients showed no effect on wellbeing at annual follow up, though sufferers spent 22 days longer in the community than the control group [26].

Information services

Although research specifically relating to the carers of elderly people is lacking, Tobin et al. [27] have shown that the knowledge that resources exist in a community to help with emergencies is itself sufficient to help families to keep impaired relatives out of institutions. Recently, Tester and Meredith [28] have shown that targeting information at the elderly population can increase the uptake of financial supplementary benefits to which they are entitled, which may also benefit carers.

Counselling education

A number of studies have evaluated the impact of counselling and/or education on carers. Horowitz [29] has shown that brief psychodynamic psychotherapy may be of benefit to carers of end-stage dementia sufferers experiencing intense anticipatory grief. Lezak [30] has shown that counselling family carers improves their adjustment and acceptance of the personality changes that accompany dementia. Counselling to promote improved family support has been attempted by Zarit [31]. Results have shown short term decline in perceived burden and emotional distress. Further evaluated programmes have been aimed at Assertion Training, Motivation Enhancement and Stress Reduction. For example, Levine [32] has reported such results after using an SET (Supporter Endurance Training) programme. Likewise, Haley [33] has reported several successful case examples indicating that caregivers treated on a one to one basis could successfully learn behavioural management strategies that were based on operant conditioning models. Linsk et al. [34] have also presented extensive data on this approach. They found that most clients improved as a result of intervention and maintained their improvement for at least six months. Recently Brodaty and Gresham [35] reported the results of a novel approach in which carers were also admitted to hospital with the dementia sufferer for a period of intensive training and education. In this controlled trial, the General Health Questionnaire (GHQ) of the control group of carers rose over time from 3.6 to 7.4 whilst the GHQ of the carers in the intervention programme fell from 6.3 to 4.7. The percentage of patients still residing at home at one-year follow up was 26 and 65 for the two groups, respectively.

Self and mutual support groups

Although these groups are now widespread and supported by a number of associations such as the Alzheimer's and Related Diseases Society, the Parkinson's Disease Society and the Chest and Heart Association, Toseland [36] comments that 'when rigorous experimental . . . designs were used and data were collected using measures with known reliability and validity characteristics . . . the outcomes of caregiver support groups were equivocal at best'. However, several less scientifically rigorous studies suggest benefit. For example, Lazarus [37] found significant positive differences between participants and non-participants in a support group. Participants indicated that they experienced a greater degree of control over their lives and expressed less dissatisfaction with changes to the family unit. The majority indicated that the group had helped in their being able to relate to, and cope with, their impaired relative.

Additional finance

There has been little research to identify the benefits of this potential strategy. However, Gray [38] reported the results of a pilot study using a randomised design to evaluate the impact of caregiver training and participation in a support group plus or minus a modest financial reimbursement to family carers. Results on several measures indicated that there were no significant differences caused by the experimental conditions of reimbursement.

Cost

No detailed information on costs is available.

Absence of resident supervision and support

Importance

In one Scottish survey of the household composition of elderly people, 30.4 per cent lived alone. Eighty per cent of those living alone were women [39]. These figures take no account of the additional times when resident carers are away from the home for employment or other purposes, though it must constitute a significant percentage of the 17.4 per cent of elderly people who live in two or three-generation households [39].

The absence of a resident carer leads to consumption of in-home community service provision. Some estimate of the need for such services can be extrapolated from the figures shown in Table 9.1, from the Scottish community survey mentioned above [39]. In this study, the population was categorised according to the interval of time during which their needs must be met. This was based on an extension of original work by Isaacs and Neville [40]. The need for, and benefit from, in-home care services would accrue most to those in the 'long interval' and 'short interval' categories, which constituted 38.8 and 9.2 respectively of the total of elderly people living alone in private households. Living alone is also a major risk factor for institutionalisation and for hypothermia, and may result in psycological and psychiatric morbidity.

Targeting/detection

The detection of those elderly people living alone is a fairly simple task in those societies with a strong, primary care base, this information usually being available from the practice records. However, the appropriate targeting of elderly people living alone for the receipt of in-home community services (one of the strategies outlined below) is one of the major outstanding practical and research issues in gerontology. This is particularly so when community services are considered an alternative to institutional care [41]. In many places, the provision of community services is demand-led. In others, provision usually depends on the need identified by elderly persons (or more commonly their families) being professionally legitimised by a care provider using some 'objective' criteria such as their ability to perform various activities of daily living. Receipt of services may also be linked to various reimbursement criteria. Consequently, the nature of the client receiving home services varies considerably from one locality to another depending on who is deemed to be 'in need' and on the resources available. Several studies suggest there is not only underprovision to those most in need but also overprovision to relatively healthy elderly people (the 'sympathy vote') which may ultimately foster their dependency.

Optimal targeting for those living alone who should receive a personal community alarm system (the other strategy outlined below) is relatively unresearched. Usually provision is based on a perception of frailty and potential for crises. It is generally believed that those with significant degrees of dementia may be excluded from alarm provision because their rate of underuse and misuse can be considerable [42].

Effectiveness

Although a number of strategies are used to supervise and assist those living alone, only two of the most commonly employed are considered in detail.

In-home community services

Research into the efficacy of in-home care services has focussed almost exclusively on the issue of whether they can substitute for, or postpone the need for, institutional care. Relatively little attention has been paid to the impact these services have on meeting client needs and improving their quality of life.

Although the subject is highly controversial, some evidence suggests that when such services are well targeted (i.e. are provided to people who in the absence of this support would definitely be admitted to institutional care), they can effectively reduce the extent of nursing home use [41, 43]. However, it is also known that some of the most difficult people to maintain in the community, even with support from these services, are those elderly people living alone who have little in the way of an *informal* support network for the formal services to complement. There is also evidence that targeting of community services can be improved by means of a care/case management system and that when the care/case manager also focusses on the psychological wellbeing and relationships of his or her clients, this can have a separate, distinct and additive effect other than that simply due to matching resources to physical needs [44].

Use of community alarm systems

Evidence from North America suggests that the use of dispersed community alarm systems may effectively reduce the need for institutional care. Ruchlin and Morris [45], using matched samples of elderly clients, found considerable reductions in use of nursing homes and in lengths of stay among alarm users, though the benefits were not shared by people who were severely functionally impaired and who were also socially isolated. Dibner [46] similarly found a

Table 9.1. *Dependency needs by living arrangements*

Dependency categories	Mobility incapacity	Self-care incapacity	Home-care incapacity	Incontinence	Mental state	Lives alone (%)	Lives with spouse (%)	Lives with others (%)
A. Independent	No difficulty with any of the *scale* activities	No difficulty with any of the *scale* activities	No difficulty with any of the *scale* activities	None	None	50.2	64.7	52.1
B. Long interval – mental only	No difficulty with any of the *scale* activities	No difficulty with any of the *scale* activities	No difficulty with any of the *scale* activities	None	Mild organic disorder or mild affective disorder or psychoneurosis	14.2	9.2	8.0
C. Long interval – functional	Difficulty with: walking outside on level surface Unable to: travel by bus	Difficulty with: washing hair dressing washing hands and face Unable to: wash hair wash or bath all over	Difficulty with: washing clothes ironing clothes preparing and cooking hot meal light housework Unable to: do heavy shopping wash clothes iron clothes	Incontinent of urine	May have mild disorder	24.8	18.9	23.7
D. Short interval – no night help	Difficulty with: walking inside on level surface Unable to: walk outside on level surface	Unable to: put on shoes and socks dress wash hands and face	Unable to: prepare and cook meals make bed do light housework	Not incontinent faeces	Not severe	9.1	5.1	10.3
E. Short interval – night help required	As short interval	As short interval *and* night help required	As short interval	As short interval	As short interval	0.1	1.0	1.0

	As independent	As independent	As independent	None	Severe organic or functional disorder
			1.1	0.2	0.7
F. Critical interval – mental independent or with long interval functional	As long interval functional	As long interval functional	As long interval functional	As long interval functional	Any
			0.7	1.0	4.3
G. Critical interval – functional Unable to: get up from chair / walk inside / Permanently or temporarily bed-fast or chair-fast	Any	Any	Any	Incontinent of faeces	Any
or Severe psychiatric disorder with short interval capacity	Short interval	Short interval	Short interval	Short interval	Severe

At A and B, E and F, all of the conditions must be satisfied. At C and D one of the incapacities listed for mobility, self-care, house-care or incontinence must be present and degree of mental impairment is a necessary condition. At G one of the mobility conditions must be satisfied or incontinence as stated.
Adapted from ref. [39].

decline of 28 per cent in hospital admissions and 29 per cent in lengths of hospital stay. These findings are supported by the work of Cain [47] and others [48, 49]. It is not known whether these results can be extrapolated to a society such as the UK, which has fewer institutional places and a 'gated' system of access to such homes. However, savings in the amount of in-home care required by alarm users have also been reported in other studies [50, 51].

Cost

In-home care services

In general terms there is a correlation between increased dependency and the cost of the in-home care services required to maintain the individuals in the community [52]. The relationship between the need for increasing levels of supervision (because of risk behaviour from dementia) and the cost of in-home service provision has been less well documented, but is likely to be similar. A cut-off point is therefore reached, beyond which it is more expensive to care for an older person in the community than to provide institutional care [53, 54].

An important question, in recent years, has been: do carefully targeted, in-home care services, provided to a minority of the elderly population, provide a cost effective alternative to institutional care? This targeting has usually been achieved through a system of community case management. The resolution of this question is still the subject of controversy and debate. The cost savings from care management depend not just on the frailty of the elderly population who are targeted but on the intensity and professionalism of the care managers themselves.

Community alarm systems

Ruchlin and Morris [45] performed a benefit–cost analysis of the *Lifeline* emergency alarm and response system. Overall, dividing estimated programme benefit by estimated programme cost yielded a benefit–cost ratio of 1.87. Of the target groups considered, the programme was not found to be cost beneficial for those with severe functional impairment and social isolation but did show a benefit–cost ratio of 7.19 for those with severe functional impairment who were *not* socially isolated and a benefit–cost ratio of 1.27 for those with social isolation who were either moderately functionally impaired or 'medically vulnerable'.

Substandard housing

Importance

Housing is a key element in providing for the health, wellbeing and independence of elderly people yet nearly half of all unfit properties are occupied by this age group [55]. Substandard housing leads to: illness from overcrowding and dampness [56]; hypothermia from inadequate heating and draughts; problems of access to, and being housebound from, adequate design for the disabled; falls and accidents from problems of layout; and to frustration and anxiety from the need for repair.

The impact of substandard housing on the health of the elderly population is, however, difficult to quantify. The causation between the health and housing relationship is difficult to establish because so many factors interplay and interact [57]. Little research has been done in this area.

Poor housing is also a primary factor in the request for allocation of sheltered housing [58]. The morbidity caused by relocation must also be taken into account [59].

Targeting/Detection

Elderly people most at risk from substandard housing are least able to seek assistance from authorities that control housing and other services. At the present time, requests for intervention from families, and home visiting by occupational therapists, community nurses and family doctors form the main means of identifying those at risk. However, no identification criteria nor any structured assessment protocol is available.

Effectiveness

Little scientific research is available in this area. The positive impact of good housing is contained mainly in case study material. Nevertheless, evidence from this and other areas lend credence to benefit from the following strategies.

Home care and repair schemes

Home care and repair schemes that assist elderly people in tackling repairs and obtaining improvements and adaptations for the disabled are widely recommended as making an important contribution to community care [60].

Staying put strategies

These include the provision in the home of personal and domestic care services, aids and adaptations and an alarm system for summoning assistance.

A housing officer with responsibility for elderly people

In public sector housing, it has been found advantageous to appoint a housing officer with a specific remit for the older population who can provide a more specialised assessment and who can liaise with social service, health care and other community service agencies.

Cost

No detailed information on costs is available.

Relocation morbidity and mortality

Importance

The extent of relocation of the elderly population to hospitals, homes and various types of housing accommodation is unknown but extensive. Considering only relocation to nursing homes, it is well to appreciate that in the USA, where there has been a relatively ungated provision of private care, although only 5 per cent of elderly people actually reside in institutional care at any one time, 25 to 40 per cent enter a nursing home at some point in their lives [61].

Major relocation is associated with psychological morbidity. There may also be a significant mortality associated with relocation, but the evidence for this is conflicting [59, 62].

Targeting

No reliable criteria are available to identify those at particular risk from relocation. The evidence suggests most adverse effects are experienced when the elderly person perceives he or she has no control, when the move is imposed and/or when it is contrary to the expressed wishes of that individual. A 'Cost of Care' Index [63] has been developed to assist in evaluating the anticipated impact of becoming involved in the caring role and may usefully be employed when considering relocating an older person into the family home to avoid later distress and recrimination.

Effectiveness

Strategies to reduce relocation morbidity remain relatively unresearched. Providing a brief nursing home visit prior to placement is associated with better subsequent adjustment. Counselling of newly admitted residents also reduces anxiety and improves the feeling of the residents' control [63]. Further strategies, such as giving the perception of choice and the perception of control in the decision making process, remain unevaluated, as do the guidelines that have been produced to promote familial harmony if an old person is moving into a relative's home [64].

Cost

No detailed information on costs is available.

Relative poverty

Importance

Despite an improvement in absolute living standards in recent years, relative poverty amongst elderly people has been well documented. Over half of those retired have been found to be in households living in poverty or on the margins of poverty [65]. In an analysis of the 1980 General Household Survey in the UK, Victor [66] found 23 per cent of the elderly persons in his study had incomes at, or below, the Supplementary Pension rate. A further 33 per cent were living at or below 1.4 times this rate.

Although average life expectancy has advanced, socioeconomic differences in mortality have persisted. For example, a recent study comparing life expectancy at birth by social class showed a difference of 2.8 years between social classes I (professional and managerial groups) and V (unskilled manual workers). In terms of morbidity, recent evidence from an analysis of two large population surveys in the USA shows that socioeconomic differences tend to be greatest in middle age and early old age and then to be smaller again amongst persons over 75 years, but nevertheless continue to show significant variance even in advanced old age [67] (see Fig. 9.3).

The existence of an association between socioeconomic status and health does not necessarily imply direct causality. Lower socioeconomic groups may be disadvantaged because of the increased association of other risk factors for morbidity and disability, such as unhealthy lifestyle behaviour, acute and chronic psychosocial stress, inadequate social relationships and support, and

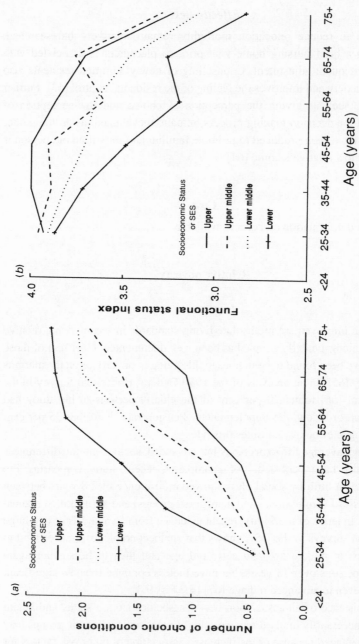

Fig. 9.3. Relationship between socioeconomic status and health at different ages. (*a*) Association of age with chronic conditions. (*b*) Association of age with functional status index. Adapted from ref. [67].

exposure to environmental risks. Additionally, Wilkinson [68], focussing on reviewing the association between life expectancy and income distribution, concluded that few countries in 1984 achieved an average life expectancy at birth of 70 years or more until gross national product per head approached a threshold of almost $5000 per year. Beyond that level, however, there was little systematic relation between gross national product per head and life expectancy.

Nevertheless, despite the long term tendency towards an improved standard of living and real income in *absolute* terms, many sociologists draw attention to the problem of the *relative* poverty of elderly people in an increasingly affluent society. This widening 'social cleavage' results in increasing social segregation and isolation in a society where conspicuous consumption is the norm. Poverty may also influence health in a number of ways. It can limit choice. It may also lead to inability or unwillingness to purchase items, such as spectacles, dentures, drugs, nutritious food or fuel for warmth, that are important to overall health. It may lead to a selection bias against those with poor financial means: for example, the private nursing home industry has been known to discriminate against those on income support rates. Even health promotional measures are negatively targeted at the poor, the group most often in need of them [69].

Targeting/detection

Primary preventive measures consist of ensuring that appropriate groups of elderly people are appropriately targeted to receive adequate job-related or governmental retirement pensions. Secondary preventive measures usually consist of means testing to identify those in need of financial support for basic needs. This screening technique requires skilled personnel, is time consuming and abhorred by many elderly people and their carers.

Effectiveness

A number of strategies have been employed.

Pension schemes

One of the most effective measures to ensure an adequate level of income for elderly people is to ensure that job-related and governmental retirement pensions maintain this population above poverty levels. This policy is difficult to achieve because considerable controversy surrounds the concept of an 'adequate' pension income (the spending needs of elderly people also lessening with age) [70] and because, in the face of other competing economic priorities, it is extremely difficult to implement these proposals politically.

Welfare benefit schemes

Intensive welfare benefit schemes targeted at elderly people have resulted in increased take up rates. This undoubtedly has led to improved health and diminished suffering/handicap in certain individuals but there is little evidence that when globally applied it leads to these benefits in the population as a whole. It is known that additional funds provided to individuals as a nutritional allowance may well be spent on non-health matters [71]. Moreover, many elderly people abhor the concept of receiving public assistance, and this aversion leads to low take up rates for supplementary funding.

Equity of payment by elderly people

Further strategies may be aimed at avoiding inequitable payments for care amongst elderly people. Examples of this would be the various attempts in the USA to introduce insurance to cover catastrophic medical costs. Much more commonly required is an equitable scheme for covering the costs of long term institutional care. At present, elderly people at poverty level may receive some financial support to defray costs. However, those just above poverty levels may have to 'spend down' their entire life's savings and assets before being eligible for such financial support [72]. Finally, if the health care of a nation's elderly population is to be increasingly underpinned by private insurance, it is important that excessive premiums, copayments and deductables be avoided and that the private insurance policies actually cover the type of chronic health problem likely to be encountered in that population. At present, many private insurance policies are deficient in this regard.

Cost

An analysis of the costs and benefits of providing pensions and various means-tested financial supplements is considered beyond the scope of this book.

Overprotection

Importance

The extent of overprotection of elderly people by well-meaning carers has not been researched or quantified. Nevertheless, it is a frequent problem. Common examples are the premature provision of community services (which fosters dependency), the imposition of unnecessary rest following minor illness (which worsens balance and mobility), and unwarranted institutionalisation (which results in loss of autonomy). Overprotection by nursing staff in hospitals and nursing homes is also common, leading to poor rehabilitation and to prolonged stays.

Detection

No reliable methods have been developed to detect this problem. Interview of the elderly person and their primary carer together and, where possible, in the home setting seems the best means currently available.

Effectiveness

Measures to counteract overprotection have not been evaluated. Family counselling can be beneficial. Overprotective care by nursing staff may be counteracted by the use of functionally orientated models of nursing practice such as that of Orem [73].

Cost

No detailed information is available.

Abuse and neglect

Importance

Abuse of elderly people can take many forms: physical, psychological or sexual abuse; financial or material exploitation; active or passive neglect; and violation of rights. The precise prevalence of abuse depends on the definition of the aspect under consideration, but surveys from the USA suggest some type, or combination of types, occur in 10 per cent of Americans over 65 years of age and about 4 per cent may be victims of moderate to severe abuse [74, 75]. Recently, Ogg and Bennett have published data for the prevalence of verbal, physical and financial abuse of the elderly British population [75a]. Abuse can occur in the community, nursing home or hospital. Detailed descriptions of the various manifestations of such abuse are provided by a number of authors [74, 76].

Detection

Abuse of elderly people is often not apparent because both the victim and the perpetrator tend to deny it or downplay its seriousness. Health professionals and society in general find it difficult to acknowledge that such abuse exists. Its identification therefore depends on an increased awareness of those dealing with elderly people and on more detailed and active case detection. Unfortunately, no validated instruments have yet been developed for screening for abuse in an elderly population. Nevertheless, a number of high risk factors have been suggested that may assist in identification [75]. These include: those elderly persons with primary carers that express frustration in dealing with care needs or who demonstrate signs of stress (particularly from external factors such as job loss, illness or other family problems); those living in families with a norm of family violence; those living in families that abuse alcohol or drugs; and those living in families with a prior history of elder abuse (the problem tends to be a recurring one) [76, 77].

Surveys indicate that elder abuse is seen by a wide range of professional and paraprofessional staff [76]. In particular, community nurses and hospital and community social service agency staff should be alert to its possible existence. The interview technique recommended is one that sees the elderly person and carer both alone and interacting together.

Effectiveness

Many strategies have been advocated to reduce abuse of the elderly population and several are actively implemented in various parts of the world. However, little research is available to validate their efficacy or effectiveness.

Organisational measures

Societal response to elder abuse has largely focussed on organisational and administrative strategies. One of the most important is the development, in a community, of an agreed multi-agency protocol for the assessment and management of suspected cases of elder abuse by a multidisciplinary team. In some societies, a 'protective services' or social services agency takes the lead role in this process. A further strategy, operational in several states in the USA, is to legislate for the compulsory reporting of all cases of elder abuse that are encountered by various professional and other groups.

Measures to reduce caregiver stress

A major strategy to reduce the risk of abuse of elderly people from their care-givers is to lessen the stress, fatigue and frustration of this latter group. Measures to identify this burden and provide assistance are discussed elsewhere.

The exploration of alternative living arrangements

The exploration of alternative living arrangements may be a worthwhile option [78], bearing in mind that the intervention should promote the least restrictive alternative. In many cases, living with the abusing caregiver may still provide the most nurturing source of long term care.

Measures to reduce crime

After surveying facts about crime that victimised elderly people in Pennsylvania, a number of recommendations were published that laid the groundwork for an effective programme to alleviate the problem [76]. They recommended the banding together of government, law enforcement organisations, business and citizens in an alliance to combat this common problem.

Fear of crime is a somewhat separate but nevertheless real issue for many elderly people. The most comprehensive review of strategies for reducing fear of crime has been presented by Henig and Maxfield [79].

Measures to reduce abuse in nursing homes

The development of a Charter of Rights or legally binding contract for elderly residents and the development of an ombudsman programme [80] to deal with complaints and act as an advocacy service are two commonly employed measures to reduce the abuse of elderly residents in long stay facilities. Traditional registration and inspection of such homes has probably had little impact on the more common non-fiscal forms of abuse. This may change with the implementation of the resident-orientated, outcome inspection protocols recommended by the Institute of Medicine in the USA [81].

Measures to reduce abuse in hospitals

Many of the strategies pertinent to the reduction of abuse of elderly hospitalised patients are considered in the section on minimising iatrogenic insult (see p. 130). Further important measures include careful patient-centred careplanning by nursing staff; ensuring that discharge plans ensure sufficient support to provide an acceptable quality of life for those with residual disability; and ensuring measures to permit death with dignity and an absence of invasive, unnecessary biomedical intervention.

Cost

No detailed information on costs is available.

References

1. Fengler AP, Goodrich N. Wives of elderly disabled men, the hidden patients. Gerontologist 1979; **19**: 175–83.
2. Rabins PV et al. The impact of dementia on the family. J Amer Med Assoc 1982; **248**: 333–5.
3. Levin E et al. The Supporters of Confused Elderly People at Home. London: National Institute for Social Work Research Unit, 1983.
4. Farkes SW. Impact of chronic illness on the patient's spouse. Health Social Work 1980; **5**: 39–46.
6. Pruchno RA, Potashnik SL. Caregiving spouses: physical and mental health in perspective. J Amer Geriatr Soc 1989; **37**: 697–705.
7. Economist Intelligence Unit Ltd. Care with dignity: analysis of costs of care for the disabled. London: The National Fund for Research into Crippling Diseases, 1977.
8. Nissel M, Bonnerjea L. Family Care of the Handicapped Elderly: Who Pays? London: Policy Studies Institute, 1982.
9. Equal Opportunities Commission. The Experience of Caring for Elderly and Handicapped Dependents. Survey Report. Manchester: EoC, 1980.
10. Brocklehurst JC, Morris P, Andrews K et al. Social effects of strokes. Social Sci Med 1981; **15A**: 35–9.
11. Archold PG. The impact of caring for an ill elderly parent on middle aged offspring. J Gerontol Nurs 1980; **6**: 78–85.
12. Rabins PV, Mace NL, Lucas MJ. The impact of dementia on the family. J Amer Med Assoc 1982; **248**: 333–5.
13. Vitaliano PP, Young HM, Russo J. A review of measures used among caregivers of individuals with dementia. Gerontologist 1991; **31**: 67–75.
14. Challis D, Davies B. Case Management in Community Care. Aldershot: Gower, 1986.
15. Gillespie JV. Night nursing service in West Fife. Health Bull (Scot) 1980; **38**: 187–93.
16. Rosenvinge GE. Personal communication, 1986.
17. Eskew R, Sexton R, Tars S, Wilcox F. Day treatment program evaluation. In: Smyer M, Gatz M (eds) Mental Health and Aging, Beverley Hills, CA: Sage, 1983.
18. Rathbone McCuan E. Geriatric day care: a family perspective. Gerontologist 1976; **16**: 517–21.
19. Sands, D, Suzuki T. Adult day care for Alzheimer patients and their families. Gerontologist 1983; **23**: 21–3.
20. Gilleard CJ, Gilleard E, Gledhill K et al. Caring for the elderly mentally infirm

at home: a survey of the supporters. J Epidem Commun Health 1984; **38**: 19–25.

21. Hartley W. A Better Way. Final report of the Senior Health Services Project. Palo Alto, CA: Mid-Peninsula Health Services Inc. and the Senior Coordinating Council Palo Alto, 1982.

22. DeLargy J. Six weeks in, six weeks out: a geriatric hospital scheme for rehabilitating the aged and relieving their relatives. Lancet 1957; **1**: 418–19.

23. Robertson D, Griffiths A, Cozin LZ. A community-based continuing care program for the elderly disabled: an evaluation of planned intermittent hospital readmission. J Gerontol 1977; **32**: 334.

24. Dunn RB, MacBeath L, Robertson D. Respite admissions and the disabled elderly. J Amer Geriatr Soc 1985; **31**: 613–16.

25. Scharlach A. An evaluation of institution-based respite care. Gerontologist 1986; **26**: 77–82.

26. Lawton MP, Brody E, Saperstein AR. A controlled study of respite service for caregivers of Alzheimer's patients. Gerontologist 1989; **29**: 8–16.

27. Tobin SS, Kulys R. The family and services. In: Eisdorfer C (ed) Annual Review of Gerontology and Geriatrics, New York: Springer, 1980.

28. Tester S, Meredith B. Ill-informed? A Study of Information and Support for Elderly People in the Inner City. London: Policy Studies Institute, 1987.

29. Horowitz A. Families who care: a study of natural support systems of the elderly. Presented at the 31st Scientific Meeting of the Gerontological Society, Dallas, TX, 1978.

30. Lezak MD. Living with the characterologically altered brain-injured patient. J Clins Psychiatr 1978; **39**: 592–9.

31. Zarit SH, Zarit JM. Families under stress: interventions for caregivers of senile dementia patients. Psychotherapy Theory Res Practive 1982; **19**: 461–71.

32. Levine NB, Dostoor DP, Gendrow GE. Coping with dementia: a pilot study. J Amer Geriatr Soc 1983; **31**: 12–18.

33. Haley WD. A family-behavioural approach to the treatment of the cognitively impaired elderly. Gerontologist 1983; **23**: 18–20.

34. Linsk NL, Pinkston E. Introducing community-based behavioural techniques to families of the impaired elderly. Paper presented at the National Conference on Social Welfare. Cleveland, OH, 1980.

35. Brodaty H, Gresham M. Effect of training programme to reduce stress in carers of patients with dementia. Brit Med J 1989; **29**: 1375–9.

36. Toseland RW, Rossiter CM. Group interventions to support family caregivers: a review and analysis. Gerontologist 1989; **29**: 438–48.

37. Lazarus LW, Stafford B, Cooper K et al. A pilot study of Alzheimer's patients relatives' discussion group. Gerontologist 1981; **21**: 353–8.

38. Gray VK. Providing support for home caregivers. In: Smyer M, Gatz M (eds) Mental Health and Ageing, pp. 197–214. Beverley Hills, CA: Sage, 1983.

39. Bond J, Carstairs V. Services for the Elderly. Scottish Health Services Studies No. 42. Edinburgh: Scottish Home and Health Department, 1982.

40. Isaacs B, Neville Y. The Measurement of Need in Old People. Scottish Health Services Studies No. 34. Edinburgh: Scottish Home and Health Department, 1975.

41. Weissert WG, Cready CM, Pawelak JE. Home and Community Care: Three Decades of Findings. In: Peterson MD, White DL (eds) Health Care of the Elderly: An Information Source Book. Beverley Hills, CA: Sage Publications, 1989.

42. Fisk MJ. Alarm Systems and Elderly People. Glasgow: The Planning Exchange, 1989.
43. Capitman JA et al. Case management in coordinated community-oriented long term care demonstrations. Gerontologist 1986; **26**: 398–404.
44. Davies B, Missiakoulis S. Heineken and Matching processes in Thanet community care project: an empirical test of their relative importance. Brit J Social Work 1987; **18**: 55–78.
45. Ruchlin HS, Morris JN. Cost benefit analysis of an emergency alarm and response system: a case study of a long term program. Health Services Res 1981; **16**: 65–79.
46. Dibner AS. Effects of a Personal Emergency Response Service on Hospital Use. Watertown, MA: Lifeline Systems Inc., 1985.
47. Cain BA. Effects of a lifeline program on hospitalisation. Masters Thesis, Department of Social Work, California State University, CA, 1987.
48. Koch JW. Response system assistance in discharge planning. Dimensions in Health Service 1984.
49. Stafford J, Dibiner AS. Lifeline programs in 1984: stability and growth. MA: Lifeline Systems Inc., 1984.
50. Dixon L. Evaluation of Electronic Call Device project. City of New York: HRA Medical Assistance Program, 1987.
51. Coordinated Care Management Corporation. Emergency Response System Demonstration Project: Preliminary Report. Buffalo, NY: 1987.
52. Duke University Center for the Study of Aging and Human Development. Multidimensional Functional Assessment: The OARS Methodology. 2nd edit. Durham, NC: Duke University Center for the Study of Aging and Human Development, 1978.
53. Wright KG. Economics and planning the care of the elderly. In: Wright KG (ed) Economics and Health Planning. London: Croom Helm, 1979.
54. Opit LJ. Domiciliary care for the elderly sick – economy or neglect. Brit Med J 1977; **1**: 30–3.
55. Department of the Environment. English House Conditions Survey Part 2. London: HMSO, 1983.
56. Platt SD et al. Damp housing: mould growth and symptomatic health state. Brit Med J 1989; **298**: 1673–8.
57. Wheeler R. Housing and health in old age: research agenda. Discussion Paper 21. Centre for Health Economics, University of York, 1986.
58. Butler A, Oldman C, Greve J. Sheltered housing for the elderly. National Institute Social Services Library No. 44, pp. 21–51. London: George Allen and Unwin, 1983.
59. Coffman TL. Relocation and survival of institutionalised aged: a reexamination of the evidence. Gerontologist 1981; **21**: 483–500.
60. Wheeler R. Don't move: we've got you covered. A study of the Anchor Housing Trust Staying Put Scheme. London: Institute of Housing, 1985.
61. Vicente L et al. The risk of institutionalisation before death. Gerontologist 1979; **19**: 361–7.
62. Kosberg J, Cairl R. The cost of care index: a case management tool for screening informal care providers. Gerontologist 1986; **26**: 273–8.
63. Dye CJ, Erber JT. Two group procedures for the treatment of nursing home patients. Gerontologist 1981; **21**: 539–44.
64. Wilcock GK, Gray JAM, Pritchard PMM. Geriatric Problems in General Practice. Oxford: University Press, 1982.

65. Whitehead M. The Health Divide: Inequalities in Health in the 1980s. London: Health Education Council 1987.
66. Victor CR, Vetter NJ. Poverty, disability and use of services by the elderly: analysis of the 1980 General Household Survey. Soc Sci Med 1986; **22**: 1087–91.
67. House JS, Kessler RC, Herzog AR. Age, socio-economic status and health. The Milbank Quarterly 1990; **68**: 383–411.
68. Wilkinson RG. Income distribution and life expectancy. Brit Med J 1992; **304**: 165–8.
69. Woolhandler S, Himmelstein DU. Reverse targeting of preventive care due to lack of health insurance. J Amer Med Assoc 1988; **259**: 2872–4.
70. Clark J, Kreps J, Spengler J. Economics of aging; a survey. J Econ Lit 1978; **xvi**: 919–62.
71. US Department of Agriculture. Food and Nutrition Service. Blanchard L, Butler JS, Doyle P et al. Food Stamp SSI/Elderly Cashout Demonstration Evaluation. Princeton, NJ: Princeton Mathematica Policy Research Inc., 1982.
72. Report to the Congress of the United States by the Comptroller General. Entering a Nursing Home – Costly Implications for Medicaid and the Elderly. Washington, DC: United States General Accounting Office (PAD–80–12), 1979.
73. Orem D. Nursing: Concepts of Practice. New York: McGraw-Hill, 1980.
74. Sub-Committee on Health and Long Term Care of the Select Committee on Aging. Elder Abuse: A National Disgrace. US House of Representatives Committee Publication 99–502, US Congress, 1985.
75. Council on Scientific Affairs. Elder Abuse and Neglect. J Amer Med Assoc 1987; **257**: 966–71.
75a. Ogg J, Bennett G. Elder abuse in Britain. Brit Med J 1992; **305**: 998–9.
76. Costa JJ. Abuse of the Elderly – a Guide to Resources and Services. Lexington, MA; Lexington Books, 1984.
77. Ogg J, Bennett G. Community care: identifying risk factors for geriatric abuse. Geriatric Medicine 1991; **21**: 11–19.
78. Seattle, Washington State Medical Association. Guidelines for Intervention by Physicians and Other Service Providers. Seattle, WA: Seattle Washington State Medical Association, 1985.
79. Henig J, Maxfield MG. Reducing fear of crime: strategies for intervention. Victimology 1978; **3**: 297–313.
80. Zischka P, Jones I. Volunteer Community representatives as ombudsmen for the elderly in long term facilities. Gerontologist 1984; **24**: 9–12.
81. Committee on Nursing Home Registration. Improving the Quality of Care in Nursing Homes. Institute of Medicine. Washington, DC: National Academy Press, 1986.

10

Summary of problems and strategies

In the previous four chapters I have identified 64 common health problems afflicting elderly people and have discussed the research evidence on the available preventive care and health promotional strategies to counter each. In this chapter I provide a summary of this evidence in tabular form.

Section A (Tables 10.1 to 10.4) contains recommendations for inclusion in a preventive care protocol. These are based on what, at the present time, seem useful, safe, simple and reasonably cost effective to apply. Section B (Tables 10.5 to 10.7) contains those strategies excluded because they are not, at the present time, considered to be so.

The conclusions drawn are personal to the author. At times, these recommendations may differ from those proposed by various professional societies or from those proposed by the US Preventive Services Task Force or Canadian Task Force on the Periodic Health Examination. Readers will need to reach their own conclusions on what is appropriate for inclusion in their daily practice based on this conflicting information, the financial resources available to their health care system and what is considered by society as usual and normal preventive care.

Notes

1. Unless otherwise stated, 'screening' implies screening of a truly *asymptomatic* elderly population.
2. The term 'relative' implies the extent of importance or cost of an issue relative to the overall burden of health problems afflicting the elderly population and the overall resources available to a society's health care delivery system to deal with these problems.
3. Strategies, or health problems which have not so far been scientifically validated may be included in a recommended preventive care protocol

either because they are simple, safe and relatively inexpensive to perform or because their exclusion would contravene the bulk of clinical experience suggesting they still constitute what is currently considered as good clinical or social preventive care practice.

Section A: Recommended protocol

Table 10.1. *Primary prevention*

Potential strategy	Target population	Anticipated benefits
Counselling to maintain exercise activity into old age	All elderly persons, in the community and in institutions	• Prevention of general deconditioning with age • Reduction in mortality and morbidity • Primary prevention of osteoporosis and hip fracture • Possible effective primary prevention of stroke disease • Possible clinically significant benefits in cognition and communication
Counselling to reduce weight	All overweight elderly persons, particularly those: – with arthritic, hypertensive or stroke disease – posing severe difficulties of attendant handling because of concomitant disability	• Primary prevention of symptomatic knee osteoarthritis • Improvement in pain control in those with existing symptomatic knee osteoarthritis • Improvement in exercise tolerance in those with cardiopulmonary complaints • Improvement in blood pressure control in hypertensive patients • The avoidance of backstrain in attendant caregivers
Counselling to quit smoking and using smokeless tobacco	All elderly smokers and users of snuff or chewing tobacco	• Improvement in life expectancy • Reduction in myocardial reinfarction rate in those with coronary artery disease • Reduction of risk of acquiring: lung (and other respiratory tract) cancers; pancreatic cancer; bladder cancer; stomach cancer; oesophageal cancer; oral tract cancers • Improvement in lung function and respiratory symptoms • Reduction in pneumonia and influenza death rates • Reduction in the risk of stroke • Reduction of fire risk for very frail or demented individuals

Intervention	Target population	Expected benefits
Counselling to use seat-belts and head restraints in motor vehicles	All elderly front and rear seat occupants of motor vehicles and their carers	• Reduction in mortality from road traffic collisions • Reduction in severe and minor injury from road traffic collisions
Counselling to avoid over-protection and unnecessary bed and chair rest	Family caregivers caring for dependent or ill elderly persons at home	• Reduction in problems of poor mobility • Reduction in falls related to poor mobility • Shortened duration of stay in institutions
Bereavement counselling	All recently bereaved elderly persons	• Improvement in sense of wellbeing • Reduction in consumption of medications • Reduction in symptoms leading to physician consultation
Preretirement counselling	All middle-aged and elderly persons in their immediate preretirement years	• Increased satisfaction of retirees • Improve adjustment and positive orientation towards leisure
Counselling at times of relocation	All frail elderly people at times of relocation: – from hospital to care home – from one care home to another – from their own home to other people's homes to live	• Reduction in anxiety • Possible reduction in inter-family conflicts
Influenza vaccination	All elderly persons omitting the most frail or ill who are on limited treatment plans	When circulating influenza A contains antigens similar to those in the vaccination: • Reduction in influenza deaths • Reduction in severity of influenzial illness • Reduction in 'flu attack rates • Reduction in need for hospitalisation
Use of low-dose aspirin	Elderly persons who: – have had a TIA – have non-rheumatic atrial fibrillation – have had a recent or remote myocardial infarction – have peripheral vascular disease	• Reduction in risk of stroke • Possible reduction in the severity of stroke • Reduction in limb amputation rates[a] • Other possible benefits include reduction in colonic cancer

Table 10.1 (*cont.*)

Potential strategy	Target population	Anticipated benefits
Provision of community services	Specific groups of elderly people in the community (see details in text)	• Reduction of handicap in domestic and social care • Delayed or postponed institutionalisation • Reduction of stress in burdened family caregivers
Provision of suitable housing and home care and repair schemes	All elderly people, particularly those in the lower socioeconomic classes and/or those who already live in substandard building stock	• Possible improvement in access to, from and in the housing • Possible reduction in fall related injuries • Possible reduction in demand for institutionalisation • Possible reduction in relocation morbidity
Legislated licence requirement to pass a direct assessment of driving ability on the road	All elderly drivers – at age 70 years, 75 years and 80 years – bi-annually thereafter	• Reduction in mortality from motor collisions • Reduction in injuries from motor collisions
Legislated requirement to plan and implement proposals for elderly and/or disabled individuals in terms of: – improved transport and access – a supportive environment – the promotion of leisure and sport – access to continuing education	Central and local planning and governmental agencies	• Improved social functioning • Improved well-being and life satisfaction

Legislated requirement to ensure that public pensions for the elderly are sufficient to keep pace with the cost of living, offer the opportunity for choice of care and detract from resulting in a society with a 'wide cleavage' between socioeconomic groups	All elderly retired persons	• Increase in life expectancy • Reduction in morbidity • Possible improvement in well being and life satisfaction

[a]Goldhaber SZ, Manson JE, Stampfer MJ et al. Low-dose aspirin and subsequent peripheral arterial surgery in the Physicians' Health Study. Lancet 1992; **340**: 143–5.

Table 10.2. *Screening*

Health problem	Detection	Timing	Frequency	Potential strategy	Comments
Breast cancer	Clinical breast examination with or without mammography	—	Every two years	Referral to surgical services of those with suspicious lesions	i) Clinical breast examination alone ensures the effective detection of a high proportion of breast cancers at a fraction of the cost of mammography but the latter may be included in societies that are sufficiently wealthy and where the expense of paying for this relatively high cost-to-benefit manoeuvre does not detract from meeting other greater health care needs of the elderly population
Cervical cancer	Pap smear in all elderly women except those on limited treatment plans	Initially at age 65 years	i) No repeat if negative in non-high-risk caucasian women ii) Every four years in other high risk groups	Referral to gynaecological services of those with suspicious lesions	i) High risk groups include those with no documented screening at a younger age, certain ethnic minority and low income groups and those who have experienced multiple sexual partners and prior venereal disease ii) Many very old women, particularly the most frail, perceive the Pap smear as an irrelevant and unacceptable manoeuvre. This must be taken into account when offering this preventive strategy
Colo-rectal cancer	Selective sigmoidoscopy or colonoscopy in high risk groups only	—	Every five years	Referral to surgical services of those with suspicious lesions	i) Flexible sigmoidoscopy more rapid and acceptable to elderly people than rigid sigmoidoscopy ii) May be supplemented by annual faecal occult blood testing but high false positive rate iii) See page 48 for discussion of high risk groups

Condition	Screening manoeuvre	Initial screening	Frequency	Action	Comments
Skin cancer	Inspection of sun exposed areas of skin in high risk groups	At times of physician contact for other purposes	Opportunistic screening only	Referral for biopsy of those with suspicious lesions	i) High risk groups include persons with a personal history of skin cancer or high exposure to sunlight ii) Complete skin examination will reveal a far greater number of melanomes and may be the detection manoeuvre of choice in those at particular risk
Oral cancer	Inspection and palpation of the oral cavity in high risk groups	At times of physician contact for other purposes	Opportunistic screening only	Referral to dental surgeon +/– biopsy of those with suspicious lesions	i) High risk groups include those who consume high quantities of alcohol and/or smokeless tobacco
Hyper-tension	Arterial blood pressure estimation by sphygmomanometry in all elderly persons	Initially at age 65 years	Annually thereafter	Anti-hypertensive therapy in those with diastolic/systolic or isolated systolic hypertension present in more than one reading obtained on each of three separate visits	i) Particular care required in selecting anti-hypertensive medication to avoid side effects ii) Blood pressure should be reduced slowly iii) End point of therapy should be higher than in younger age groups iv) Particular caution should be exercised in reducing blood pressure in those with multi-infarct dementia or severe bilateral carotid occlusive disease
Anaemia	Haemoglobin or haematocrit estimation only in selected, symptomatic elderly persons	At time of physician contact for other purposes	Opportunistic screening only	Appropriate investigation and therapy as indicated	Symptomatic elderly persons include those with the typical symptoms and signs of anaemia plus those with many non-specific presentations such as lethargy, declining function and increasing difficulty in maintaining an independent existence at home

Table 10.3. *Tertiary preventive care*

Health problem	Detection	Timing	Frequency	Potential strategy	Comments
Hypo-thyroid-ism	Serum TSH esti-mation in selected groups of elderly persons	Initially at age 75 years	Biannually thereafter	Subsequent treatment with L-thyroxine supplements	Selective groups of elderly persons include frail people presenting to health services because of vague, chronic unexplained disability, depression or mental impairment
Oral and dental problems	Semi-structured interview and examination protocol	At time of physician contact for other purposes	Opportunistic screening only	i) Counselling on preventive care and oral hygiene ii) Referral to dental surgeon where appropriate iii) Ensure individual marking and ultrasound cleansing of dentures in institutionalised populations	
Problems with feet	Inspection of feet of all elderly persons particularly those with – diabetes mellitus – peripheral vascular disease	Initially at age 65 years	Biannually to age 75 years annually thereafter	i) Nail clipping and buffing to improve foot comfort and hygiene ii) Implementation of a structured foot care programme to reduce amputation rates in diabetics iii) Referral for specialist chiropody treatment where appropriate	

Condition	Procedure	Timing	Intervention	Notes
Pressure ulcers	Use of validated rating scale to predict pressure sore development in high risk groups	At the start of the illness, disablement or institutionalisation itemised opposite	With each worsening of patient status until preventive strategies are being employed	i) Employment of low pressure mattresses and cushions ii) Protection of heels by the use of low pressure devices, foot cradles and, where appropriate, the wearing of shoes	i) High risk groups include those who are sufficiently ill or disabled to be bedfast or chair-fast; those newly admitted to institutional care; and recent stroke, amputee and hip fracture patients
Alcohol dependence	Use of brief structured screening for alcohol dependency in selected groups of elderly patients	At time of physician contact for other purposes	Opportunistic screening only	i) Referral to alcohol dependency treatment programme ii) Environmental manipulation such as voluntary visiting or social care to lessen precipitating factors of loneliness or depression	i) Selected groups of elderly patients include those presenting with depression, suicidal intent, unexpected adverse effects of medication, the consequences of home or motoring accidents and unexplained recurrent acute confusional states
Memory impairment	Use of abbreviated mental test score on all elderly persons	Initially at age 65 years	Biannually to age 75 years, annually thereafter	For those with significant cognitive impairment: i) More comprehensive assessment of functional status and behaviour ii) assessment and amelioration of stressors on care givers iii) Prescription of appropriate social supports	i) Ensure that any degree of deafness, language difficulty, depression or lack of motivation, is taken into account in interpreting the score ii) More complex psychometric testing for 'early' or mild cognitive impairment is considered counterproductive except for research purposes at the present time

Table 10.3. (cont.)

Health problem	Detection	Timing	Frequency	Potential strategy	Comments
Memory impairment (cont.)				iv) Counselling to avoid relocation where possible and the maintenance of a regular routine v) Discussion and counselling on issues of autonomy, protection and the appropriate extent of future care vi) Reduction of risk factors in those with multi-infarct dementia e.g. antihypertensive treatment, quit smoking, prescribe aspirin vii) Further diagnostic investigations for the small minority with short, rapid or atypical onset of memory loss	

Condition	Screening method		Frequency	Intervention	Notes
Poor mobility	Use of structured measure of mobility status – on all elderly persons – recurrent fallers and those with H/O stroke, arthritis, hip fracture or unstable gait	Initially at age 70 years. At times of physician contact for other purposes	Biannually to age 80 years, annually thereafter plus opportunistic screening	i) Rehabilitation where appropriate. ii) Reduction of handicap by use of walking aids, raised seats etc. iii) Counselling of caregivers to avoid overprotection iv) Use of functionally orientated models of nursing care in hospitals and other institutions	i) More detailed targeting strategies are referred to in Chapter 8
Inability to perform the Activities of Daily Living	Use of short structured questionnaire on personal and domestic ADL status – on all elderly persons – recurrent fallers and those with stroke, arthritis, hip fracture or unstable gait	Initially at age 70 years or at time of presentation for condition mentioned	Every five years	i) The provision of appropriate aids ii) The provision of domestic, bathing or meal services in the home as appropriate	i) More frequent screening unnecessary provided strategy of further functional assessment carried out when memory impairment and/or poor mobility detected ii) Community care/case management policies may improve targeting of resources

Table 10.3. (*cont.*)

Health problem	Detection	Timing	Frequency	Potential strategy	Comments
Feeding/ eating depend- ency	Observational monitoring by care attendants of feeding/eating abilities in high risk groups in institutional care	Initially at time of admission to institutional care	Monthly	i) Personal assistance in feeding by care attendants to supplement residents' efforts	i) High risk groups include those with severe dementia, disabling stroke disease, Parkinsonism and those with extreme frailty ii) Effectiveness of strategies may be constrained by ethical considerations
Poor vision	Questioning and testing of near and distance vision using print charts and test cards	At 70 and 75 years	Annually after 75 years	i) Referral for specialist ophthalmo- logical evaluation and treatment if vision significantly impaired or worsening ii) The provision of improved level of ambient lighting in domestic or work environment iii) The provision of low-vision aids where appropriate	i) Suggested cut-off points for specialist referral suggested in Chapter 8 ii) The inclusion of routine tonometry for the detection of glaucoma is not currently recommended

Deafness	Test hearing of all elderly persons using one of the following: – free field voice voice testing – Hearing Handicap Inventory questionnaire – Welch–Alyn audioscope	At 70 and 75 years	Annually after 75 years	i) Removal of ear wax where appropriate ii) The provision of a hearing aid iii) The provision of communication and environmental aids	
Imposed burden on family carers	Interview supplemented by a structured rating scale to assess extent of stress and burden on high risk groups of carers	Upon identification of existence of a caring role either from patient/carer contacts or from patient records. At times of patient or carer contact with physician for other purposes	Annually thereafter. Opportunistic screening may permit for more frequent monitoring	i) The provision of in-home domestic or personal care services to the elderly person to lessen caregiver input ii) The provision of a dispersed community alarm to the elderly person living alone to reduce caregiver anxiety iii) The provision of in-home, day care or institutional respite	i) High risk groups of carers include those who are themselves elderly disabled or ill; those with competing domestic or occupational demands on their time; those who express fatigue, stress, anger or resentment in the caring role; those in whom the premorbid relationship with the person cared for was poor; those caring for elderly persons who are restless or demanding by night or are severely physically disabled or who are suffering from brain damage (from dementia, stroke or Parkinsonism) particularly if there are behavioural or personality changes or if there are problems of communication ii) Interview of the caregiver should be conducted after the establishment of rapport and in privacy away from the person cared for

Table 10.3. (cont.)

Health problem	Detection	Timing	Frequency	Potential strategy	Comments
Imposed burden on family carers (cont.)				iv) Counselling and education v) Referral to self-help or mutual support group where appropriate	
Sub-standard housing	Inspection during home visit on all elderly persons	Initially at age 75 years	Opportunistically thereafter	i) Use of home care repair schemes ii) Provision of aids and adaptations in the home iii) Use of dispersed community alarm systems	i) Home assessment visit may best be conducted by occupational therapist or nursing members of the primary health care team

Table 10.4. *Other tertiary preventive care strategies*

Health problem	Target population	Strategy	Anticipated benefit
The sequelae of herpes zoster	Elderly persons in the early stages of herpes zoster irrespective of the dermatome affected	•Course of acyclovir therapy	•Modification of the rash, toxaemia and acute pain of herpes zoster
Recurrent falls	Elderly persons presenting after one or more syncopal or non-syncopal fall	•Professional assessment and treatment of underlying cause •Reduction of medication likely to precipitate falls •Elimination of home hazards •Use of dispersed community alarm systems to minimise complications of a 'long lie' •Improved supervision by staff in institutions	•Reduction in fall injuries •Reduction in complications from fall injuries e.g. hypothermia, pressure ulcers etc. •Maintenance of independent mobility •Reduction in carer stress •Reduced demand for institutionalisation •Reduced complaints and litigation from families of those who fall in institutions
Incontinence of urine	Elderly persons presenting with persistent incontinence of urine	•Professional assessments and treatment with range of treatments including drugs; hormonal therapy, pelvic floor exercises and surgery •Implementation of certain toilet training schedules •Provision of various continence aids and devices	•Reduction in the frequency of incontinence •Reduction of social handicap from persisting incontinence •Reduction in carer stress

Table 10.4 (cont.)

Health problem	Target population	Strategy	Associated benefit
Nocturia	Elderly persons presenting with troublesome nocturnal frequency of micturition	• Prescription of a range of possible drug therapies predominantly to reduce uninhibited bladder contractions	• Reduction in nocturnal frequency of micturition • Improved sleep pattern • Reduction in nocturnal falls • Reduction in carer stress
Constipation	Elderly persons with verified slow bowel transit or hard stools	• Bran supplements or supplementation of diet • Avoidance of constipating drugs • Maintenance of an adequate fluid intake • Maintenance of physical activity	• Shortened bowel transit times and bulkier softer stools • Reduction in faecal impaction with or without overflow incontinence • Possible reduction in problems with haemorrhoids and diverticular disease
Insomnia	Elderly persons presenting with insomnia	• Implementation of comfort measures at night • Avoidance of early evening napping • Maintenance of day time activity • Prescription of hypnotic agents only on a short-term basis at times of illness and crises	• Improved nocturnal sleep pattern • Reduction of carer stress

Section B: Exclusions

Table 10.5. *Exclusions from primary prevention*

Health problem	Potential strategy	Reason(s) for exclusion
Colorectal cancer	Dietary modification	Current lack of evidence on efficacy from prospective randomised controlled trials in elderly populations
	Aspirin use	Current lack of evidence on efficacy from prospective randomised controlled trials in elderly populations
		Unknown risk–benefit ratio
Stroke	Widespread low dose aspirin use in the healthy elderly population	Proven inefficacy in younger age groups
	Carotid endarterectomy in asymptomatic persons with carotid bruits	Lack of evidence of efficacy
Hypothermia	Provision of free heating in homes	Proven to be ineffective
	Financial supplementation for heating	Lack of corroborating evidence to suggest its efficacy
	Health education of the elderly public on dangers of hypothermia	Proven to be ineffective
	Counselling by family doctors on dangers of hypothermia	Proven to be of very limited benefit
Pneumococcal pneumonia	Pneumococcal vaccination	Questionable efficacy in the populations most at risk. Relative cost
Tetanus	Widespread tetanus toxoid administration to the elderly population	Relative unimportance of the problem. Relative cost
An 'unhealthy lifestyle'	Health education of the elderly population	Questionable efficacy except for quitting smoking and maintaining regular physical activity
The ageing processes	Miscellaneous anti-ageing cures	None currently of proven efficacy

Table 10.6. *Exclusions from screening*

Health problem	Detection manoeuvre	Reason(s) for exclusion
Colorectal cancer	Faecal occult blood testing	Poor quality of the detection manoeuvre available Positive tests mandate an invasive investigative workup Lack of evidence of definitive proof of efficacy from randomised controlled trials (see note at the foot of this table) *See colorectal screening for high risk groups elsewhere in this chapter
Prostatic cancer	Prostatic specific antigen **or** Prostatic acid phosphatase **or** Digital rectal examination	Poor quality of the detection manoeuvres available Lack of evidence of efficacy of screening or early intervention influencing outcomes
Lung cancer	Chest x-ray + sputum cytology	Screening shown to be ineffective in influencing outcomes in younger age groups Relative cost and resource use
Endometrial cancer	Pap smear **or** Transvaginal ultrasonography with colour flow imaging	Poor quality or lack of experience with detection manoeuvres available Lack of evidence of efficacy of screening influencing outcomes in any age group Relative importance
Ovarian cancer	Pelvic examination **or** Serum CA125 + transvaginal ultrasonography with colour flow imaging	Poor quality or lack of experience with detection manoeuvres available Lack of evidence of efficacy of screening influencing outcomes in any age group
Gastric cancer	Endoscopy **or** Double contrast barium meal examination	Poor quality of the detection manoeuvres available Lack of evidence of efficacy of screening influencing outcomes in Western societies in any age group *Selective endoscopic screening of new-onset symptomatic elderly individuals may be a worthwhile strategy but awaits the outcome of further research

Condition	Detection manoeuvre	Comments
Bladder cancer	Dipstick urinalysis for haematuria	Poor quality of detection manoeuvres available Lack of evidence of efficacy of screening influencing outcomes in any age group
Pancreatic cancer	Ultrasonography **or** serological markers	Poor quality of the detection manoeuvre available Dubiety about the benefit of early treatment
Hyperlipidaemia	Serum cholesterol	Lack of evidence of efficacy of screening influencing outcomes in elderly people Dubiety about the risk–benefit ratio of screening younger age groups Relative cost
Abdominal aortic aneurysms	Ultrasonography	Poor quality of the detection manoeuvre available Lack of evidence of efficacy of screening influencing outcomes in any age group Risk–benefit ratio and acceptability of early treatment unknown
Anaemia	Haemoglobin or haematocrit estimation	Relative importance Early treatment of asymptomatic younger individuals shown to be ineffective *Opportunistic screening of *symptomatic* elderly individuals is considered a worthwhile strategy for inclusion in a preventive care protocol – see elsewhere in this chapter
Open angle glaucoma	Tonometry **or** ophthalmoscopy	Poor quality of the detection manoeuvres available Dubiety about the benefit of screening in any age group
Bacteriuria	Urine culture **or** visual appearance + dipstick testing for nitrite and leucocyte esterase	Relative importance Dubiety about the efficacy of screening influencing outcomes in elderly people

Table 10.6 (*cont.*)

Health problem	Detection manoeuvre	Reason for exclusion
Benign prostatic hypertrophy	Symptom scoring + Transrectal ultrasonography	Quality of detection manoeuvres unknown Dubiety about the benefit of early surgical treatment *Screening for BPH may become a worthwhile manoeuvre for inclusion in a preventive care protocol not only as evidence improves on the quality of the detection manoeuvres but as medical therapies become available for the early treatment of this condition
Diabetes mellitus	Oral glucose tolerance test **or** Fasting plasma glucose	Poor quality of the detection manoeuvres available Lack of evidence of efficacy of screening influencing outcomes in any age group
Hypothyroidism	TSH estimation	Relative importance Lack of evidence of efficacy of screening influencing outcomes *Selective screening of certain elderly subpopulations is considered a worthwhile strategy and is described elsewhere in this chapter
Subnutrition	Nutritional Risk Screening Questionnaire **or** Clinical assessment	Relative importance Poor quality of the detection manoeuvres available Lack of evidence for food supplementation influencing outcomes in elderly people *See however screening for eating/feeding dependency elsewhere in this chapter
Osteoporosis	Measurement of bone mineral density **or** The Singh Index	Poor quality of the detection manoeuvres available Dubiety about the efficacy and risk–benefit ratio of HRT in very old populations Relative cost *An effective therapy may soon be recommended with the rapid development of research evidence for an older age group (see text pp. 134–141)

| Depression | Screening questionnaire (e.g. MAST, UMAST, CAGE) | Poor targeting for use of detection strategy with resultant impracticability of screening all individuals at potential risk
Lack of evidence on improved outcomes with regard to alcohol dependence |
| Abuse | Interview and clinical assessment | Lack of available, good quality detection manoeuvres available
Lack of evidence of efficacy of screening influencing outcomes |

Note: A very recent study of faecal occult blood testing by Mandel et al. (N Engl J Med 1993; **328**: 1365–71), in which 46 551 participants aged 50 to 80 years were randomly assigned to screened and unscreened groups, showed a significant decrease of 33 per cent in the cumulative mortality in colorectal cancer in the screened group. However, this decrease was shown only in those screened annually, and not in those screened every two years. In view of this, the fact that only about one in ten of the screened individuals had the possibility of a neoplastic lesion, and taking into account the other comments on the screening test described in Chapter 6, routine screening is still not recommended at this time.

Table 10.7. *Exclusions: tertiary prevention*

Health problems	Strategy	Reason for exclusion
Complications from silent gallstones	Ultrasonography and elective surgery	Relative unimportance due to the benign natural history of the condition Evidence from decision-analysis models that favour expectant versus interventional management
Recurrent falls	Formal fall rehabilitation programmes	Evidence that such intervention is ineffective

11

Tailoring strategies to individuals

When the specific strategies outlined in the previous chapters are applied, they should be tailored to meet the needs and wishes of elderly individuals according to the following broad principles.

Time the intervention precisely

There is a 'critical intervention time' or 'window' during which various types of support should be provided. A patient's functional status may deteriorate slightly for several years, with the impairment being noticeable only to the family. A crisis may then develop during which the situation deteriorates rapidly. If support is added too late, institutionalisation is often the outcome. If it is provided too early, however, it merely fosters dependency, wastes resources, is costly to society, and is considered by many elderly people to be an intrusion on their privacy.

Intervention of any sort, whether it be the relocation of an elderly person into specialised housing or the provision of a community service, must, therefore, be timed precisely if it is to be effective and to avoid detriment. Many caring professionals, however, will be tempted to prescribe unnecessary supports for the elderly during the early phase of functional decline because of their own anxieties and pressure from anxious family members. There is, for example, evidence from the UK [1, 2] that a significant proportion of social service 'home help', 'meals on wheels' and home aid allocation is given to those elderly people who are relatively fit and who are not strictly in need of the service. These allocations appear to be made because of inflexibility in the system, the services provided being 'the next best thing' to what is really wanted. On many occasions services are allocated simply because the recipient is perceived as being frail. This engenders a humane feeling of wanting to help and hence the allocation of services is made as a 'sympathy vote' [2]. If

265

community service organisations are to target those truly in need of assistance more effectively and to use their resources more efficiently, such emotive pressures will have to be combatted.

Case example 1: Premature institutionalisation

Mrs P.J., of 84 years, began causing anxiety because of dizziness and an unsteady gait. She lived alone in fairly isolated circumstances. Her family (who lived abroad) spent one Christmas with her, and during this time exerted strong pressure on her to go into a residential care home both for her protection and also for their own peace of mind. They would be unable to travel frequently back and forth if she got into trouble. Within a few weeks, she was placed in a local home of high standard and the family breathed a sigh of relief that a crisis had been averted. Although Mrs P.J.'s health and mobility actually improved, the family began receiving letters from her a few weeks later with numerous complaints about the way the home was run. After several more of these letters, the family, through the assistance of a local lawyer, moved her to another pleasant residential home. Within a few weeks the same complaining letters started again. The manager of the home eventually asked the local social worker to call. After a lengthy series of interviews she found that Mrs P.J. was very unhappy, not because of the home itself but because she disliked being in the company of others (always having been a bit of a loner) and hated the loss of personal freedom that had accompanied the move away from her own home. After a family counselling session, Mrs P.J. was eventually resettled in a groundfloor flatlet in her local community. She was supplied with some home services to assist with shopping and the heavier domestic chores, and was given a dispersed alarm system for wearing round her neck that she could use if she had further falls and required help. In this state she lived contentedly with almost no further problems or concerns until she suddenly died three years later, at home, of a massive stroke.

Minimise unnecessary disruption to lifestyle

A number of health maintenance measures have the potential for disrupting an elderly person's lifestyle. The prescription of low-sodium or weight-reduction diet or advice on stopping smoking are some common examples. All of these measures have a place in the management of selected groups of elderly people, but it must be appreciated that in old age, when the scope for prolongation of life becomes limited, issues concerned with the quality of life become more relevant, and to many of the elderly restriction of diet or the cessation of smoking may seriously affect what little enjoyment they have left. Therefore, while it is appropriate to encourage elderly people who can exercise choice to adopt preventive measures, their impact on life satisfaction must be weighed against theoretical advantages to health in those who cannot express their wishes or opt to continue their existing lifestyle. If elderly people living in the community perceive the equation to be unequal they can opt out by non-compliance. The institutionalised elderly population are less fortunate, being a captive audience at particular risk of inappropriate and zealous application of preventive strategies.

Case example 2: Disruption to lifestyle of antihypertensive measures

Mr J.R., a hypertensive man of 69, had been in a local residential home for over two years when a new family practitioner became very concerned with the level of blood pressure. Accordingly, Mr J.R. was placed on a diuretic and a low-sodium diet. Difficulty in obtaining advice on correct dietary intake and poor compliance with this diet led to his being moved from the local home to a nursing home some distance away. Over the next seven months, he expressed dissatisfaction with the fact that fewer visitors came to see him. He regularly complained that his food had no taste and he developed mild transient hypoanatraemia attributed in part to his concomitant diuretic therapy. His blood pressure remained significantly elevated. Eventually his doctor placed him on a calcium-channel blocker for his hypertension with satisfactory results. He was also taken off his low-salt diet with no significant change to his blood pressure. Mr J.R. remained a resident in the nursing home until his death 18 months later of bronchopneumonia.

Respect the older person's autonomy

As elderly people age, they become subject to increasing risk at home because of physical and mental disability. This generates considerable anxiety among families, neighbours, and friends, which in turn results in demand on health and social service providers to offer community service support or an institutional bed. This anxiety and pressure is most commonly seen in those carers coming from a distance who are able to see their loved ones only intermittently. The anxiety is also most acute in carers who have only a short time themselves in which to 'get something done' or who secretly feel guilty about the situation in which they have had to leave the elderly person.

Many of the above requests for help are in accordance with the older persons' wishes. Often, however, this is not the case, and attempts are made by well-meaning caregivers to intervene despite an old person's expressed wishes not to be institutionalised or to have no further help in the house. Even regular surveillance may be considered by them as an intrusion on their privacy.

At these times, although maintenance of the elderly person's health may require additional support or intervention, the professional caregiver must ultimately respect their right to self determination. The only exception to this is the mentally incompetent patient, although even here the presence of senile dementia does not necessarily imply incompetence. This discrepancy in views between the elderly person and the health or social work provider occurs frequently.

Case example 3: Ultimately respecting the older person's autonomy

Mrs B.H., 89 years, a hospital inpatient, was being rehabilitated after a severe stroke. Although she had made some progress, some months later she still remained in a dependent condition. She required assistance dressing herself, she was regularly incontinent of urine, and most distressingly, she was virtually immobile, being able to transfer to bed or commode from her wheelchair only after the most precarious shuffling procedure that, in the eyes of the rehabilitation team, placed her regularly at risk of falling. Despite this, Mrs B.H. claimed she had had enough of hospitals and irrespective of the risks wished to be allowed back to her own home. She refused to contemplate the alternative of ongoing institutional care. The situation was complicated by the presence of a naturally anxious daughter who wasn't at all sure that it would be correct to let her mother go home and who was unable to take her to live with her. Eventually, after much discussion and soul searching, Mrs B.H. was discharged home with the maximum amount of support possible and with her daughter calling several times a day to check that all was well. Five months later Mrs B.H. did indeed fall as had been feared, lay for some time on the floor on a cold winter's night and succumbed to a combination of hypothermia and bronchopneumonia. On hearing about the death, the original hospital physician and his team were deeply concerned and discussed at length whether or not they had been correct to discharge her from their care. A few days later, however, they received a letter from the originally anxious daughter saying how grateful she was that she had been persuaded that her mother should go home. The older woman had apparently been very glad to be there and, despite many minor daily problems, had been very content living in familiar surroundings frequently claiming that whatever happened to her it would have been worth it because she had been allowed a little longer in her own home to be with the fond memories that surrounded her. The daughter also felt that assisting her mother over the last few months had emotionally brought them even closer together.

Recognise that death is a legitimate 'end-point'

An elderly patient's right to live and benefit from the developments of medical science is incontestable, but at some point in the life cycle an elderly person also has the right to die peacefully and with dignity. This is particularly true for those suffering from irremediable disease. Health promotion of elderly people, therefore, has as its principal goal not the prolongation of life, but an improvement in the quality of that life. It therefore behoves the professional attempting to implement health promotional measures to take cognisance of the elderly individual's existing state of health, their future prognosis, their likely quality of life if the latter is extended, their prior wishes about what should happen to them in these circumstances or, failing this, some substituted judgement on this issue from family or other carers.

If *treating* an elderly individual for an acute illness, the above issues would involve the health professional in considering the existence of a 'Living Will' [3] and in confirming 'Do Not Resuscitate' orders [4]. With *health promotion* the situation is also complex, involving an attempt to gain insight into the older person's values, not just about using biotechnology to maintain life, but about the less extreme issues of balance between length of life and quality of life. This may involve explicitly identifying that a proportion of the most frail and dependent elderly population are on 'Limited Treatment Plans' [5, 6].

Case example 4: Influenza vaccine and limited treatment plans

Mrs M.G., 74 years, was newly admitted to nursing home care. As part of the home's official policy all residents were persuaded to receive annual flu vaccination. This engendered concern in Mrs M.G.'s family who asked for an interview with her doctor. At this meeting they expressed surprise that such a measure was being considered for their mother in view of her current frailty. They wondered if this reflected a policy to keep their mother alive 'at all costs' and said they hoped she would be allowed to 'slip away peacefully' without too much further intervention. This led to a staff conference, where it became clear that many of the nurses sympathised with the family's views, particularly as Mrs M.G. was severely demented, rarely recognising her family or attendants, and was bedridden with contractures and pressure sores. Some of the nurses also claimed that other families had expressed feelings similar to those of Mrs M.G.'s. The doctor concerned again met with Mrs M.G.'s relatives and agreed to omit the annual flu vaccination. During conversation, the use of a number of other potential medical interventions were discussed and agreement reached about the limits that all considered appropriate. The range of this simple 'limited treatment plan' were then conveyed to the nursing staff. Over the next two years this individualised policy for influenza vaccination gradually became the norm within the nursing home.

References

1. Challis D, Davies B. Case Management in Community Care. Aldershot: Gower, 1986.
2. Carpenter M. A study of community care services and their relevance to the elderly. MSc. Thesis. London: School of Policy Studies, 1984.
3. Lazaroff AE, Orr WF. Living wills and other advanced directives. In: Jahnigen DW, Schrier RW (eds) Clinics in Geriatric Medicine: Ethical Issues in Care of the Elderly, vol. 2, pp. 521–34. Philadelphia, PA: WB Saunders, 1986.
4. Evans AL, Brodie EA. The do-not resuscitate order in teaching hospitals. J Amer Med Assoc 1985; **253**: 2235–9.

5. Volicer L. Need for hospice approach to treatment of patients with advanced progressive dementia. J Amer Geriatr Soc 1986; **34**: 655–8.
6. Brennan TA. Ethics committees and decisions to limit care. J Amer Med Assoc 1988; **260**: 803–7.

12

Targeting, screening and surveillance
in primary care

Within the UK, preventive care for elderly people has historically centred around population screening and surveillance by the family doctor and his primary care team. In this chapter, therefore, I look at the primary care services as a resource for this older age group, review in detail the value of such screening, consider more efficient methods of targeting the frail elderly and discuss the implications of recent government legislation mandating an annual health check being offered to those over 75 years.

Primary care as a resource for elderly people

In the community, primary care services usually consist of family practitioners or other 'generalist' doctors who serve as first point of contact for elderly patients and who provide comprehensive, ongoing care. Community nurses also figure prominently in community care, either being directly employed by the family doctor's practice or liaising closely with it. Primary care is also represented by a wide range of other health professionals who work as part of a multidisciplinary team, or network, with the practice. In some countries, family doctors have a statutory responsibility to consider their patients' social needs and to make referral through the appropriate social services [1].

Some countries still have problems in providing geographically and financially accessible care to their older populations or in making this readily available on a 24-hour, 7-day week basis. However, in the UK, where these problems have been overcome, the family doctor and his or her primary care team constitute the single most important health resource for elderly people. Over 90 per cent of elderly people are registered with a general practitioner and the vast majority of very old patients come into contact with that doctor or his primary care team at least once a year [2]. General practitioners have the highest professional contact rate with frail elderly people in the community

271

[3] and, in the UK, more than half of these contacts are made in the patients' home [4]. Elderly people rely heavily on general practitioners as their first professional source of information and assistance. For many years, use has been made of this invaluable resource by many primary care practices carrying out preventive care programmes, not just for those patients attending with intercurrent illness, but for those currently fit individuals who are nevertheless still registered with that practice. These programmes have usually taken the form of screening and case finding with the elderly population.

Screening and surveillance

The existence of a reservoir of unreported health problems in elderly people is well documented and for many years family practice surveys have identified large numbers of previously unrecognised disorders [5–22]. Evidence of the continuance of this state of affairs is still being produced [23–26]. Traditionally, this has been considered to reflect serious unmet or unvoiced 'need' in the elderly population and a positive approach to seek out such problems before they presented as crises has been developed in the form of screening and surveillance programmes. More recently, however, doubt has been cast on the significance of these previously unreported problems. Doubt has also been cast on the benefits of population-wide screening in terms of the resources used. These concerns will become apparent after reviewing the input and outcomes of these activities.

Who has done the screening?

In the UK, a wide variety of personnel including doctors [20, 22], nurses [23, 24] and even trained lay volunteers [27] have been utilised in screening the elderly population. By far the greatest involvement has been with nursing staff of all grades, from the health visitor (a community nurse with specific training and responsibility for promoting health), to less trained grades of community and practice nurses. No information is available as to the relative efficacy of screening amongst this skill mix. The heavy involvement of nursing staff in screening is a reflection in part on the constraints on physicians' time and on the strong functional and 'social' component in British screening programmes for the older population.

However, the average nurse will not be willing or able to undertake such screening unless he or she has been adequately trained and prepared. Luker [28] points out that, in contrast to the situation for infants and young children, for whom there exists a structured developmental model from which to work, the preventive approach to elderly people has not been well defined or documented. As a consequence, nurses may dislike visiting elderly people because of the lack of an appropriate frame of reference. This may, in part, explain the relatively small amount of time spent by health visitors with the elderly population in the UK. Nevertheless, a number of structured screening protocols have been devised. Using these, it has been shown that nurses may achieve results comparable to those obtained by physicians, the exception being with regard to psychiatric illness [29, 30]. The additional inclusion of formal scoring systems for cognitive deficit [31] and for functional psychiatric illness [32, 33] may go some way toward resolving these difficulties in this elderly population.

What have been the implications on workload?

There are difficulties in translating manpower experience from one country's health care system to another, but a number of reports clearly indicate the additional staffing required to conduct screening and surveillance of elderly people living in the community. The most detailed account is that of Barber [34], from a Scottish practice, who estimated that 18 hours per week would be required to set up a full screening and assessment programme over a one-year period for patients 75 years and over in a defined population, of all ages, of 4000. The time required to continue the programme in subsequent years was calculated at 11 hours per week. Barber's screening programme, like many others, used the skills of the community nursing service to a considerable extent. A recent joint statement from the Health Visitors' Association and British Geriatrics Society recommended the need for a further 18 000 health visitors in England and Wales if such a programme of screening were to be implemented [35].

What has been the content and methodology of the screening?

The issue of what constitutes appropriate screening content has been the subject of much variation and debate. Brodsky et al. [36] have described and compared this content in a number of British screening programmes. The results are shown in Table 12.1.

It should be noted that British authorities tend to recommend fewer laboratory tests than do health providers in other countries and the emphasis in most screening programmes in the UK is still on functional status and available social support. This has usually been conducted by means of a questionnaire

Table 12.1. *Comparison of screening protocols used in several British screening programmes for elderly people*

	The Glasgow Woodside geriatric assessment form	Pike's screening approach	William's survey of people over age 75	Currie's screening of patients age 70–72	Lowther's examination of high risk elderly	Freedman's screening project for patients over 65	Tulloch's trial of geriatric screening in patients over 70	The Kilsyth questionnaire
History taking and physical exam								
Blood pressure	+	+		+	?		+?	+
Hearing assessment	+	+	+	+	+		+	+
Vision assessment	+	+		+			+	
Eye condition	+		+	+	+	+	+	
Weight measurement				+		+		+
Height measurement				+				
Assessment of nutrition diet	+							
Assessment of social and psychiatric function	+	+	+	+		+	+	+
Assessment of dementia and memory loss	+		+	+			+	+
Oral cavity exam.	+	+		+				
Breast exam.	+			+		+		+
Mobility exam.	+	+	+	+	+	+	+	+
Oedema in ankles	+	+	+	+		+		+ᵃ
Performance/IADL	+		+				+	+
Medications taken				+			+	
Hypothyroidism	+							
Heart and lungs	+ᵇ	Lungs +	+	+	+	+	+	+
Urinary system	+	+	+	+	+		+	+
Alimentary system	+	+	+	+	+		+	+

Muscles and joints	Pains in joints +		+		+		+	+
Nervous system	+		+		+		+	
Rectal exam.			+	Only when necessary +				
Pelvic or genital exam.			+	Only when necessary +			+	
Skin exam.	+	+	+			+	+	
Other exam.			Neoplasms +			Abdomen +	Feet: drug problem +	
Pap smear								
Chest X-ray		+			+			
Laboratory tests								
Blood haemoglobin concentration	+	+	White cell count, iodine +	+	+		+	
Serum protein concentration	Blood abnormalities +	Bio-chemical profile +	Albumin phosphatase calcium +				+	
Blood sugar	+		+					
Cholesterol			urea +					
Occult blood in stool								
Urinalysis	+	+	+	Glucose, albumin +	+	Albumin, sugar, blood +		
Tuberculin sensitivity test								
Influenza immunisation								

Table 12.1 (*cont.*)

	The Glasgow Woodside geriatric assessment form	Pike's screening approach	William's survey of people over age 75	Currie's screening of patients age 70–72	Lowther's examination of high risk elderly	Freedman's screening project for patients over 65	Tulloch's trial of geriatric screening in patients over 70	The Kilsyth questionnaire
Tetanus/diphtheria immunisation								
EKG								
Counselling								
Daily oral hygiene								
Alcoholism, smoking		Assessment only +						
Accident prevention	+							
Nutrition and diet counselling				+				

A plus sign indicates the parameter is assessed in the protocol

[a] Also assesses performance in ADL (i.e. dressing, bathing, etc.)

[b] Urinary system and alimentary system are checked as examinations. These may not necessarily be performed by the doctor, if no need is found for it by the questionnaire or other tests.

Adapted from ref. [36].

checklist, which has then led to varyingly intensive degrees of physical examination and laboratory investigation.

How well has screening been accepted?

There are conflicting reports on the acceptability of screening programmes to elderly people. Some authors report high acceptance rates of 83 per cent when a general medical examination was offered as part of a screening procedure, and acceptance rates of over 90 per cent have been found when nurses have been used to screen for a more general assessment of health and social need. Others report a fall-off in acceptance rates in old age. This has been shown both for breast cancer screening programmes and for use of the Hemoccult test as a screen for large bowel cancer. It is also possible that the likelihood of accepting an invitation to be screened is inversely related to the risk factors or problem concerned. This has been shown for cardiovascular health checks in general practice for a middle aged population [37]. Therefore many factors, apart from age, seem to influence compliance with screening. These include the relevance and benefit of the programme as perceived by the participants, the disruption and inconvenience in undertaking the programme, the extent to which it is integrated with primary care services, and perhaps most of all, the relationship in terms of empathy and trust between the health professional and the older person.

What benefits have accrued from screening?

Many descriptive studies have drawn attention to the large number of previously unrecognised disorders that have been identified through screening. Several studies have also described resolution of many of these problems at follow up. Not surprisingly, many of these authors have the impression that their screening activities have been beneficial.

More recently however, a number of controlled trials [38–41] and randomised controlled trials [42, 42a, 42b, 42c] of screening have provided a more detailed and critical appraisal of this strategy. In the following sections I summarise this information.

Amelioration of disease

In one of the first randomised controlled trials of screening and surveillance of an elderly population from family practice, Tulloch and Moore [42] noted that many more patients in the control group were free of medical disorders or suffered from only one condition at the end of a two-year period. This difference was statistically significant ($P < 0.011$). However, the number of patients with two disorders was greater in the study group and this pattern was repeated for those with three or more conditions although the differences were not significant. Of 144 previously unrecognised medical conditions found in this study, one-third were resolved, one-third were improved, and one-third were unchanged by the end of the study. In another controlled trial of screening, McEwan et al. [42a] found no evidence that this strategy resolved the number of physical problems experienced by the intervention group. In contrast, in their randomised controlled study, Carpenter and Demopoulos [42b] found the number of falls reported in their control group doubled whilst those in the study group remained unchanged.

Mortality rates

Evidence from the literature on the effect of screening on mortality rates is conflicting. Pathy et al. [42c] in a surveillance programme of patients aged 65 and over, using a postal questionnaire and nurse intervention, found that mortality was significantly lower in the intervention group (18%) than in the control group (24%). In a three-year interventional study with three-monthly visits and screening by nurses, Hendriksen [38] found 56 deaths in the intervention group and 75 in the control ($p < 0.05$). In a similar study, Vetter [41] found a difference in the number of deaths significant at the one per cent level from one of two randomised control groups, but found no difference between the intervention and second control groups. Contrarily, Carpenter and Demopoulos [42b], in their randomised controlled study, found no difference in mortality between the screened and control groups.

Functional status

Five studies have examined the effects of health maintenance screening programmes on functional status in the elderly. Tulloch and Moore [42], using a domestic care rating (i.e. whether or not they were dependent on others), found differences between control and treatment groups, but these were marginal and not statistically significant. In an 18-month controlled intervention study in Norway among people aged 80 and over, Ro [39] showed no improvement in functional ability in the intervention group. Vetter [41], in Denmark, using the Townsend index of physical disability, showed no significant differences between control and intervention groups. In a randomised, controlled study of an elderly English population, Carpenter [42b] found no difference between the screened and unscreened groups in their activity of daily living scores. Likewise McEwan [42a], considering a number of functional parameters, was unable to demonstrate any significant improvement in the screened group.

Quality of life

Tulloch and Moore [42], like many others, believed their patients benefited from a screening and surveillance programme and reported a perceived increase in patient morale and esteem. Similarly, in McEwan's study [42a], 20 months after screening, the intervention group scored significantly better than the control group on the Philadelphia Geriatric Center Morale Scale. However, these findings have not been borne out in other studies. Vetter [41], measuring the patients' change in their perceived 'subjective view of life overall' reported a higher quality of life than controls, but the differences were not significant at the five per cent level. In a more precise study, Luker [40] used the Neugarten Life Satisfaction Index (LSI) and found no statistically significant difference between control and intervention groups. In Pathy's randomised trial of case finding in general practice [42c], quality-of-life measures revealed no between-group differences though self-rated health status was superior in the intervention group. Screening and surveillance programmes for elderly people seem therefore to have at best a marginal and transient effect on the quality of life.

Service utilisation

Most screening programmes of elderly people report a wide-ranging increase in utilisation of community services. Tulloch and Moore [42] found an increase in referrals for physical therapy and chiropody services. Vetter [41] reported an increase in the use of home helps and an increased attendance at luncheon clubs, although there were only minor differences in the provision of mobile meal services. Hendriksen [38] found an increase in the supply of home equipment and adaptations. Two other reports comment on hospital workload. Tulloch and Moore [42], from a study of general practice, found an increased number of outpatient clinic referrals, 37 versus 21 per 100 patients in their study group. Hendriksen [38], however, found a lower use of the emergency medical service in the intervention group ($p < 0.05$). Although Pathy et al. [42c] found an increase in visits to the general practitioner, this was largely offset by a lower number of home visits being required.

Extent of institutionalisation

Although further clarification is required, it would seem that certain types of screening and health maintenance programmes may reduce rates of institutionalisation. In a three-year randomised controlled trial to assess whether scheduled medically and socially preventive intervention would influence the numbers of admissions to hospitals and nursing homes, Hendriksen [38] found 209 hospital admissions in the intervention group and 271 among the controls, or 4884 bed days in the intervention group and 6442 in the control group ($p < 0.01$). There were 20 and 29 admissions to nursing homes in the intervention and control groups, respectively, but this did not reach statistical significance. In another study, Ro [39], after an 18-month intervention study, found a 25 per cent reduction in hospital bed days in the intervention group. Tulloch and Moore [42] found their study group patients spent less time in hospital, 407 versus 288 bed days per 1000 patients. In this study, however, they also reported an increased admission rate of 29 versus 19 per 100 patients, although this did not reach statistical significance because of the small numbers involved. Similarly, Carpenter [42b] found that, although their control group spent 33 per cent more days in institutions, the screened group were admitted to hospital *more* often than controls (335 occasions versus 252). Pathy et al. [42c] found that the total number of hospital admissions did not differ between intervention and control groups, but that the duration of hospital stay of patients aged 65 to 74 years was significantly shorter in the intervention group.

The degree of institutionalisation must, in the final analysis, depend on the experience and efficacy of the health professionals acting as gatekeepers to these resources. Their level of experience, their degree of biomedical orientation, and their confidence in dealing with disability in the community will all affect institutionalisation rates.

Costs

Hendriksen [38], subsequent to his screening programme, gave a rough calculation of an expenditure of 2 480 812 Danish kroner against 5 018 800 kroner, but pointed out that the savings in bed days, which in large part formed the gains, would not necessarily be realised if the beds were filled with other patients. Therefore, there might be no short term gains, and long term gains would be obtained only by a contraction in bed availability. This in turn would dictate the need for more stringent admission criteria.

Why the relatively unimpressive outcome?

Screening of elderly people living in the community may result in slight but inconclusive improvements in morbidity and mortality. The effect on quality of life is marginal, and no effect has been shown on functional status. Screening may reduce rates of institutionalisation, but referrals for hospital clinic attendance may increase. These results are achieved with fairly significant effort and use of resources. Cost savings seem unlikely in the short term. Screening the elderly may therefore work, but the results are not particularly impressive. The following are some suggestions why greater improvements have not been demonstrated.

1. Screening and case finding may not be an effective strategy.
2. The assessment instruments used in evaluation (for example the life satisfaction scales) may be insufficiently sensitive to measure change.
3. Elderly people may adapt to their disabilities and problems, making it difficult to show subjective improvement. Tulloch and Moore [42] specifically commented 'the . . . profile of social and functional and medical problems found after intensive review . . . did not always reflect accurately the health status of individual patients unless account was taken of the patients' adaptability. In fact, 88 per cent of patients were held to be well adapted as they had come to terms with their problems to the point where the effect on the quality of life was minimal'.
4. One illness or problem detected and resolved by preventive strategies may rapidly be replaced by another, so perceived benefit is minimised.
5. Many of the screening and case-finding programmes have lacked clear objectives and descriptions of the methodology by which the health problems were detected and resolved.
6. It may be too late in life to improve some well-established health problems. Preventive strategies may need to be employed earlier in life.

Targeting

In view of the debate about the value, relative to the resources used, of screening the whole of an elderly population, attempts have been made to establish other methods of screening that identify subgroups for whom this strategy would be of particular benefit [43]. A simplified list of these selective strategies is shown in Table 12.2.

Screening and case finding in selected patient groups

Self selection

Elderly people may select themselves for further attention. For instance, a postal questionnaire has been used to allow those fit enough and with no significant problems to exclude themselves from further study. By using this self-report technique, about one-fifth of a screening workload was avoided

[44]. Since then, it has been shown that the letter's efficiency can be increased by varying the number of questions. This has led to a number of experimental schemes in which variants of the screening letter have been tested. One of the most notable of these is the Edinburgh Birthday Card Scheme [45], in which a screening letter is attached to a birthday card and sent to patients on their 65th, 70th, 75th, 80th and 85th birthdays.

Risk groups

Another method is to select only those elderly patients perceived to be 'at risk'. This concept has at least two problems. The first is that the term 'at risk' has been used variously to imply a risk of death, of increased morbidity, of being institutionalised, and of stressing family caregivers. Also, 'at risk groups', as defined in the world literature, have failed to show that any of the risk indicators is particularly effective in terms of case finding. One of the few attempts to validate these groups has been carried out by Taylor et al. [46]. In their study they tested the hypothesis that certain groups 'at risk' might contain a high proportion of patients with unreported and untreated illness. Eleven such groups were examined:

(1) The very old (80 years and over).
(2) The recently widowed.
(3) The never married.
(4) Those living alone.
(5) Those socially isolated.
(6) Those without children.
(7) Those in poor economic circumstances.
(8) Those recently discharged from hospital.
(9) Those who had recently moved to another dwelling.
(10) Those divorced or separated.
(11) Those in the lowest social classes.

When these groups were correlated with various parameters of health and psychosocial wellbeing, it was found that those recently discharged, those moved, the divorced or separated, and the very old constituted those at greatest risk, but when the groups were considered in terms of their efficiency for case finding, none was particularly efficient. Concentrating on health and psychological function, the domains of most relevance to health professionals, it was found that the proportion of all cases accounted for by any one group never rose about 0.26 (those recently discharged).

Moreover, Taylor et al. [46] have also found considerable mismatch between those in these groups receiving surveillance and those in need of such

Table 12.2. *Targeting strategies*

Whole population screening
Screening of selected groups
• Self-selection
• 'At Risk' Groups
    The very old (> 80 years)
    The recently widowed
    The never married
    Those living alone
    Those 'socially isolated'
    Those without children
    Those in poor economic circumstances
    Those recently discharged from hospital
    Those recently moved to another residence
    Those divorced or separated
    Those in the lowest social class
• Prior to long-term institutionalisation
Opportunistic screening and case finding

---

surveillance as estimated by a range of health and psychosocial variables. In all parameters measured, the number of false positive results was greater than the false negative results, suggesting that much of the visiting was unnecessary. With more refined criteria for identifying those at risk, more effective use might be made of existing resources by reallocating manpower to those truly in need.

More recently, Iliffe et al. [46a] tested the hypothesis that elderly people living alone were an 'at risk' group and found that they did not have an excess of morbidity compared with elderly people living with others. As such they did not seem to merit specifically targeted assessments.

Screening those in institutional care

Results of numerous *preadmission* screening programmes both within the UK and abroad suggest that referral for long stay institutional care is a time and an opportunity for the instigation of health maintenance measures as part of a multidimensional assessment [47–51]. Apart from bringing to light undetected disease, the subsequent rehabilitation and provision of home supports can do much to avert and delay institutionalisation and allow resettlement at a lesser level of care. Acknowledgement of the value of preadmission screening has been reflected by its inclusion in the recommendations of the recent Griffiths report on community care. Considerable controversy surrounds the issue of whether preadmission screening is a *cost effective* strategy for rationing long term care. The detail of this subject is beyond the scope of this book.

There have been relatively few evaluative studies on *post-admission* screening of nursing home populations despite the large numbers of elderly people domiciled there. However, in the USA, Irvine et al. [52] found that approximately half of the annual screening examinations produced either a new finding or a revision of an old problem. These were then assessed independently for their degree of importance by the primary care physician concerned in the patients' care. They estimated that 3.4 per cent were of major importance, 26.8 per cent were of intermediate importance, and 69.8 per cent were of minor importance. Irvine's [52] conclusion was that the results provided only modest support for endorsing annual medical examinations for nursing home residents. Similar conclusions were reached by Gambert [53] in an academically affiliated Veterans' Administration nursing home. Findings on the annual examinations were compared with the most recently formulated problem list. This revealed a total of only eight previously unknown abnormalities in 96 male patients. It was concluded that ongoing health care as part of an academic geriatric programme might obviate the need for annual examinations. No detailed analysis was made of the workload required in these studies, though the authors comment that the evaluations were time consuming and costly in terms of manpower. In the USA, some surveys of nursing homes have shown over half of them have laboratory-testing protocols, with 90 per cent of these employing screening tests [54]. The value of such routine annual laboratory screening of institutionalised elderly residents has, however, been evaluated [55]. The results suggest that the annual performance of a large 'panel' of lab tests is not indicated, with most of the abnormalities that lead to resident benefit being identified by a complete blood count, electrolyte determinations, renal and thyroid function tests and a urinalysis.

Caution should be exercised before transporting these results from the USA to other health care settings. It should be remembered that in the USA there is a relatively strict code of medical practice in these nursing homes, with physicians requiring to see their patients and/or review their medications several times per year. The supervisory role of the nursing home medical director is also relatively well developed. This should be contrasted with the UK, where there is no compulsion on physicians to visit their nursing home patients. Consequently, in some areas only 13 per cent of patients received regular review and 19 per cent had not been seen since admission [56].

Opportunistic case finding

Probably the most favoured method of reaching the target population in the UK has been by opportunistic screening and case finding, i.e. seeking out unreported illness during normal doctor/patient relationships. In the setting of the National Health Service, this has considerable scope, for more than 90 per cent of the elderly patient population make contact with some member of the primary health care team over a one-year period [2]. Furthermore, in a well-organised practice, the practitioner will already have a considerable knowledge of the patient's problems and functional status [57]. The results of several studies have also shown that elderly non-attenders [2, 58–60] or refusers [61, 62] or elderly patients not known to their general practitioner [63] are a relatively healthy group who are at no greater risk of illness or disability. Opportunistic screening and case finding offer both a challenge and an opportunity to primary care providers by removing the artificial dichotomy between preventive and traditional medical care. Health maintenance and traditional medical care become integrated and the medical process serves as a major channel for the delivery of preventive health services.

The annual health examination

Despite the debate about the relative merits of whole population screening and the shift in emphasis towards more selective measures by primary care providers, some countries still require an annual health check for their elderly population. Notably, the British government, in its terms of service for doctors in general practice [1], has recently stipulated that each over 75-year-old patient be offered a home visit and have certain health checks carried out at yearly intervals if the practitioner is to qualify for additional capitation payments.

In the general practitioners' contract with the UK government there is little guidance on the goals and content of the health checks. However, these issues are described in detail in *Care of Old People: A Framework for Progress* (Royal College of General Practitioners, 1990) and, more recently, members of the Royal College of General Practitioners have developed a detailed protocol for use in health checks in people aged 75 years and over. The health check (apart from a review of medication by the doctor) can be carried out by a nurse or other professionally qualified person, though the doctor retains ultimate responsibility for the patient and must ensure that the person to whom he or she delegates screening responsibility has the necessary skills and training. There is also widespread acceptance of the need for these health checks to be staged: stage 1 is a brief assessment to discriminate as far as possible between the majority of older people who are fit and the minority who have significant health problems; stage 2 is a more detailed assessment of that minority, perhaps using more structured assessment and measurement instruments; and stage 3 is a further specialist or multidisciplinary assessment of the small percentage who still require this level of evaluation.

Further guidance on strategies for the various components of these health checks is provided in the above reference and also in this book as follows:

- vision, pp. 199–203
- hearing, pp. 203–206
- mental condition, pp. 174–177
- continence, pp. 193–197
- mobility and other functions, pp. 179–183
- 'social environment', pp. 229–230
- use of medicines, pp. 146–149

Recent reports [64, 65] on the first year of implementation of this strategy suggest that general practitioners remain uncertain of the purpose and content of these health checks, although uptake and patient satisfaction with them was high. Substantial amounts of unmet needs were identified in one of these studies [64]. Whilst there is likely to be ongoing debate about whether an annual health check per se improves outcome for the elderly recipients, it is likely that the organisational and clinical effort involved in the process may have other advantages. Screening or case-finding programmes for elderly people are an excellent means of identifying unmet need in this population and setting priorities for the allocation of resources. The data from annual health checks may therefore make an invaluable contribution to the assessment of need in a local community. These programmes are also useful as a means of collecting normative data for this age group and can provide a valuable educational resource for teaching about elderly people living in the community. Perhaps the most important outcome of the mandatory offer of a health check is that, in many cases for the first time, family doctors are seriously beginning to review their services and consider improved ways of promoting the health of this previously relatively neglected population.

References

1. Department of Health. Terms of Service for Doctors in General Practice. London: DoH, 1989.
2. Williams EI. Characteristics of patients aged over 75 not seen during one year in general practice. Brit Med J 1984; **288**: 119–21.
3. Hunt A. The Elderly at Home. A Study of People Aged Sixty Five and Over Living in the Community in England in 1976. Department of Health and Social Security. OPCS. London: HMSO, 1978.

4. Royal College of General Practitioners. Care of Old People: A Framework for Progress. occasional Paper 45; 1990.
5. Anderson WF, Cowan NR. A consultative health centre for older people. Lancet 1955; **2**: 239–40.
6. Bendkowski B. Incapacitating diseases in the elderly: a survey in General Practice. J Amer Geriatr Soc 1968; **16**: 1340–5.
7. Burns C. Geriatric care in General Practice. J Roy Coll Gen Prac 1969; **18**: 287–96.
8. Carey GCR. Undisclosed morbidity in persons aged over 70 in a Belfast General Practice. In Report of a Symposium on Early Diagnosis. J Roy Coll Gen Prac 1967; **14** (Suppl 2): 43–53.
9. Dunn TB. The Redbridge Scheme for routine medical examination of elderly people. Modern Geriatr 1971; **1**: 261–30.
10. Fairley HF. Unrecognised disease among the elderly in a General Practice. Practitioner 1967; **199**: 215–17.
11. Fry J. Care of the elderly in General Practice. Brit Med J 1957; **2**: 666–700.
12. Hay EH. Geriatric Survey in General Practice. Practitioner 1976; **216**: 443–70.
13. Hiscock E, Prangnell DR, Wilmot JF. A screening survey of old people in a General Practice. Practitioner 1973; **210**: 271–7.
14. Lowther CP, MacLeod RDM, Williamson J. Evaluation of early diagnostic services for the elderly. Brit Med J 1970; **3**: 275–7.
15. Meyrick RL. Geriatric survey in General Practice. Lancet 1962; **2**: 393–5.
16. Currie G, MacNeil RM, Walker JG et al. Medical and social screening of patients aged 70 to 72 by an urban general practice health team. Brit Med J 1974; **778**: 108–11.
17. Paulett JB, Buxton JD. Pilot study of old age pensioners. Brit Med J 1969; **1**: 432–6.
18. Pike LA. Screening the elderly in General Practice. J Roy Coll Gen Prac 1976; **26**: 698–703.
19. Taylor GF, Eddy TP, Scott DL. A survey of 216 elderly men and women in General Practice. J Roy Coll Gen Prac 1971; **21**: 267–75.
20. Thomas P. Experiences of two preventive clinics for the elderly. Brit Med J 1968; **2**: 357–60.
21. Williams EI, Bennett FM, Nixon JV et al. Socio-medical study of patients over 75 in General Practice. Brit Med J 1972; **2**: 445–8.
22. Williamson J, Stokoe IH, Gray S et al. Old people at home: their unreported needs. Lancet 1964; **1**: 1117–20.
23. Harrison S, Rous S, Martin E, Wilson S. Assessing the needs of the elderly using unsolicited visits by Health Visitors. J Roy Soc Med 1985; **78**: 557–61.
24. McIntosh IB, Young M, Stewart T. General Practice geriatric surveillance scheme. Scot Med J 1988; **73**: 332–3.
25. Young MG, Chamove AS. Screening evaluation of the elderly. Scottish Medicine 1989; **9**: 10–11.
26. Farquhar M, Bowling A. Older people and their GPs. J Brit Soc Gerontol 1991; 7–10.
27. Carpenter GI, Dmopoulous GD. The use of a disability rating questionnaire in a case-controlled screening surveillance programme. In: Taylor RC, Buckley EG (eds) Preventive Care of the Elderly: A Review of Current Developments. Occasional Paper 35. London: Royal College of General Practitioners, 1987.
28. Luker KA. The role of the Health Visitor in screening and surveillance of the

elderly. In: Kinnaird J, Brotherstone J, Williamson J (eds) The Provision of Care for the Elderly. New York: Churchill Livingstone, 1981.

29. Powell C, Crombie A. The Kilsyth questionnaire: method of screening elderly people at home. Age Ageing 1974; **3**: 23–8.

30. Williamson J, Lowther CP, Gray S. The use of Health Visitors in preventive geriatrics. Gerontol Clin 1966; **8**: 362.

31. Pfeiffer E. A short portable mental status questionnaire for the assessment of organic brain deficit in elderly patients. J Amer Geriatric Soc 1975; **23**: 433.

32. McNab A, Phillip AE. Screening an elderly population for psychological well-being. Scot Health Bull 1980; **38**: 160.

33. Pfeiffer E. The psycho-social evaluation of the elderly patient. In: Busse DW, Blazer DG (eds) Handbook of Geriatric Psychiatry, pp. 275–84. New York: Van Nostrand Reinhold, 1980.

34. Barber JH. An assessment programme in Glasgow: screening and surveillance of the elderly. In: Kinnaird J, Brotherston J, Williams J (eds) The Provision of Care for the Elderly. London: Churchill Livingstone, 1981.

35. Barley S. An uncompromising report on health visiting for the elderly. Brit Med J 1987; **294**: 595–6.

36. Brodsky J, Haron T, Catch H, Loval NO. A look at screening content in preventive health examinations of elderly. World Health Organisation January 1986. WHO Advisory Group on the effectiveness of health promotion for the elderly. Paper presented Hamilton, Ontario, April 1986.

37. Waller D, Agass M, Mant D et al. Health checks in General Practice: another example of inverse care? Brit Med J 1990; **300**: 1115–18.

38. Hendriksen C, Lund E, Stromgard E. Consequences of assessment and intervention among elderly people: a 3 year randomised controlled trial. Brit Med J 1984; **289**: 1522.

39. Ro OC, Biering K, Bjornsen LE et al. Eldreomsorgens Nye Giv-et Eksperiment Med Styrkat Innsats i Primaertjenesten i Oslo Rapport Nr 6. Oslo: Gruppe for Helsetjenesteforskning, 1983.

40. Luker KA. Health visiting and the elderly. Nursing Times 1981; **77**: 137–40.

41. Vetter NJ, Jones DA, Victor CR. Effect of health visitors working with elderly patients in General Practice: a randomised controlled trial. Brit Med J 1984; **288**: 369.

42. Tulloch AJ, Moore V. A randomised controlled trial of geriatric screening and surveillance in General Practice. J Roy Coll Gen Pract 1979; **29**: 733.

42a. McEwan RT, Davison N, Forster DP et al. Screening elderly people in primary care: a randomized controlled trial. Brit J Gen Pract 1990; **40**: 94–7.

42b. Carpenter GI, Demopoulos GR. Screening the elderly in the community: controlled trial of dependency surveillance using a questionnaire administered by volunteers. Brit Med J 1990; **300**: 1253–6.

42c. Pathy MSJ, Bayer A, Harding K, Dibble A. Randomised trial of case finding and surveillance of elderly people at home. Lancet 1992; **340**: 890–3.

43. Taylor RC, Buckley EG (eds). Preventive Care of the Elderly. A Review of Current Developments. Occasional Paper 35. London: Royal College of General Practitioners, 1987.

44. Barber JH. An assessment programme in Glasgow: screening and surveillance of the elderly. In: Kinnaird J, Brotherston J, Williamson J (eds) The Provision of Care for the Elderly. London: Churchill Livingstone, 1981.

45. Porter AMD. Postal screening survey: the Edinburgh birthday card scheme. In: Taylor RC, Buckley EG (eds) Preventive Care of the Elderly. A Review of

Current Developments. Occasional Paper 35. London: Royal College of General Practitioners, 1987.

46. Taylor R, Ford G, Barber H. The elderly at risk: a critical review of problems and progress in screening and case finding. Research Perspectives on Ageing 6. London: Age Concern Research Unit, 1983.

46a. Iliffe S, Tai SS, Haines A et al. Are elderly people living alone an at risk group? Brit Med J 1992; **305**: 1001–4.

47. Lowther A, McLeod H. Admission to a welfare home. Health Bull (Scot) 1974; **32**: 14–18.

48. Cobb JS. Medical screening of old people. Lancet 1978; **2**: 676.

49. Brocklehurst JC. Medical screening of old people accepted for residential care. Lancet 1978; **2**: 141–3.

50. Gibson P, Robertson K, Power M. Multidisciplinary assessment for residential accommodation. Practice 1988; **2**: 85–92.

51. Rafferty J, Smith RG, Williamson J. Medical assessment of elderly persons prior to a move to residential care: a review of seven years' experience in Edinburgh. Age Ageing 1987; **16**: 10–12.

52. Irvine PW, Carlson K, Adcock M, Slag M. The value of annual medical examinations in the nursing home. J Amer Geriatr Soc 1984; **32**: 540.

53. Gambert SR, Duthie EH, Wiltzins F. The value of yearly medical evaluation in a nursing home. J Chron Dis 1982; **35**: 65.

54. Joseph C, Lyles Y. Routine laboratory assessment of nursing home patients. J Amer Geriatr Soc 1992; **40**: 98–100.

55. Levinstein MR, Ouslander JG, Rubenstein LZ, Forsythe SB. Yield of routine annual laboratory tests in a skilled nursing home population. J Amer Geriatr Soc 1987; **258**: 1909–15.

56. Hepple J, Bowler I, Bowman CE. A survey of private nursing home residents in Weston-Super-Mare. Age Ageing 1989; **18**: 61–3.

57. Hooper J. Case finding in the elderly: does the primary care team already know enough? Brit Med J 1988; **297**: 1450–2.

58. Dr. Stringfellow's team. Prevention for patients over 75: is it worth the bother? Brit Med J 1986; **292**: 1243–4.

59. Rossow CS, Kirkevy OJ, Fossum S. Medical screening of 70-year-old patients without regular contact with General Practitioners. Nortidsskr Nor Laegeforen 1985; **105**: 1240–2 + 1254.

60. Ebrehim S, Hedley R, Sheldon M. Low levels of ill health among elderly non-consulters in General Practice. Brit Med J 1984; **289**: 1273–5.

61. Akhtar AJ. Refusal to participate in a survey of the elderly. Gerontol Clinica 1972; **14**: 208.

62. Milne JS, Maule M, Williamson J. Method of sampling in a study of older people with a comparison of respondents and non-respondents. Brit J Prev Soc Med 1971; **25**: 37.

63. Williams ES, Barley NH. Old people not known to the General Practitioner: low risk group. Brit Med J 1985; **291**: 1251–4.

64. Brown K, Williams EI, Groom L. Health checks on patients 75 years and over in Nottinghamshire after the new GP contract. Brit Med J 1992; **305**: 619–21.

65. Tremellen J. Assessment of patients aged over 75 in general practice. Brit Med J 1992; **305**: 621–4.

13

Practical aspects of implementation

In this chapter I consider some of the practical aspects of incorporating preventive care and health promotional strategies for elderly people into existing health and social care delivery systems. An overview will be given of the implications for both the providers and purchasers of health. It is assumed that the majority of purchasers will be governments and also health insurance companies and other third-party payers who commonly meet the costs of provision on behalf of the older population. It is also assumed that the purchasers of health care have (or should have) a close liaison with public health professionals and that the latter will guide purchasers in formulating a strategy and setting quality standards. In the discussion that follows, the boundaries between the provision of certain health care services and health promotional strategies will be deliberately blurred because the distinction between the two is artificial and counterproductive.

Public health

Assist purchasers on appropriate health services

An essential task for public health professionals is to assist health purchasers in buying an appropriate mix of health services that will have maximum impact on the health of an older population. Often the health services available to a local population have arisen because of historical precedent and the interests of the people working within the system. Much money is often spent on high technology aspects of biomedical care that at times have marginal benefit. Some aspects of intensive care and oncology treatments are examples of this. This is often done at the expense of failing to provide simpler, but equally important, broader based treatments, for example hearing aids or adequate rehabilitation services. It is the responsibility, therefore, of public health to consider the needs of the elderly population in holistic terms and to convert this to advice to the purchasers of health services on buying not merely treatment modalities for disease states, but also the services necessary to minimise the functional consequences and to ensure an adequate system of support that will provide a reasonable quality of life for older persons and for the family caring for them.

Reorientate resources towards the pursuit of health

Purchasers of health are largely preoccupied with the purchase of health services. Yet many would contend that some of the greater gains in health promotion (for example reduction in smoking) lie outwith the health service delivery area. It is therefore a justifiable task of public health professionals to scrutinise these potential benefits and encourage a shift in resourcing towards these goals, if necessary by moving funding away from the health (service) purchaser to other agencies.

However, in considering a shift of funds for elderly people away from traditional health service delivery towards health promotion it is necessary to consider three things. Firstly, relatively little funding goes towards the more chronic care of the elderly population and a small reduction in an annual budget could result in a severe reduction in the coverage and intensity of existing services. Secondly, the potential benefit of the health promotional strategy must have withstood the rigours of scientific scrutiny and should not merely be a proposal based on emotive, political or influential views on elderly people. Thirdly, shifts in funding away from existing services may not only be difficult to achieve but may be unwanted by the population for which they are being proposed. This concern has recently been reinforced with the outcome of Oregon's more logical approach to rationing health resources. This approach (which admittedly focussed on health service provision rather than health promotion) initially proceeded with a strategy based on the cost effectiveness of services. However, the resulting list was considered unacceptable in certain areas because it denied the emotive and intuitive 'Rescue Drive' [1] of human beings to help those in immediate suffering. It may therefore be difficult to shift too many resources away from services that give immediate succour to a more long range and less certain investment in health. Elderly people themselves may not wish this, and they should be polled on their opinions.

Develop local community health strategies

The health of elderly people depends on the activities of many professional and voluntary organisations other than health and social service agencies. Public

Health should therefore assume some responsibility for drawing them together, along with local government, in developing broad local community health strategies. As a focal point for this process, a five-yearly summary statement might be published on the current position and intended developments for the following strategies for the elderly population:

- improving transport and access
- ensuring a supportive and enabling environment
- promoting leisure and sports facilities
- providing continuing education opportunities

Promote health education for the elderly population

A final task for public health is the promotion of health education aimed at engendering healthy behaviour and lifestyles. There are three main target audiences.

Health professionals

This category includes doctors, nurses and, to a lesser extent, care/case managers and certain social service providers. The purpose here is to increase the awareness and inclusion of health promotional strategies in their daily work (for example flu vaccination) and to increase their counselling skills (for example in advising elderly people on how to quit smoking). A further aim is to ensure they display appropriate health educational materials in the facilities over which they have control.

Families and other carers

Education of this group would have the goals of ensuring they are aware of:

- the dangers and threat to the autonomy of elderly individuals by over-protection
- the availability and procedures for obtaining services that would either improve the quality of life of elderly persons and/or assist in reducing carer burden
- the benefits to the people for whom they care of early referral and the dangers of late referral for treatment and assistance

The elderly themselves

Education of this group would aim to make them aware of:

- the benefits of early referral and the dangers of late referral for treatment and assistance

- the importance of sustaining exercise into old age, including reference to the range of locally organised activities whereby it is possible for this age group to incorporate exercise into its daily routine
- accident prevention
- those self care and healthy lifestyle practices relevant to the elderly population
- strategies for coping with retirement and financial affairs
- the range of locally available leisure activities, social events, crafts, hobbies and continuing education opportunities specifically geared for an older population that permit them to continue their self development and improve their quality of life.

Health providers

Range of services

It is pointless to introduce health promotion strategies to an elderly population if, after identifying a problem, there are inadequate services to treat, rehabilitate, support or enable an older person to achieve greater health. Even worse is to raise expectation (and the elderly population is becoming increasingly educated about its health) and then have inadequate services even to begin identifying such a problem.

Preventive care and health promotional strategies must therefore be linked to the availability of resources. To implement all the measures in the protocol outlined in Chapter 10 each locality will need a comprehensive range of services for elderly people [2].

Access

In addition to being available, services must also be accessible in geographical, financial and administrative terms. When trying to promote the health of an often disabled, relatively poor elderly population, it is essential that organisations providing health care establish their services close to the communities they serve, ensure that the charges for their services are within the reach of the significantly reduced income of the older person and that the avenues for obtaining these services are well publicised, simple and easy to understand.

Reorientation of existing services

Health care providers need to respond to the public and to health purchasers' pressures to reorientate their services away from the marginal benefits of some aspects of high technology care towards providing a broader and more adequate range of strategies that will impact on the less 'glamorous' health problems afflicting the elderly population.

Managing health promotion into the system

Because of the tendency of many health care institutions (and to a lesser extent many social service organisations) to focus only on presenting crises and problems (and the many pressing and time consuming priorities surrounding such issues), it is unrealistic to expect the average health or social service provider to implement much health promotion into their daily routine unless there are strong financial incentives to implement such measures or unless someone acts as a focus to manage such strategies into the existing health care system.

It is, therefore, recommended that full-time trained members of staff should be employed to facilitate the promotion of health for older people in each locality. Such facilitators are already being employed in the UK and the USA. Whilst they may not be the most cost effective way of putting across certain preventive measures to primary care physicians [3], and while some concern has been expressed that they must focus on measures of proven efficacy, nevertheless several reports have shown that they are effective in increasing the rates of cancer screening [4], counselling and other [5] preventive care measures by family physicians.

These health promotion facilitators do not personally carry out such activities, but act as catalysts, educators and managers ensuring that health promotion is integrated into the agenda and daily practice of other health (and social service) professionals. The health promotion facilitator would:

- Promote the introduction of preventive care strategies (such as the protocol in Chapter 10) into primary care settings, including the development of appropriate data sets and preventive care cards)
- Act as a resource and teacher for community nursing and social service staff, assisting them to introduce health promotional strategies into their assessment procedures and routine work
- Assist staff in the implementation of ongoing health promotional

programmes for those elderly people in long stay hospitals, nursing and residential homes and other types of continuing care facility.

• Train staff in local day care facilities in simple assessment and health promotional techniques for their elderly clients
• Monitor and audit the extent of coverage and penetration of health promotional strategies within the local elderly population.

Other requirements

Other requirements for providing health promotional services are beyond the scope of this book. They are, however, far ranging and might include some of the following examples.

• The development of an explicit (and if possible common) policy on the containerisation and labelling of drugs for elderly patients by hospital and all community pharmacy services. This policy should contain an agreed prescribing procedure for patients being admitted to and discharged from hospital
• Improved access and counselling facilities for the take up of welfare benefits
• Home care and repair schemes with the availability of suitable adaptation grants
• Accessible, available home aids and equipment for the disabled at affordable prices
• The provision of no-smoking policies in hospital and residential facilities and, whenever this restriction is considered inhumane (see p. 266), the provision of both smoking and non-smoking lounge areas in these facilities
• The establishment of relatives or carers committees to enable feedback and input from the families and friends of elderly residents in continuing care facilities
• The establishment of an ombudsman scheme to deal with the concerns and complaints of residents in continuing care facilities

Health professionals

The development of a pertinent data set

The traditional biomedical model of health care unfortunately tends to minimise consideration of the broader health problems afflicting elderly people. Thus, concerns about functional dependency and social support are often overlooked by physicians. It is known, for example, that there is significant underdiagnosis and underrecording of incontinence [6, 7], impaired cognition [8, 9], and caregiver stress. It is likely, therefore, that in the conventional setting many tertiary strategies of prevention (minimising disability or handicap once it has developed) will remain unused even after an elderly person has come into contact with a health care provider.

The method of ensuring that professionals take cognisance of these health problems is to provide a structured assessment protocol for any elderly individual. Details of such an assessment are beyond the scope of this book, but if health promotional measures are to be fully implemented any assessment should include, as a minimum, an accurate measurement of mental functioning, of key physical functioning and of the social support available. The specific measures chosen will depend on the purpose and location of the assessment. Several comprehensive texts are available for assisting in their selection.

Whatever choices are made, they should, as an approximate guideline, be used on everyone over 74 years and in selected individuals of 65 to 74 years. The measurements should also be displayed prominently in the files and records.

Structured evaluation instruments can be rapidly incorporated into a traditional approach to assessing an elderly individual. It should be remembered, however, that very short consultations mitigate against considering the social aspects of care [10]. Contrarily, scheduling a few minutes more for each consultation has been shown to increase the extent of health promotional strategies employed [11].

Health professionals should also adopt a problem orientated approach to summarising the range of problems identified during assessment. One such example of a multidimensional problem list is shown in Table 13.1. In this table, health problems are categorised into three domains: traditional medical problems; problems of mental and physical functioning; and problems with the social support system.

Consideration should also be given to incorporating and displaying the above information into the numerous computerised clinical information software systems currently in use for resource management, audit and quality assurance. It is particularly important that the software in use by family practitioners and by primary care services contain such information displays.

A further refinement of the health promotional database would be to develop a 'preventive care card' (akin to the immunisation card [12] used for children) that explicitly identifies the nature, timing and frequency of health promotional

Table 13.1. *Conceptual framework for information display*

Problems	Examples
Medical	
Physical	Acute myocardial infarction
	Bronchopneumonia
Psychiatric	Reactive depression
	Senile dementia of Alzheimer type
Psychological	Dependent personality
Pharmacological	Poor medication compliance
	Excessive medications
Functional	
Mental (a) Cognition	Poor memory, confusional state
(b) Behaviour	Restlessness, paranoia
Mobility	Inability to rise and transfer
	Inability to walk
	Recurrent falls
Continence and excretion	Incontinence of urine/faeces
	Nocturia
	Constipation
Activities of daily living	Difficulty with PADL[a]
	Difficulty with DADL[a]
Hearing and vision	Deafness
	Poor vision
Communication	Dysphasia
	Dysarthria
Other	Insomnia
Support	
People	No resident attendant at home
	Potential withdrawal of family support
Places	Demanding home environment
	No longer fulfils criteria for placement at current level of care
Provisions	Wrong height of walking aid
	At poverty level
Policies of care	Over-protection
	Abuse

[a]PADL, personal activities of daily living;
DADL, domestic activities of daily living.

measures appropriate to the individual and identifies whether or not they have been undertaken by the professionals concerned. Such a card might be retained by some fitter elderly individuals, or by their carers, and taken with them when they attend for any intercurrent health problems.

Skill training

There are many implications for education and training if preventive care measures and health promotion are to be fully implemented. The following are some of the more important.

- The expertise of selected social service providers and care/case managers should be expanded to include a knowledge of effective health promotional measures for elderly people that might be considered when assessing their clients, particularly those referred for day care or long term institutional care
- The skills of all community nursing staff (not just those with a specific remit in health promotion) should be extended to include:
  techniques for screening visual ability in the elderly (see p. 200)
  techniques for screening hearing impairment in the elderly (see p. 203)
  techniques for assessing cognitive status (see p. 174)
  techniques for assessing physical functioning (see p. 181)
  techniques for evaluating dysphoria and depression (see p. 143)
  techniques for assessing carer burden and fatigue (see p. 219)
- A good chiropody service is a major boon to an elderly population. However, in some areas the more mundane and simple tasks such as nail clipping receive low priority from chiropodists. These tasks are nevertheless essential to the wellbeing of many elderly people, for they often cannot bend down far enough to reach their feet, or their toenails may be too thick to cut. A more effective coverage and intensity of service might be achieved by training a limited number of community and institutional nursing staff to assess and manage simple nail and foot care problems as a part of their work. These latter skills would need to be developed in conjunction with adequately trained chiropodists, ultimately developing a cadre of trained nurse 'footcare assistants' that would work as part of a team responsible to a chiropodist acting as team leader).
- A similar model may be adopted for simple oral and denture problems experienced by older people. Basic assessment and management skills (see pp. 66 and 112) can be taught by qualified dental staff to experienced nurses who can then exercise their new skills in the course of their daily duties, reporting back to designated qualified dental staff
- Bereavement counselling skills should be a required part of training for many community staff and for key personnel working in long term institutions where death is commonplace
- Facilities specialising in promoting the functional abilities of elderly

patients should ensure that the nurses employed are conversant in the practice of functionally orientated care that enables elderly patients to relearn prior functional skills, rather than traditional supportive care that merely helps elderly people in their disability. Certain models of nursing practice, for example Orem's Self Care Deficit Theory [13], are more conducive to this than others and should be more widely taught.

Collaboration in care

The health needs of elderly people are broad and constantly changing. Inter-agency and professional boundaries, particularly between health and social service providers can be detrimental. The promotion of health for this older population depends on close inter-agency planning and service delivery. A number of practical health promotional issues with which health and social service agencies can collaborate are therefore outlined.

- All admissions to long term care institutions, whether under the aegis of social or health care agencies, should undergo a multidimensional assessment, part of which should consist of an appropriate medical screen [14–17]. Experience has shown that such a procedure reveals significant illness and dependency that with treatment and/or rehabilitation can benefit the potential resident. If the assessment is conducted outwith the auspices of the future long stay facility, the results can give much reassurance to family carers and help to assuage some of the guilt surrounding the placement of a loved one. The health promotional component of this screening assessment should be explicit and based on the protocol outlined in Chapter 10 and elsewhere.
- Once in care, health promotional protocols should be developed for the commonest health problems afflicting the residents of such homes. Staff should be made conversant with these through their incorporation in in-service training programmes. In parts of the USA, through an expansion of a Minimum Data Set, some progress is being made towards incorporating health promotion into explicit protocols for care in long stay institutions. It should be remembered, however, that devotion to such protocols may be a cumbersome, poor and equally expensive substitute for the regular input of skilled professionals poorly funded within the existing system.
- An application for social or community day care may also be considered an opportune time for a health maintenance check. The screening measures might be conducted by a range of health or social service

personnel, provided that an explicit protocol is adhered to. At times, community day care is an extremely informal process and as such may be unable to cope with the practicalities of such a health promotional component. However, for more formally structured day care, or for day hospital care, a health promotional input should be considered a routine part of good practice. The inclusion of health promotional measures by a day care facility should be a condition for funding or the placing of a contract by any health or social service purchaser.

- Most cadres of home or community care assistants are nowadays being developed with a flexible remit to include a range of domestic, personal care and health care tasks. Any organisation or organisations involved in this process should ensure that, whatever the label attached to these carers, they become a vehicle for the introduction of certain simple health promotional strategies. These should be made explicit in their job description and their training should incorporate appropriate knowledge and skills in this area.

- Abuse of elderly people in its various forms is an increasingly recognised problem [18]. Any department of protective services having responsibility for minimising the problem should recognise that its detection and prevention spans professional boundaries. Any protocol for dealing with elder abuse should therefore be drawn up in collaboration with other agencies. It should then be widely disseminated, particularly to relevant health and social service professionals.

Methods of delivering care

There is increasing evidence that the method by which routine health care and social support is delivered can have a significant impact on promoting health. This is particularly so when the manner of health care delivery is personalised and provides the elderly individual with the perception of control and choice. Two such examples are illustrated here.

Care management

In recent years, the concept of care management (often referred to as case management outside the UK) has been introduced as a more effective and efficient technique of delivering community care. It is one of the policy cornerstones upon which the British Government has based the future of community care. Its essential features include: a comprehensive assessment of needs; one individual (the care manager) taking responsibility to orchestrate the necessary care planning; a flexible (though capped) budget devolved to the control of the care manager; a more individually tailored and imaginative package of care; and monitoring and review. The emergence of care management is resulting in a developing cadre of specialist workers, in social service and health care organisations having to face the realities of devolved managerial responsibility and in detailed costing exercises for community services.

Although proof of the efficacy of care management is beset with methodological problems and problems of targeting, evidence suggests it may have the following distinct benefits [19]:

- a reduction in the probability of admission to long term care
- an increase in the probability of continuing to live at home
- improved self perception of wellbeing
- improved objective rating of health
- a reduction in the probability of death at one and three years
- a reduction in informal carers' burden and in the costs incurred by them in their caring role.

The key worker principle and primary nursing

Primary nursing, and its social service equivalent the key worker principle have been shown in institutionalised care to improve staff/resident interaction, improve choice, promote a more personal caring approach and to promote functional independence when compared with more traditional task orientated approaches to care [20]. This technique, emphasising a personal approach to the resident and individualised care planning provides an important contribution to promoting the health of elderly institutionalised individuals.

References

1. Hadorn DC. Setting health care priorities in Oregon: cost-effectiveness meets the rule of rescue. J Amer Med Assoc 1991; **265**: 2218–25.
2. Horrocks P. The components of a comprehensive district health service for elderly people – a personal view. Age Ageing 1986; **15**: 321–42.
3. Cockburn J, Ruth D, Silagy C et al. Randomised trial of three approaches for marketing smoking cessation programmes to Australian general practitioners. Brit Med J 1992; **304**: 691–4.
4. Dietrich AJ, O'Connor GT, Keller A et al. Cancer: improving early detection and prevention. A community practice randomised trial. Brit Med J 1992; **304**: 687–91.
5. Fullard E, Fowler G, Gray M. Promoting prevention in primary care. Brit Med J 1987; **294**: 1080–2.

6. Ouslander JG, Kane RL, Abrass IB. Urinary incontinence in elderly nursing home patients. J Amer Med Assoc 1982; **248**: 1194–8.

7. Thomas M, Plymat KR, Blannin J et al. Prevalence of urinary incontinence. Brit Med J 1980; **281**: 1243–6.

8. Brody DS. Physician recognition of behavioural, psychological and social aspects of care. Arch Intern Med 1980; **240**: 126–8.

9. Garcia CA, Tweedy JR, Blass JP. Underdiagnosis of cognitive impairment in a rehabilitation setting. J Amer Geriatr Soc 1984; **32**: 339–42.

10. Morrell DC, Evans ME, Morris RW et al. The 'five minute' consultation: effect of time constraint on clinical content and patient satisfaction. Brit Med J 1986; **292**: 870–3.

11. Wilson A, McDonald P, Hayes L, Cooney J. Health promotion in the general practice consultation: a minute makes a difference. Brit Med J 1992; **304**: 227–30.

12. Grundy R, Dwyer DM. Preventive care card for General Practice. J Roy Coll Gen Pract 1989; **39**: 15–16.

13. Orem D. Nursing: Concepts of Practice. New York: McGraw Hill, 1980.

14. Brocklehurst JC. Medical screening of old people accepted for residential care. Lancet 1978; **2**: 141–3.

15. Lowther A, Mcleod H. Admission to a welfare home. Health Bull (Scot) 1974; **32**: 14–18.

16. Cobb JC. Medical screening of old people accepted for residential care. Lancet 1978; **2**: 676.

17. Rafferty J, Smith RG, Williamson J. Medical assessment of elderly persons prior to a move to residential care: a review of seven years' experience in Edinburgh. Age Ageing 1987; **16**: 10–12.

18. Council on Scientific Affairs. Elder abuse and neglect. J Amer Med Assoc 1987; **257**: 966–71.

19. Challis D, Davies B. Case Management in Community Care. Aldershot: Gower Publishing, 1986.

14

The costs of preventive care and health promotion

It is generally believed that, in addition to its obvious health benefits, prevention costs less than cure and that because the potential savings are so great, more attention should be given to prevention simply on the grounds that it saves money. For example, President Jimmy Carter of the USA wrote that prevention 'can substantially reduce both the suffering on our people and the burden on our expensive system of medical care' [1]. Likewise, in outlining a four point programme to control Medicare costs in the USA, Somers [2] commented how distressing it was to see continued lack of attention on prevention which was 'potentially the most effective of all cost-control strategies'. The situation is much more complex, however, and careful economic analysis suggests a different picture. In reviewing a variety of health promotional strategies for all age groups, Russell [3] concludes that 'even when financial cost of the preventive measure looks small, careful evaluation often shows that the full costs are rather large, larger than any savings'.

In this chapter, therefore, I look at the nature of the costs of health promotion, summarise current information on the magnitude of these costs to individuals and to society, describe some of the ways in which costing techniques may be biased against elderly people, emphasise the lack of current funding on health promotion and suggest ways in which potential purchasers might get the best value for their money.

Types of costs

In Chapter 2, the World Health Organization definition of health was given as 'a state of complete physical, mental and social wellbeing'. It was, however, considered somewhat impractical and utopian. This is because it represents the elusive concept of *perfect health*. Not only is this extremely rare, but most people would not even try to achieve perfect health for the reason that

303

improvements in health status are not costless. Most people prefer to achieve *optimum health* where the cost of any further improvement outweighs the value attached to that improvement. For each individual this optimum depends on perceptions on both the desirability of being healthy and the sacrifices involved in improving health [4]. In other words, elderly individuals will trade off a degree of health against a degree of cost.

These costs can take many forms. At their simplest level they may involve the sacrifice of pleasure such as giving up smoking or eating excessively. Costs can also be represented by inconvenience: the inconvenience of disrupting a fixed lifestyle; the inconvenience of committing time and energy to regular exercise; the psychological inconvenience and anxiety of having expectations raised when submitting to preventive screening programmes.

Traditionally, however, costs are represented in financial terms. Elderly individuals may pay directly for preventive services or they may incur hidden costs in other ways such as taking lower wages for a safer job or paying the subscription rate for a health club. Of increasing importance, however, is the extent to which society as a whole has to pay the costs of trying to achieve *perfect* health for its individual members. This issue has particular relevance to an elderly population with relatively low income and high need for financial subsidy to fund the care it requires.

The rest of this chapter now focuses on a range of issues predominantly surrounding the financial costs of preventive and health promotional programmes.

The magnitude of costs

Review of the data in previous chapters suggests quite significant, explicit costs attached to many health promotional or preventive strategies for elderly people. For example, the costs per quality adjusted life year in old age have been calculated variously as Canadian $520 000 for tetanus immunisation, US $993 700 for cholesterol screening and US $1411 for smoking reduction.

Attempts have also been made to cost *packages* of preventive services as well as individual items. Eddy [5], listing the tests and procedures used for the *detection* of cancers in asymptomatic people and assuming their use once every year on the approximately 80 million adults over age 40 in the USA, has calculated that the direct financial cost would be over $20 billion each year. The cost of further diagnostic tests in persons who have false positive tests would add another $5 billion to $10 billion per year. By contrast, the total direct financial cost (physicians, hospital and out patient fees) for the *treatment* of all cancers was estimated in 1975 to be $5.3 billion. When the indirect costs of

Table 14.1. *1988 yearly fees (US$) for preventive services*

	With less frequent services		With more frequent services	
	Total fees per male	Total fees per female	Total fees per male	Total fees per female
Age group (years)				
0–4	107	102	107	102
5–18	4	4	7	7
19–29	20	22	45	52
30–49	17	30	44	51
50–64	16	88	45	128
>65	72	105	81	155
All persons with family coverage	24	37	41	55
Per family coverage	79		125	
Per single coverage	28		56	
Medicare	82		105	

Adapted from ref. [6].

disability and premature death are added ($12.4 billion), the total costs were estimated to be about $17.7 billion. Thus an 'ideal' programme designed for the early detection of cancer might eliminate about one-tenth to one-third of cancer mortality and extend the average person's life by about 200 days. However, it would cost between 1.4 and 1.7 times the overall costs for all cancers and, as the total cost of all medical care in the USA in 1978 was estimated to be about $192.4 billion, would consume 10 to 15 per cent of all the financial resources put into all diseases.

A more detailed but complex approach to costing preventive care services is to quantify the costs of insuring them for a given population. Chu and Trapnel [6] have estimated these in relation to implementing the recommendations of the US Preventive Services Task Force. They firstly considered the costs in absolute terms assuming full 'take up' of the services offered. They then considered the insurance costs that would reflect likely utilisation levels for these services. These latter data they obtained from the INSURE Project [7] (funded by insurance companies, private foundations and the Federal Government to study preventive services as a health insurance benefit), the National Health Interview Survey and the 1985 Immunisation Survey. The yearly fees for the preventive services recommended by the US Preventive Services Task Force and the monthly costs reflecting utilisation rates are shown in Tables 14.1 and 14.2.

Table 14.2. *1990 total monthly costs (US$) of preventive services under insurance plans*

	Less frequent services	More frequent services
Self-insured plans		
Family	4.35	6.89
Single	1.21	2.41
Other insurance plans		
Groups of 25 or more employees		
Family	4.35–4.68	6.89–7.41
Single	1.21–1.30	2.41–2.59
Individual insurance		
Family	4.57–6.09	7.24–9.65
Single	1.27–1.69	2.53–3.37
Medicare	3.99	5.10

Costs include claims processing, sales costs, premium taxes and profit. Costs for self insured plans include claims processing only.
Adapted from ref. [6].

Finally, consideration must be given to the possible impact of successful preventive and health promotional measures, not just on individuals but on the overall or 'macro-economy' of a nation as a whole [4].

In previous decades, the major preventive impact has been on reducing communicable disease with increased life expectancy for infants and children, the majority of whom would then grow into healthy and economically productive adults. The current situation is quite different. Current preventive measures would firstly increase the labour supply at a time when there is less and less work to do. This would result in many adults, and particularly elderly adults, who are often discriminated against in the job market, requiring some form of public subsidy to exist. The second result of current preventive measures would be to extend the lives of retired people. Some of these would be relatively fit, but would require a pension. Others would be more dependent and require more public resources for their care and management. There is therefore at least a potential for current preventive practices to actually harm the 'macro-economy' of a nation. Some studies suggest this to be so. For example, Gori and Richter [8] have estimated that if the USA could achieve the mortality rates from preventable diseases of the countries with even the second lowest rates in the industrialised world, then life expectancy at age 60 would increase by two years. When these and other age-specific increases were then put into the Wharton economic forecasting model, it was shown that if the increase in population was phased in over a 25 year period the Gross National

Product (GNP) would increase by \$20 billion, but if the increase in the population was immediate the GNP would fall by \$106 billion (1972 prices) [8]. Highly successful prevention policies that produce immediate and dramatic results may therefore adversely affect a nation's economy.

Costing techniques

In order to assist in making rational choices about how to spend resources on preventive strategies and health promotion, economists have developed quantitative methods that compare them in terms of costs and benefits. The two most common forms of such economic appraisal are known as Cost–Benefit Analysis (CBA) and Cost–Effectiveness Analysis (CEA). In CBA, the costs and benefits are expressed in comparable monetary units. In CEA, the benefits are usually expressed in more clinical terms such as the reduction in the number of cigarettes smoked or the number of years of life gained. In a variant of CEA known as Cost–Utility Analysis (CUA), benefits are expressed in terms of the Quality Adjusted Life Years (QALYs) gained.

It is important to appreciate that these new techniques, despite having many advantages, are considered by many to be intrinsically ageist, carrying with them a discriminatory bias against the elderly population [9–11]. The reasons for this are complex, but revolve around methodological issues, the apparent devaluation of life in old age and around the principle of using an economic model for intergenerational resource allocation.

There are numerous methodological concerns surrounding the calculation of QALYs. The data on health status have usually been obtained from self reporting questionnaires, yet elderly people are known to report erroneously in this way, particularly about disability, as often as 30 per cent of the time. Some of the estimates of QALYs gained have been based on the views of healthy populations and not the views of the persons concerned. Even a quality adjustment for the ageing process itself was based on the views of young university undergraduates [12]. Another methodological concern is that the two-dimensional classification system, based on disability and distress, which is currently used in the UK as a tool for calculating QALYs, was developed without consideration of the specific attributes of a frail elderly population. In particular, Donaldson et al. [14] have expressed concern that QALYs are insensitive to changes in the health status of elderly people in long term care when compared with other measures of quality of life that are frequently used in studies of older people. They recommend that QALYs should be based on attributes appropriate to the groups studied, otherwise certain groups may be discriminated against owing to the use of an insensitive measure of outcome.

The techniques upon which CBA and CEA are based may inherently devalue life in old age. For example, one of the basic measures of benefit is founded on the concept of 'human capital'. In this method, the projected lifetime earnings of a person are calculated from data on average earnings at various ages in the lifespan. The worth of an elderly person who stops work at retirement in old age drops dramatically in this way [15]. A second technique of estimating benefit is known as 'willingness to pay'. Here, the benefit of a health-related strategy is measured by asking people how much money they would be willing to spend to achieve a particular outcome. This method also contains a subtle bias against elderly people, for it has been shown that it is difficult to compare hypothetical spending decisions between groups of people of different economic status [9]. Because elderly people will have markedly reduced income from their retirement pensions, they may also be relatively unwilling to make hypothetical payment for avoiding certain health outcomes because of a desire to spend cautiously, fearing a need to save their money for crises such as needing to go into institutional care [9].

Another example of the ageist nature of economic comparisons lies in the concept of the QALY. Economic value of a strategy becomes greater if there are a large number of years of life to be gained. Because of the position of elderly people in the age spectrum this gain is unlikely. Strategies will also appear of increasing worth if there is a high gain in the elderly person's quality of life. In contrast to younger age groups, there is usually multiple pathology in the older population. Effective prevention of one problem may still leave them afflicted with another with a consequent lesser gain in overall quality of life.

From the above discussion it can be seen that few, if any, interventions directed at elderly people can stand up favourably from an economic viewpoint against programmes for younger people based on current techniques. The figures from CBA and CEA for the preventive strategies quoted in various parts of this book should be critically reviewed with the above concerns and caveats in mind. There should also be a very justifiable reluctance to use a purely economic model to decide on intergenerational resource allocation for preventive care and health promotional programmes.

Current funding of health promotion

Regan [16] has attempted to identify current funding spent on health promotional and disease preventive activities in the USA, and Cohen [4] has attempted to do the same for the UK. Both have found it extremely difficult to provide an accurate estimate for they faced many problems: funding for these services is fragmented amongst the public and private sectors and amongst charitable and voluntary organisations; budgetary accounting often fails to identify separately preventive expenditures; budgets for preventive programmes may overstate expenditure on prevention as they may also be concerned with treatment; and many budgets (e.g. for improved housing) are not considered in the total for preventive programmes yet have a strong 'preventive element'. The topic is sufficiently complex that the Department of Health and Social Security in the UK has stated that 'a meaningful estimate of the total sum spent on prevention cannot be achieved' [17].

Perhaps the only firm conclusion that can be drawn is that, in comparison with 'acute' services for treatment and cure, preventive services in general receive only a small proportion of the total expenditure on health care of any nation. Cohen and Henderson [4] estimated that in the UK in 1980–81 the expenditure on preventive services in the National Health Service (£550 million) was about 4.6 per cent of its total costs. They also estimated that a further £417 million was spent outwith the National Health Service on health promotional activities.

Amidst these complexities, it is even more difficult to be certain of the extent of funding for preventive services specifically for elderly people. Certainly, they seem to receive only a small proportion of the preventive care budget. Nations also limit their expenditures on preventive services to elderly people in different ways. For example in the USA, Medicare, the largest Federal programme benefitting the elderly, is explicitly prohibited by law from paying for routine preventive services such as physical examinations or immunisations (with the exception of pneumococcal vaccination). Alternatively, in the UK where annual screening of older people by family practitioners is a requirement to qualify for additional capitation fees [18], preventive services may then be limited by the existence of waiting lists or by non-availability of local services to which they might be referred.

There is therefore a further danger that inadequate funding of preventive services may lead to 'reverse targeting' of preventive care. Populations at high risk of morbidity and mortality (as frail elderly people are) will be least likely to receive adequate preventive care. Such 'reverse targeting' has already been described for a middle aged population by Woolhandler and Himmelstein [19]. They consider this another demonstration of the psychosocial phenomenon known as the Matthew effect – 'Unto every one that hath shall be given . . . but from him that hath not, shall be taken away even that which he has' (St Matthew xxiv, 40).

Thus, despite both the UK and the US Governments having espoused an overall comprehensive prevention policy as the way forward in trying to reduce morbidity and mortality, relatively little is being achieved for elderly people. This may reflect a genuine scepticism about the value of various preventive services for such an age group, since it is only in recent years that scientific data have been available to clarify the situation. Alternatively, the lack of funding may reflect ignorance about what can be achieved, or may imply an ageist bias in society, or may indicate society's reluctance to shift resources away from services that 'rescue' individuals from acute illness.

Obtaining value for money

Elderly people themselves may wish to purchase health promotional and preventive services directly out of pocket. Of greater magnitude, governments, health insurance companies and other third-party payers may wish to purchase these services on behalf of the older population. What is certain is that these purchasers have a difficult task in front of them, being faced with a wide variety of preventive strategies yet having limited resources with which to implement them. The following suggestions may assist in obtaining the best value for money spent.

Face reality

Selecting health promotional and preventive strategies is not a costless decision. It will therefore be very difficult to obtain funding for them when they are placed in competition with the need for other health services. Indeed, Thwaites [20] describes the public's expectations for health care treatment as increasing exponentially and running away from the supply of available resources. Potential purchasers of preventive services will thus have an increasingly difficult task to set aside funds for this purpose in the years ahead. The marketers of health promotion for elderly people should not weaken the case for a health promotional strategy by falsely claiming it will save money. Instead it should be promoted solely for the benefit it will contribute to the older population.

Identify priority areas for prevention

Local planning, purchasing and public health agencies need to collaborate in formulating a prevention strategy for each age group. This should include elderly people. Priorities should be identified within the prevention strategy based on the importance of the health problem (in a holistic sense) and the suitability, effectiveness and cost of the proposed preventive measure. Much of this book has been devoted to a consideration of this, and the summary 'package' of strategies recommended in Chapter 10 should serve as a sound basis for consideration.

Ensure the preventive strategy is effective

The next step is to ensure that the preventive measure or health promotional strategy to be purchased has been subjected to scientific scrutiny and has been shown to be effective. This is *not* to say that every measure must have been subjected to the ideal of a randomised controlled trial, but it must have been subjected to critical appraisal and must not merely be purchased as an emotive response to a superficially good idea. In Chapter 5 I provided further details on this and the contents of the protocol in Chapter 10 lists what appear as reasonably effective strategies.

Simplify the strategy

There are several preventive and health promotional strategies for elderly people that will incur significant additional costs. Many of these relate to cancer detection and prevention. One strategy to minimise such costs is to simplify the health promotional strategy, lessening the technological input. For example, 90 per cent of the costs of breast screening are due to the costs of the mammogram; if this procedure were dropped altogether, with reliance being placed solely on breast examination by a health professional, 63 per cent of the effectiveness of the programme would be retained at less than 10 per cent of the cost.

Use an efficient protocol for implementing the strategy

A further method of minimising costs is to ensure an efficient protocol for implementing the preventive strategy. For example, it is clear that virtually all of the benefit of an annual or biannual protocol for the screening of cervical carcinoma would be preserved with screening every three or four years, but at a greater than fourfold reduction in costs [5]. Likewise, the natural history of colonic polyps and cancer appears to be such that screening with sigmoidoscopy every four years would deliver about 94 per cent of the effectiveness of an annual protocol [5]. This will only occur, however, if patients faithfully follow their physicians' recommendations, and it is known that many people find the policy of an annual sigmoidoscopy unacceptable. If around 0.2 per cent of persons who reject an annual protocol accept a four-year protocol, the net effect of reducing the frequency would be positive. The cost would also be cut by a factor of about four [5].

Ensure accurate targeting

A further means of maintaining opportunities whilst reducing costs is to improve the targeting of those at risk. An example of this has previously been given where the conventional 'at risk' groups for the community-living elderly were found to be inefficient means for screening and case finding [21]. By using more refined classification criteria for identifying those at risk, resources could be used more effectively by allowing the reallocation of manpower to those truly in need.

Integrate health promotion through quality standards

Many preventive strategies for elderly people are inexpensive and incur only minimal additional costs. They do require, however, that health professionals discipline themselves into considering them part of good practice and integrating them into their routine care plans. These strategies may best be achieved by working them explicitly into quality assurance standards and into the process of Continuous Quality Improvement. Purchasing organisations should expedite this process by insisting on their inclusion when placing contracts with provider agencies.

Integrate health promotion through explicit planning

Many other health promotional measures can be achieved at little cost by organisations other than health services organisations. It does, however, require many public service organisations to include specific, explicit planning for elderly people into their social policies. Some examples are given on p. 192.

Use implicit rationing whenever possible

No matter how efficiently resources are used, it is unlikely that funding will be available for all proposed preventive strategies. A form of rationing will therefore need to be implemented. Aaron and Schwartz [22], in an analysis of the British and the US health care systems, identified clear benefit in difficult rationing decisions being tied up implicitly in 'clinical judgement'. This produced tensions for the provider practitioners, but appeared to allow a system to operate with lower levels of resource than would otherwise have been possible. It is therefore important that every health practitioner should be aware of what can, *and cannot*, be afforded in the way of preventive services by their local purchasers, so that they can integrate appropriate measures into their clinical management plans. It is also a further reason why health promotion should not be artificially segregated from the mainstream of health care delivery.

Ensure the consumer viewpoint in explicit rationing models

In many health care systems, rationing is moving towards a more explicit model where the purchasers and providers of health care have to make clear precisely what they are able to offer an elderly public. Within these explicit rationing models, it is important to develop a prominent consumer feedback mechanism so that elderly people themselves can express their views, firstly about possible shifts in resources from treatment to preventive services and, secondly, about the type of health promotional strategies they truly value. In particular, their views should be sought on the proportionate funding that should be spent between biomedical preventive care, for example cancer screening, and other types of health promotional strategies, such as functional restoration and the maintenance of an adequate system of social support. For this sort of consumer feedback to be meaningful, the elderly public must firstly be educated and informed about the issues in question.

Ensure some flexibility in the system

Whilst some form of rationing will always be important for the bulk of publicly funded preventive care, some flexibility should be retained for wealthy elderly individuals to purchase, or obtain through private insurance, those health promotional strategies that they consider of value.

In conclusion, the future success of preventive care and health promotional strategies for older people will depend on strong advocacy coupled with the advocates themselves being willing to put aside biased and adversarial viewpoints, accept economic reality and welcome critical appraisal of their work.

References

1. President Jimmy Carter. In: Foreword to 'Healthy People; The Surgeon General's Report on Health Promotion and Disease Prevention'. Washington, DC: Government Printing Office, 1979.
2. Somers AR. Why not try preventing illness as a way of controlling Medicare costs? N Engl J Med 1984; **3**: 853–6.

3. Russell LB. Is Prevention Better Than Cure? Washington, DC: Brookings Institution, 1986.
4. Cohen DR, Henderson JB (eds). Health, Prevention and Economics. Oxford: University Press, 1988.
5. Eddy DM. The economics of cancer prevention and detection. Cancer 1981; **47**: 1200–9.
6. Chu RC, Trapnell GR. Costs of ensuring preventive care. Inquiry 1990; **27**: 273–80.
7. Logsdon DN, Rosen MA, Demak MM. The INSURE project on life cycle preventive health services: cost-containment issue. Inquiry 1983; **20**: 121–6.
8. Gori GB, Richter BJ. Macro-economics of disease prevention in United States. Science 1978; **200**: 1124–30.
9. Avorn J. Benefit and cost analysis in geriatric care. N Engl J Med 1984; **310**: 1294–301.
10. Whitaker P. The inherent ageism of health economics. Geriatric Med 1991; **21**: 57–9.
11. Harris J. QALYfying the value of life. J Med Ethics 1987; **13**: 117–23.
12. Vaupel JW. Early death: an American tragedy. Law Contemp Probl 1976; **40**: 73–121.
13. Rosser RM, Kind P. A scale of evaluation of states of illness: is there a social consensus? Int J Epidemiol 1978; **7**: 347–57.
14. Donaldson C, Atkinson A, Bond J, Wright K. QALYS and long term care for elderly people in the UK: scales for assessment of quality of life. Age Ageing 1988; **17**: 379–87.
15. Dolan TJ, Hodgson TA, Wun WM. Present values of expected life time earnings and housekeeping services. Bethesda, MD: National Center for Health Statistics, 1980.
16. Regan PJ. Federally funded preventive health programs. In: Russell LB (ed) Is Prevention Better Than Cure? Washington, DC: Brookings Institution, 1986.
17. Department of Health and Social Security. Prevention and Health. London: HMSO, 1977.
18. Department of Health (UK). Terms of Service for Doctors in General Practice. London: HMSO, 1989.
19. Woolhandler S, Himmelstein DU. Reverse-targeting of preventive care due to lack of health insurance. J Amer Med Assoc 1988; **259**: 2872–4.
20. Thwaites B. The NHS: the end of the rainbow. Southampton: Institute for Health Policy Studies, 1987.
21. Taylor R, Ford G, Barber H. The elderly at risk: a critical review of problems and progress in screening and case finding. Research Perspectives on Ageing 6. London: Age Concern Research Unit, 1983.
22. Aaron HJ, Schwartz WB. The Painful Prescription: Rationing Hospital Care. Washington, DC: The Brookings Institution, 1984.

Index